Quick Reference to Outbreak Investigation and Control in Health Care Facilities

Kathleen Meehan Arias, MS, CIC

Manager
Infection Control Department
Sinai Hospital of Baltimore
Baltimore, Maryland

AN ASPEN PUBLICATION®
Aspen Publishers, Inc.
Gaithersburg, Maryland
2000

The author has made every effort to ensure the accuracy of the information herein. However, appropriate information sources should be consulted, especially for new or unfamiliar procedures. It is the responsibility of every practitioner to evaluate the appropriateness of a particular opinion in the context of actual clinical situations and with due considerations to new developments. The author, editors, and the publisher cannot be held responsible for any typographical or other errors found in this book.

Library of Congress Cataloging-in-Publication Data

Arias, Kathleen Meehan.
Quick reference to outbreak investigation and control in health care facilities / Kathleen Meehan Arias.
p. cm.
Includes bibliographical references and index.
ISBN 0-8342-1179-3
1. Health facilities—Sanitation Handbooks, manuals, etc.
2. Nosocomial infections—Prevention Handbooks, manuals, etc.
3. Cross infection—Prevention Handbooks, manuals, etc. I. Title.
[DNLM: 1. Health Facilities Handbooks. 2. Infection Control—
methods Handbooks. 3. Disease Outbreaks Handbooks.
4. Epidemiologic Method Handbooks. WX 39 A696q 1999]
RA969.A736 1999
614.4'4—dc21
DNLM/DLC
for Library of Congress
99-33381
CIP

Copyright © 2000 by Aspen Publishers, Inc.
A Wolters Kluwer Company
www.aspenpublishers.com
All rights reserved.

Orders: (800) 638-8437
Customer Service: (800) 234-1660

About Aspen Publishers • For more than 40 years, Aspen has been a leading professional publisher in a variety of disciplines. Aspen's vast information resources are available in both print and electronic formats. We are committed to providing the highest quality information available in the most appropriate format for our customers. Visit Aspen's Internet site for more information resources, directories, articles, and a searchable version of Aspen's full catalog, including the most recent publications: **www.aspenpublishers.com**

Aspen Publishers, Inc. • The hallmark of quality in publishing
Member of the worldwide Wolters Kluwer group.

Editorial Services: Kate Hawker
Library of Congress Catalog Card Number: 99-33381
ISBN: 0-8342-1179-3

Printed in the United States of America

1 2 3 4 5

For my wonderful husband, Bob,
Who did my share of the cooking while I worked on "the book."

Table of Contents

Contributors

Kathleen Meehan Arias, MS, CIC
Manager
Infection Control Department
Sinai Hospital of Baltimore
Baltimore, Maryland

Georgia Phelps Dash, RN, BSN, MS, CIC
Director
Epidemiology/Infection Control Department
Medical College of Pennsylvania Hospital
Philadelphia, Pennsylvania

Lorraine Messinger Harkavy, RN, MS, CIC
Vice President, Infection Control and Epidemiology
    Programs
Integrated Health Services, Inc.
Owings Mills, Maryland

Deborah Y. Phillips, RN, MPH, CIC
Infection Control Coordinator
Infection Control Department
Parkland Health and Hospital System
Dallas, Texas

Robert L. Sautter, PhD
System Microbiologist
Point of Care Medical Director
Pinnacle Health
Harrisburg, Pennsylvania
Clinical Assistant Professor of Pathology
Milton S. Hershey Medical Center
Pennsylvania State University College of Medicine
Hershey, Pennsylvania
Adjunct Faculty
Department of Continuing Education
Pennsylvania State Capital College
Middletown, Pennsylvania
Adjunct Faculty
Mathematics, Science and Allied Health Division
Harrisburg Area Community College
Harrisburg, Pennsylvania

Preface

Societal, technological, and environmental factors continue to have a dramatic effect on infectious diseases worldwide, facilitating the emergence of new diseases and the re-emergence of old ones, sometimes in drug-resistant forms. Modern demographic and ecologic conditions that favor the spread of infectious diseases include rapid population growth; increasing poverty and urban migration; more frequent movement across international boundaries by tourists, workers, immigrants, and refugees; alterations in the habitats of animals and arthropods that transmit disease; increasing numbers of persons with impaired host defenses; and changes in the way that food is processed and distributed.

Centers for Disease Control and
Prevention. Preventing emerging
infectious diseases: a strategy for the
21st century. Overview of the
updated CDC plan. *MMWR Morb
Mortal Wkly Rep.* 1998;47(RR-15):1.

In the past two decades, the world has witnessed the emergence of new microbial agents, such as the human immunodeficiency virus, *Clostridium difficile, Candida,* and *Cryptosporidium,* and the development of antibiotic resistance in pathogens such as *Staphylococcus aureus, Mycobacterium tuberculosis,* and *Streptococcus pneumoniae.* Many of these organisms have been responsible for causing endemic and epidemic infections in health care facilities. Considerable progress has been made in understanding the nature, sources, reservoirs, and modes of transmission of infectious agents. Much of this knowledge has been gained through the use of descriptive and analytical epidemiology, the application of new laboratory techniques for identifying organisms, and the use of molecular epidemiology in investigating outbreaks. By studying the reports of these outbreaks, health care personnel can expand their knowledge of the epidemiology of nosocomial infections and apply this knowledge toward preventing future infections.

The field of health care epidemiology was initially concerned with infection surveillance, prevention, and control in acute care hospitals. However, this focus has moved beyond the hospital to include the long-term care and ambulatory care settings and has expanded beyond infections to include the use of sound epidemiological principles in studying noninfectious outcomes of medical care. This book was written for infection control professionals, health care facility epidemiologists, quality management personnel, clinical laboratory scientists, students, and educators—those who are interested in using epidemiologic methods to monitor health care outcomes. Its purpose is threefold:

1. to explain epidemiologic principles as they apply to the health care setting
2. to serve as a quick reference for published reports pertaining to the identification, investigation, and

control of outbreaks in a variety of health care settings

3. to present practical guidelines for identifying, investigating, and controlling outbreaks caused by either infectious or noninfectious agents

Chapter 1 defines terms used in epidemiology, describes the different types of epidemiologic studies used in the health care setting, and addresses the concepts of association and causation. Chapter 2 outlines the components of effective surveillance programs for a variety of health care settings—programs that are necessary to recognize a potential outbreak or occurrence of adverse events. Chapters 3–7 review reports of outbreaks and pseudo-outbreaks that have occurred in acute care, long-term care, and ambulatory care facilities. By studying these reports, health care personnel can expand their knowledge of the epidemiology of nosocomial outbreaks to identify and implement effective interventions to control such outbreaks or to prevent them from occurring. Examples of both infectious and noninfectious outbreaks are included to demonstrate how epidemiologic principles can be used to monitor and identify a variety of outcomes.

Chapter 8 presents practical guidelines for recognizing, investigating, and controlling an outbreak in a variety of health care settings. Chapter 9 gives useful tips on conducting a literature search—how to identify sources of information, how to conduct an electronic search, and when to use the Internet. Chapter 10 explains basic statistical terms and concepts used in outbreak investigation so the reader can recognize how and when to apply these methods to describe an outbreak, to perform a case-control study, to analyze findings, and to test the hypothesis generated to identify the likely cause of an epidemic. Chapter 11 outlines the key role that the laboratory plays in the diagnosis and surveillance of nosocomial infections and in outbreak investigations. This chapter gives practical information on when and how to collect cultures from personnel, patients, equipment, or the environment, and reviews the various typing methods currently available to provide evidence that organisms are related. Finally, Chapter 12 gives practical information on collecting, organizing, and displaying epidemiologic data using tables, graphs, and charts.

The appendixes contain a glossary of terms used in the practice of epidemiology in the health care setting, case definitions for infectious diseases, sample forms that can be used as templates to develop facility-specific data collection tools for routine surveillance and outbreak investigation, and infection control guidelines related to outbreak investigation and control.

I am indebted to the contributing authors (colleagues and friends who graciously shared their expertise) and to their families, who were understanding of the time it takes to prepare a manuscript. I wish to acknowledge Kalen Conerly at Aspen Publishers, Inc., who patiently guided me through the publication process. Special thanks go to my husband Bob, who cooked many dinners and persevered through many solitary walks and bicycle rides while I worked on the manuscript.

The authors would like to thank the following for reviewing sections of the manuscript and for providing constructive criticism: Robert P. Arias; Joanne Balderson; Colleen Clay; Lee Cook; Dawn Ernest; Jeremy Gradon, MD; Cindy M. Gross; Patricia Hnatuck; William D. Lebar; James Lubby, MD; Andrew R. Mayrer, MD; Barbara Moody; and James VanDerslice, PhD. Thanks also go to Lillian Himes and the staff of the Sinai Hospital of Baltimore Medical Library, and to Libby Coldsmith, Laurie Schwing, and Sherry A. Fletcher in the Pinnacle Health System Library.

Lastly, I would like to thank Emily Rinehart for her thoughtful and expert review of the manuscript and her many helpful suggestions.

Kathleen Meehan Arias

CHAPTER 1

An Introduction to Epidemiology

Kathleen Meehan Arias

One of the continuing perplexities of medicine is the nature of epidemics. The epidemic diseases themselves are no longer much of a mystery. Their causes (microbial, fungal, metazoal), their modes of transmission (by respiration, by ingestion, by insect or animal bite), and the means of controlling their spread (immunization, sanitation, isolation) have all been pretty well established. What still remains to be fathomed is the dynamics of the interplay of pathogenic virulence and human susceptibility that determines their comings and goings.
   Berton Roueché, *The Medical Detectives**

For 50 years, Berton Roueché fascinated readers of *The New Yorker* magazine with his detailed accounts of the investigations of unexplained illnesses. Stories from his classic "Annals of Medicine" series have been compiled into several volumes, which are frequently used as unofficial textbooks for epidemiology courses (see Suggested Reading). This chapter provides, in five sections, information needed to investigate outbreaks in health care facilities and to fathom "the dynamics of the interplay of pathogenic virulence and human susceptibility that determines their comings and goings."[1]

*Source: Reprinted with permission from B. Roueche, In the Bughouse, from *The Medical Detectives, Vol. II,* p. 212, published by Washington Square Press/Pocket Books, February 1986, first published in *The New Yorker,* 1965.

DEFINITIONS USED IN HEALTH CARE EPIDEMIOLOGY

The term "epidemiology" is derived from three Greek words: *epi,* on or among; *demos,* people; and *logos,* the study of. Although many definitions can be found, the following is appropriate for use in the health care setting: Epidemiology is the study of the distribution and determinants of health-related states and events in defined populations, and the application of this study to the control of health problems.[2]

In other words, epidemiology is used to describe what, where, when, why, and to whom disease and other health-related problems occur so that control measures can be identified and implemented. The information in this chapter focuses on the basic principles of epidemiology as they are applied to the surveillance, prevention, and control of nosocomial infections and other adverse events in health care facilities.

The terms defined in the following list are used in this text to describe the occurrence of disease. (The word "disease" is used throughout the text in a broad sense to include health-related conditions and events such as accidents, adverse drug reactions, and injuries.) In addition to these definitions, a glossary can be found in Appendix A.

- **endemic**—The usual or expected number of cases of disease within a specific geographic location or population.
- **epidemic**—The occurrence of more cases of disease than expected in a given area or specific population over a specified period of time.

- **pandemic**—An epidemic that affects several countries or continents.
- **incidence**—The number of new cases of disease in a particular population during a specified period of time.
- **prevalence**—The number of existing cases (both old and new) of disease in a particular population during a specified period of time.
- **community acquired**—A disease that results from exposure to physical, chemical, or biological agents in the community.
- **nosocomial**—A disease that results from exposure to physical, chemical, or biological agents in the health care setting.

A HISTORICAL PERSPECTIVE: SOME EPIDEMIOLOGICAL TIDBITS

Epidemiologic principles have long been used to determine the suspected cause of diseases so that control measures can be identified and implemented to prevent their spread. The Bible indicates that lepers were isolated from society (c. 1400 BC) to prevent the spread of leprosy (". . . he shall dwell alone . . ." Lev 13:46). In the Mosaic code, the consumption of pork was forbidden ("The swine . . . is unclean to you." Lev 11:7), and this prohibition still exists today in some cultures. Around 400 BC, Hippocrates wrote his famous treatise, *The Airs, Waters, and Places*, in which he associated disease occurrence with environmental factors such as air, water, and places rather than with supernatural causes. In the Dark Ages (c. AD 500–1400), diseases were thought to be caused by miasmas or rising vapors, such as those from marshes, which were thought to infect the air. The word "quarantine" comes from 14th century Italy where sailing vessels were detained for 40 days (*quaranta giorni*) before travelers could disembark. This precaution was taken to prevent the spread of plague. This practice carries over to modern-day maritime regulations in the United States where a vessel, upon arrival from a foreign port, is required to display a square yellow flag until permission is granted to land.[3] The yellow signal flag represents the letter "Q" in the international code of flags, which is used by ships around the world.

In the 16th century, the Italian physician and poet Girolamo Fracastoro recognized that there were three modes of transmission (person to person, air, and objects) and in his 1546 work, *De Contagione et Contagionis Morbis*, he suspected that minute agents caused disease.

The word "malaria" can be traced back to the 18th century and comes from the Italian *mala aria* or "bad air." This alludes to the former belief that malaria was spread by foul air from swamps. In the late 1700s, the British physician Edward Jenner observed that dairy workers who had contact with cows having cowpox did not succumb when exposed to smallpox. He discovered that individuals could be protected from smallpox if they were inoculated with cowpox—thus giving us the word "vaccine," which is adopted from the Latin *vaccinus* for cow.

In 1846, Panum noticed that if measles were introduced to a population there were fewer cases if some of the population previously had measles. He was the first person to scientifically explain herd immunity (i.e., the resistance of a population to invasion and spread of an infectious agent because many in the population are immune). In the 1840s Ignaz Phillipp Semmelweis noticed that there appeared to be more deaths from puerperal (childbed) fever in the first division of the Vienna Lying-In Hospital than in the second division. He reviewed the literature on the purported causes of puerperal fever, observed the practices in both divisions, and carefully collected data on the numbers of deaths and possible risk factors, such as exposure to different types of medical personnel. After comparing mortality rates and risk factors between the two divisions, he formed the hypothesis that cadaveric material on the hands of medical students was somehow responsible for causing puerperal fever. Semmelweis then required students and physicians to wash their hands in chlorinated lime after performing autopsies prior to attending a patient. Semmelweis was able to demonstrate a dramatic decrease in maternal mortality rates after mandating hand disinfection.[4]

Florence Nightingale began her reformation of the British army medical system by introducing sanitary practices, such as environmental cleanliness and safe food and water, during the Crimean War (1853–1855). After the war, she collaborated with the British statistician William Farr to study mortality rates in British hospitals. Using carefully collected epidemiologic data, they were able to show that many deaths were caused by communicable diseases, and they used this information to lobby for further improvements in hospital sanitation.[5]

In his well-known epidemiological studies conducted in the 1850s, the anesthesiologist John Snow investigated the occurrence of cholera in the Golden Square area of London and deduced that the water supply coming from the Broad Street pump was associated with development of the disease.[6] Based on his findings, Snow supposedly removed the handle of the water pump, thus ending the cholera outbreak. John Snow is known as the "father" of field epidemiology because his studies classically illustrate the use of the epidemiologic principles used today to investigate and control outbreaks. It should be noted that Jenner, Panum, Semmelweis, Nightingale, and Snow used imagination, logic, and common sense to determine the most likely factors causing disease and to develop preventive measures—and all worked before the French chemist Louis Pasteur developed his germ theory in the late 1800s.

Any discussion of the evolution of epidemiology would be incomplete without mentioning Robert Koch (1843–1910), who won the Nobel Prize for his studies in microbiology. Among other things, Koch established techniques for growing microorganisms in pure culture and studied the relationship between *Mycobacterium tuberculosis* and tuberculosis. He developed four postulates, now known as Koch's postulates, that he believed were necessary to prove that an organism was the cause of a disease:

1. The organism must be associated with all cases of a given disease.
2. The organism must be isolated in pure culture from persons with that disease.
3. When the pure culture is inoculated into a susceptible person or animal, it must cause the same disease.
4. The organism must then be isolated in pure culture from the person or animal infected by this inoculation.

Although Koch's postulates cannot be used to establish the etiological relationship of some organisms, such as viruses and noncultivable agents, to the disease they are thought to cause, he created a scientific standard for establishing disease causation.[7]

THE MULTIFACTORIAL NATURE OF DISEASE

Etiologic Agents of Disease

It is now recognized that diseases are multifactorial. That is, a disease cannot be attributed to any one factor because there is a complex interrelationship between various agents, a host, and the environment—a concept known as the epidemiologic triangle. Epidemiology was originally concerned with the study of infectious disease, and thus the epidemiologic triangle of agent, host, and the environment is the traditional model used to explain disease causation. Because epidemiologic principles are now applied to the study of noninfectious conditions as well, the concept of the causative agent has been expanded beyond biological agents to include chemical and physical agents. Exhibit 1–1 provides examples of the various etiologic agents of disease.

Exhibit 1–1 Examples of Etiologic Agents of Disease

Biological Agents	Examples
Bacteria	*Staphylococcus, Pseudomonas, Mycobacterium, Campylobacter, Clostridium, Ehrlichia*
Fungi	*Candida, Aspergillus, Cryptococcus, Histoplasmosis*
Viruses	Hepatitis, human immunodeficiency virus, herpes, influenza, measles, Norwalk, rotavirus
Protozoa	*Plasmodium* (malaria), *Cryptosporidium, Giardia, Pneumocystis, Toxoplasma*
Metazoa	*Trichinella*; *Necator* and *Ancylostoma* (hookworm)
Rickettsiae	*Rickettsia*
Arthropods	*Sarcoptes* (mites); *Dermacentor, Amblyomma,* and *Ixodes* (ticks)

Chemical Agents	Examples
Organic chemicals	Aldehydes (e.g., gluteraldehyde), disinfectants
Inorganic chemicals	Heavy metals
Pesticides	DDT, sterilants (e.g., ethylene oxide)
Food additives	Monosodium glutamate
Pharmaceuticals	Antibiotics, analgesics, psychotropics
Occupational exposure	Industrial/laboratory reagents, silica, asbestos, latex

Physical Agents	Examples
Thermal extremes	Heat, cold
Light	Ultraviolet, laser, lightning
Noise	Music
Ionizing radiation	X-rays
Moving objects	Cars, bicycles, bullets
Physical forces	Repetitive motion, lifting, falls

Biological Agents

There is a long list of biological agents that either have been newly recognized or have re-emerged since 1970, and many of these have caused outbreaks in the community and in health care facilities (see Table 1–1). In addition, several well-known organisms have developed drug resistance and have caused serious epidemics: methicillin-resistant *Staphylococcus aureus* (MRSA), vancomycin-resistant *Enterococcus* (VRE), and multidrug-resistant *Mycobacterium tuberculosis* (MDR-TB). MRSA and VRE have now become endemic in some health care facilities.

Chemical Agents

Many chemical agents can cause adverse reactions in humans. Personnel in health care facilities have developed dermatitis and other allergic reactions follow-

Table 1–1 Part 1: Examples of Emergent Bacteria, Rickettsiae, and Chlamydiae

Agent	Related Diseases/Symptoms	Mode of Transmission
Aeromonas species	Areomonad gastroenteritis, cellulitis, wound infection, septicemia	Ingestion of contaminated water or food; entry of organism through a break in the skin
Borrelia burgdorferi	Lyme disease: rash, fever, neurologic and cardiac abnormalities, arthritis	Bite of infective *Ixodes* tick
Campylobacter	*Campylobacter enteritis*: abdominal pain, diarrhea, fever	Ingestion of contaminated food, water, or milk; fecal-oral spread from infected person or animal
Chlamydia pneumoniae (TWAR strain)	TWAR infection: fever, myalgias, cough, sore throat; pneumonia	Inhalation of infective organisms; possibly by direct contact with secretions of an infected person
Chlamydia trachomatis	Trachoma, genital infections, conjunctivitis; infection during pregnancy can result in infant pneumonia	Sexual intercourse
Clostridium difficile	Colitis: abdominal pain, watery diarrhea, bloody diarrhea	Fecal-oral transmission; contact with the organism in the environment
Ehrlichia chaffeensis	Ehrlichiosis; febrile illness (fever, headache, nausea, vomiting, myalgia)	Unknown; tick is suspected vector
Escherichia coli O157:H7	Hemorrhagic colitis; thrombocytopenia; hemolytic uremic syndrome	Ingestion of contaminated food, especially undercooked beef and raw milk
Haemophilus influenzae bio-group *aegyptius*	Brazilian purpuric fever: purulent conjunctivitis, high fever, vomiting, and purpura	Contact with discharges of infected persons; eye flies are suspected vectors
Helicobacter pylori	Gastritis, peptic ulcer, possibly stomach cancer	Ingestion of contaminated food or water, especially unpasteurized milk; contact with infected pets
Legionella pneumophila	Legionnaires' disease: malaise, myalgia, fever, headache, respiratory illness	Air-cooling systems, water supplies
Listeria monocytogenes	Listeriosis: meningoencephalitis and/or septicemia	Ingestion of contaminated foods; contact with soil contaminated with infected animal feces; inhalation of organism
Mycobacterium tuberculosis	Tuberculosis: cough, weight loss, lung lesions; infection can spread to other organ systems	Exposure to sputum droplets (exhaled through a cough or sneeze) of a person with active disease
Staphylococcus aureus	Abscesses, pneumonia, endocarditis, toxic shock	Contact with the organism in a purulent lesion or on the hands
Streptococcus pyogenes (Group A)	Scarlet fever, rheumatic fever, toxic shock	Direct contact with infected persons or carriers; sometimes ingestion of contaminated foods
Vibrio cholerae	Cholera: severe diarrhea, rapid dehydration	Ingestion of water contaminated with the feces of infected persons; ingestion of food exposed to contaminated water
Vibrio vulnificus	Cellulitis; fatal bacteremia; diarrheal illness (occasionally)	Contact of superficial wounds with seawater or with contaminated (raw or undercooked) seafood; ingestion (occasionally)

continues

Part 2: Examples of Emergent Viruses

Agent	Related Diseases/Symptoms	Mode of Transmission
Bovine spongiform encephalopathy (BSE) agent	Bovine spongiform encephalopathy in cows	Ingestion of feed containing infected sheep tissue
Chikungunya	Fever, arthritis, hemorrhagic fever	Bite of infected mosquito
Crimean-Congo hemorrhagic fever	Hemorrhagic fever	Bite of an infected adult tick
Dengue	Hemorrhagic fever	Bite of an infected mosquito (primarily *Aedes aegypti*)
Filoviruses (Marburg, Ebola)	Fulminant, high-mortality hemorrhagic fever	Direct contact with infected blood, organs, secretions, and semen
Hantaviruses	Abdominal pain, vomiting, hemorrhagic fever	Inhalation of aerosolized rodent urine and feces
Hepatitis B	Nausea, vomiting, jaundice; chronic infection leads to hepatocellular carcinoma and cirrhosis	Contact with saliva, semen, blood, or vaginal fluids of an infected person; mode of transmission to children not known
Hepatitis C	Nausea, vomiting, jaundice; chronic infection leads to hepatocellular carcinoma and cirrhosis	Exposure (percutaneous) to contaminated blood or plasma; sexual transmission
Hepatitis E	Fever, abdominal pain, jaundice	Contaminated water
Human herpesvirus 6 (HHV-6)	Roseola in children, syndrome resembling mononucleosis	Unknown; possibly respiratory spread
Human immuno-deficiency viruses		
HIV-1	HIV disease, including acquired immune deficiency syndrome (AIDS): severe immune system dysfunction, opportunistic infections	Sexual contact with or exposure to blood or tissues of an infected person; vertical transmission
HIV-2	Similar to above	Same as above
Human papillomavirus	Skin and mucous membrane lesions (often, warts): strongly linked to cancer of the cervix and penis	Direct contact (sexual contact/contact with contaminated surfaces)
Human parvovirus B19	Erythema infectiosum: erythema on face, rash on trunk; aplastic anemia	Contact with respiratory secretions of an infected person; vertical transmission
Human T-cell lymphotropic viruses (HTLV-I and HTLV-II)	Leukemias and lymphomas	Vertical transmission through blood/breast milk; exposure to contaminated blood products; sexual transmission
Influenza	Fever, headache, cough, pneumonia	Airborne, especially in crowded, enclosed spaces
Lassa	Fever, headache, sore throat, nausea	Contact with urine or feces of infected rodents
Measles	Fever, conjunctivitis, cough, red blotchy rash	Airborne; direct contact with respiratory secretions of infected persons
Norwalk and Norwalk-like agents	Gastroenteritis; epidemic diarrhea	Most likely fecal-oral; alleged vehicles of transmission include drinking and swimming water, and uncooked foods
Rabies	Acute viral encephalomyelitis	Bite of a rabid animal
Ross River	Arthritis, rash	Bite of an infective mosquito
Rotavirus	Enteritis; diarrhea, vomiting, dehydration, and low-grade fever	Primarily fecal-oral; fecal-respiratory transmission can also occur
Yellow fever	Fever, headache, muscle pain, nausea, vomiting	Bite of an infective mosquito (*Aedes aegypti*)

Part 3: Examples of Emergent Protozoans, Helminths, and Fungi

Agent	Related Diseases/Symptoms	Mode of Transmission
Anisakis	Anisakiasis: abdominal pain, vomiting	Ingestion of larvae-infected fish (undercooked)
Babesia	Babesiosis: fever, fatigue, hemolytic anemia	Bite of an *Ixodes* tick (carried by mice in the presence of deer)

continues

Table 1–1 continued

Agent	Related Diseases/Symptoms	Mode of Transmission
Candida	Candidiasis: fungal infections of the gastrointestinal tract, vagina, and oral cavity	Endogenous flora; contact with secretions or excretions from infected persons
Cryptococcus	Meningitis; sometimes infections of the lungs, kidneys, prostate, liver	Inhalation
Cryptosporidium	Cryptosporidiosis: infection of epithelial cells in the gastrointestinal and respiratory tracts	Fecal-oral, person to person, waterborne
Giardia lamblia	Giardiasis: infection of the upper small intestine, diarrhea, bloating	Ingestion of fecally contaminated food or water
Microsporidia	Gastrointestinal illness, diarrhea; wasting in immunosuppressed persons	Unknown; probably ingestion of fecally contaminated food or water
Plasmodium	Malaria	Bite of an infective Anopheles mosquito
Pneumocystis carinii	Acute pneumonia	Unknown; possibly reactivation of latent infection
Strongyloides stercoralis	Strongyloidiasis: rash and cough followed by diarrhea; wasting, pulmonary involvement, and death in immunosuppressed persons	Penetration of skin or mucous membrane by larvae (usually from fecally contaminated soil); oral-anal sexual activities
Toxoplasma gondii	Toxoplasmosis: fever, lymphadenopathy, lymphocytosis	Exposure to feces of cats carrying the protozoan; sometimes foodborne

Source: Reprinted with permission from J. Lederberg, R.E. Shope, and S.C. Oaks, Jr., *Emerging Infections, Microbial Threats to Health in the United States*, pp. 36–41. Copyright 1992 by the National Academy of Sciences. Courtesy of the National Academy Press, Washington, D.C.

---

ing exposure to gluteraldehyde and latex, and patients have experienced hearing loss after therapy with gentamycin.

Physical Agents

Physical agents such as heat, cold, electricity, light, or ionizing radiation may cause injuries in the health care setting (e.g., lasers have caused burns when they malfunctioned during surgery; ultraviolet [UV] light has caused conjunctivitis in exposed personnel). Health care workers are also at risk for back injuries from lifting patients and from percutaneous injuries caused by needles and sharp instruments.

Host Factors Affecting Disease

Conditions that affect an individual's risk of exposure and resistance or susceptibility to disease are called host factors. They include intrinsic factors such as age, sex, genetic composition, or race. Age is one of the most important host factors because it affects both risk of exposure and immunologic status. Factors that influence a person's risk of exposure to disease-causing agents include socioeconomic status, lifestyle behaviors, occupation, and marital status. Factors that influence a person's susceptibility or resistance to disease include immuno-

logic and nutritional status, underlying disease, severity of illness, and psychological state.

Environmental Factors Affecting Disease

Environmental factors are extrinsic factors that affect either the agent or a person's opportunity for exposure to the agent. Factors that affect a person's risk of exposure to nosocomial events include hospitalization or residing in a long-term care facility. Crowding, sanitation, and living in a rural versus urban area are all environmental factors. In some instances, it is difficult to determine whether a particular factor should be classified as agent or environment. For instance, factors such as intravenous therapy, mechanical ventilation, surgery, and invasive diagnostic procedures all affect a patient's risk of exposure to both biological and physical agents; these procedures are also associated with the environment of health care.

Although the epidemiologic triangle may not be appropriate for illustrating disease causation in many noninfectious conditions, it can facilitate understanding of the many interrelated factors that affect the occurrence of infectious diseases. This is an important concept that must be recognized when investigating outbreaks of disease.

STUDY METHODS USED IN EPIDEMIOLOGY: THE FIVE W'S—WHAT, WHO, WHERE, WHEN, AND WHY

Epidemiology is used to understand the causes of a disease (what) by studying its distribution (who, where, and when) and its determinants (why). This helps to characterize the natural history of a disease so that prevention and control measures can be identified. Note that a major purpose of epidemiology is to develop intervention and prevention programs rather than to find a cure.

Epidemiology is a population-based science. Many disciplines contribute to the knowledge of human health and disease—the basic sciences (such as microbiology and biochemistry), the clinical sciences (such as infectious diseases, pediatrics, and internal medicine), and population medicine (such as community medicine and public health)—and all are highly interrelated. The major difference between clinical medicine and population medicine is that the former focuses on an individual person (e.g., a patient with a respiratory disease) while the latter focuses on the community as a whole (e.g., an influenza outbreak). Epidemiology is a science of comparison and rates. The epidemiologist looks for groups with high or low rates of disease so that reasons for disease and freedom from disease can be postulated.

There are three types of epidemiologic studies: descriptive (or observational), analytic, and experimental. Descriptive and analytic studies are used to observe the natural course of events (e.g., an outbreak of food poisoning or the course of the HIV epidemic); however, in an experimental study, the investigator studies the impact of varying some factor under his control (e.g., clinical trials of products or therapeutic agents).

Descriptive Epidemiology: Who, Where, and When

Descriptive studies are used to identify individuals and populations at greatest risk of acquiring a disease, to determine clues as to the etiology of disease, and to predict disease occurrence through knowledge of association of a disease with some risk factor. In descriptive epidemiology, the focus of study is on the incidence (rates) and distribution (population at risk) of disease. Data are organized according to the variables of person, place, and time to identify factors that may be causally related to disease incidence.

Person

Age. Age is considered the most important factor among the personal variables because it affects a person's potential for exposure (e.g., school children are exposed to childhood diseases and adults are exposed to occupational diseases), immune status (e.g., infants have poorly developed immune systems; the elderly have decreased resistance to many infections), and mental and physical condition (e.g., the elderly are generally more prone to falls than the young).

Sex. Males have higher incidence rates for some diseases and conditions than females (e.g., HIV infection), while females have higher rates for others (e.g., breast cancer).

Socioeconomic status. Variables such as social class, occupation, lifestyle, educational level, and family income affect nutritional status, access to health care, and environmental living and working conditions—all of which influence a person's susceptibility or resistance to disease and risk of exposure to various agents and physical injury.

Ethnic and racial groups. Cultural and religious differences can affect a person's risk of exposure to various agents, such as types of food eaten and methods of preparing it.[8]

Genetic variables. Variables associated with genetic composition can affect susceptibility to some diseases, such as sickle cell, Tay-Sachs and Kaposi's sarcoma.

Place

Depending on the event being studied, place may be characterized by birthplace, residence, school, hospital unit, place of employment, restaurant, and so forth. Place can also be defined by political boundaries such as country, state, city, county, or parish or natural boundaries such as mountains, valleys, or watersheds. Some diseases are associated with the place where they were first recognized, such as Lyme disease with a town in Connecticut.

In the health care setting, surveillance data are usually collected and analyzed by the number of cases or the incidence rates in a specific place or area (e.g., the incidence of intravenous therapy–related phlebitis on 3 West, patient falls in the North Wing, or nosocomial bloodstream infections in the intensive care unit [ICU]).

Many health departments use counties, census tracts, and ZIP codes to report statistics on injuries, illnesses, or communicable diseases (Table 1–2). Those responsible for infection control and other quality management programs in health care facilities should use this type of information to identify populations at risk for disease. Since exposure to many infectious diseases occurs both in the health care setting (through infected patients, residents, visitors, or personnel) and in the community (through infected relatives, friends, co-workers, classmates, etc.), outbreaks in health care facilities often reflect what is occurring locally. For example, community outbreaks of pertussis, chicken pox, rotavirus, tuberculosis, and influenza have caused simultaneous outbreaks in area hospitals and long-term care facilities.[9–12] In addition, community disease profiles should be used to conduct an assessment of the risk of health care workers' exposure to diseases such as tuberculosis.[13]

Time

Surveillance data are collected and analyzed over time for evidence of change in the incidence of an event (such as nosocomial infections or medication errors). These data are often shown on a graph with the number of cases or the incidence rate on the vertical axis (y-axis) and time on the horizontal axis (x-axis) (see Figure 1–1). The time periods depicted on the x-axis may be hours, days, weeks, months, quarters, or years, depending on the event described.

Table 1–2 Percentage of Cases with Penicillin Nonsusceptible and Highly Resistant *S pneumoniae* isolates, by County of Residence, Baltimore Metropolitan Area, January 1, 1995–June 30, 1997

County	Total Tested	No. (%) Nonsusceptible	No. (%) Highly Resistant
Anne Arundel	120	32 (27)	20 (17)
Baltimore City	885	107 (12)	43 (5)
Baltimore County	324	45 (14)	20 (6)
Carroll	54	15 (28)	10 (18)
Harford	61	10 (16)	5 (8)
Howard	50	12 (24)	9 (18)
TOTAL	1494	221 (15)	107 (7)

Source: Reprinted from *HIV/AIDS Update,* Spring 1998, State of Maryland, Department of Health & Mental Hygiene.

Epidemic period. An epidemic is the occurrence of more cases of disease than expected in a given area or population over a specified period of time. For some diseases, a graph of an epidemic period, called an epidemic curve, can be used to provide insight into the time of exposure, the mode of transmission, and the agent causing the outbreak (Figure 1–2). Information on constructing and using epidemic curves can be found in Chapters 8 and 12.

Secular (long-term) trends. Surveillance data can be graphed over a period of years to show trends occurring over long periods of time. This information can be used to monitor the efficacy of infection control and quality management programs in health care facilities and in the public health sector. For example, Figure 1–3 is a graph of the incidence of tuberculosis (TB) reported in the United States for the period from 1975 to 1996. It illustrates the increasing incidence that occurred from 1985 through 1992 and the decline that followed through 1996.[14] According to the Centers for Disease Control and Prevention (CDC), factors that were associated with the resurgence of TB included the AIDS/HIV epidemic; immigration of persons from countries where incidence rates are 10 to 30 times higher than in the United States; transmission of TB in settings such as hospitals, homeless shelters, and prisons; and declines in resources for TB control.[15] The downward trend that began in 1993 has been attributed to the implementation of stronger TB control programs that emphasize prompt identification of persons with TB, initiation of appropriate therapy, and completion of therapy.[16]

Seasonal occurrence. Some diseases have a characteristic seasonal pattern. For instance, in the United States the common cold caused by rhinovirus in adults occurs most frequently in the fall and chicken pox occurs most frequently in winter and early spring. In temperate climates, outbreaks of influenza generally occur in winter. Information such as this can be used to recognize the possible causative agent of an outbreak of respiratory disease in a health care facility and to target the timing of influenza immunization campaigns.

Analytic Epidemiology: Why

When conducting an outbreak investigation, descriptive epidemiology is used to describe the outbreak or the cluster of events (i.e., the population involved,

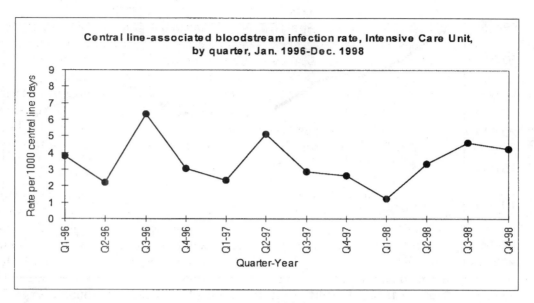

Figure 1–1 Surveillance Data Showing Nosocomial Infection Rates over Time.

the time, and the place), and then attack rates are calculated to identify the population with the highest rate of disease. The next step in the investigation is to use analytic methods to search for a probable cause by mathematically comparing risk factors (attack rates) between the population with the disease and the population without the disease. The statistical methods used are discussed in Chapter 10.

Two important concepts used in analytic epidemiology are cause and association. A cause is a factor that directly influences the occurrence of a disease. Reduction or elimination of the factor in a population will re-

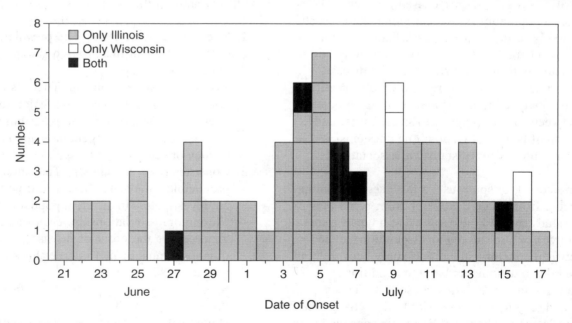

Figure 1–2 Onset of Fever among Triathlon Athletes, by Date—Madison, Wisconsin, and Springfield, Illinois, June 21–July 17, 1998. *Source:* Reprinted from Outbreak of Acute Febrile Illness among Athletes Participating in Triathlons—Wisconsin and Illinois, 1998, *Morbidity and Mortality Weekly Report,* Vol. 47, No. 28, p. 586, 1998, Centers for Disease Control and Prevention.

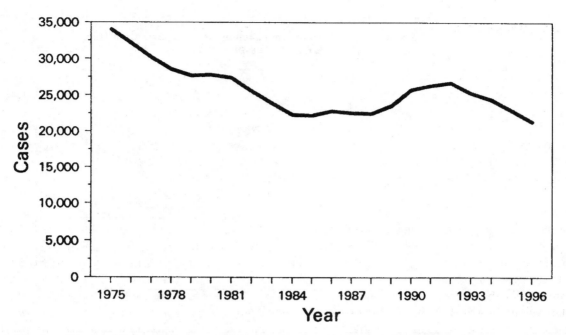

Figure 1–3 Number of Reported Tuberculosis Cases—United States, 1975–1996. *Source:* Reprinted from Tuberculosis Morbidity—United States, 1996, *Morbidity and Mortality Weekly Report,* Vol. 46, No. 30, p. 695, 1997, Centers for Disease Control and Prevention.

duce or eliminate the occurrence of the disease in that population. An association is a statistical relationship between two or more variables.

It is commonly said that statistics cannot be used to prove that a particular factor caused an event. Therefore, when a population with a particular characteristic is more likely to develop a disease than a population without that characteristic, the characteristic is said to be associated with the occurrence of the disease.[17] In analytic epidemiology, the results of observational studies are analyzed to determine (1) if an association exists between a factor (exposure) and a disease and (2) the strength of that association if one does exist.

There are three types of statistical associations:

1. Artefactual, or spurious—a false association that occurs from chance alone or from some bias in the study method (also known as a type I error).
2. Indirect, or noncausal—an association that occurs between a factor and a disease only because both are related to some underlying condition.
3. Causal—factor "A" truly causes "B." This occurs if, and only if, A occurs prior to B; a change in A correlates to a change in B; and this correlation is not the consequence of both A and B being correlated with some prior C.

Criteria for Judging Causality

The following criteria provide a basis for judging if an association is causal, that is, the suspected factor is the likely cause of the event:[18]

1. Strength of association. The prevalence of disease is higher in the exposed group than in the nonexposed group.
2. Dose-response relationship. There is a quantitative relationship between the factor and the frequency of disease, for example, those with the most exposure to the agent have the greatest frequency or severity of illness.
3. Consistency of association. The findings are reproducible—they have been confirmed by different investigators in different populations.
4. Chronological relationship. Exposure to the factor precedes the onset of disease. This criterion obviously must be met in order for a factor to be able to cause a disease.
5. Specificity of association. If the factor occurs, disease can be predicted.
6. Biologically plausible. The findings are coherent with existing information. They are acceptable in light of current knowledge.

Establishing Causal Relations

Two types of observational studies are used to determine causal relations: case control and cohort. Case-control studies compare groups of people who have a disease (the cases) with groups from the same population who are not ill (the controls). In cohort studies the subjects are categorized based on their exposures to specific risk factors and they are then observed to determine if they develop a disease.

The case-control study. The case-control study is the most commonly used method for testing causal associations when investigating outbreaks in the health care setting. In a case-control study, cases are identified (i.e., persons identified as having a disease or condition) and compared with controls (i.e., persons from the same population who do not have the disease or condition). Case-control studies can be used to investigate outbreaks of either infectious or noninfectious events.[19,20] A statistical analysis is conducted to determine if the two groups differ in the proportion of persons who were exposed to a specific factor.

Case-control study is a retrospective method because it compares cases and controls to an exposure that has already occurred. For example, the microbiology laboratory in a hospital reports to the Infection Control Department that it has isolated *Burkholderia cepacia* from the respiratory secretions of seven patients in the intensive care unit (ICU) in the past month. A review of microbiology reports for the previous 6 months reveals only one prior isolate of *B cepacia*. Despite reinforcement of appropriate hand-washing practices, the organism is isolated from the respiratory tract of two more patients in the ICU in the next 2 weeks. A case-control study could be designed to evaluate exposures among cases (those from whom *B cepacia* is isolated) and controls (patients in the ICU at the same time as the cases but who do not have a positive culture for *B cepacia*) in order to determine which risk factors (exposures) are associated with the occurrence of *B cepacia*.

Information on designing, conducting, analyzing, and interpreting a case-control study can be found in Chapter 10.

The cohort study. In a cohort study, a defined group of individuals (a cohort) is studied to determine if specified exposures result in disease. Cohort studies may be conducted prospectively or retrospectively. A prospective cohort study begins with a group of subjects who are free of a given disease. The cohort is divided into groups, one of which is exposed to a potential risk factor and one of which is not. The groups are then followed over time (prospectively) to determine if there are differences in the rates at which disease develops in relation to the risk factor. The Framingham Study, conducted by the National Heart, Lung and Blood Institute in Massachusetts, is a well-known example of a long-term prospective study. Some of the subjects in this study have been followed for almost 40 years.[21]

By contrast, a retrospective cohort study can be used to analyze an outbreak in a small, well-defined population. For example, many of the 29 attendees of a luncheon at a long-term care facility are reported to have developed nausea, vomiting, and abdominal cramps within a five-hour period following the luncheon. A few have diarrhea. A case definition for gastrointestinal illness should be developed and, using the methodology of a cohort study, the 29 attendees could be identified and questioned to determine whether or not they had become ill after attending the luncheon. An attack rate (the percentage of persons who became ill) could then be calculated. If the investigator found that 11 persons fit the case definition, this would be an attack rate of 38 percent (11 ill/29 total attendees × 100). Since it is unusual for 38 percent of the attendees at a meal to develop these symptoms in such a short time period, it would be possible to develop a preliminary hypothesis that the attendees may have developed an acute foodborne illness following the consumption of a contaminated food or beverage at the luncheon. At this point, a retrospective cohort study could be designed to investigate possible associations between exposures to specific foods and the development of a gastrointestinal illness, as discussed in Chapter 10.

Experimental studies. Although experimental studies are not used in the investigation of outbreaks (and will not be covered in this text), infection control professionals, hospital epidemiologists, and quality management personnel frequently review published experimental studies before making decisions about the merits of a new device, product, or procedure. Therefore, they need to be familiar with the principles, problems, and pitfalls in the design and interpretation of experimental studies. For information on conducting and interpreting experimental studies, refer to the Suggested Reading list at the end of this chapter. In addition, several articles about critically reviewing the results of clinical trials are listed in the reference section.[22–26]

THE EPIDEMIOLOGY OF INFECTIOUS DISEASES

As most outbreak investigations in health care facilities involve infectious diseases, this section will describe the spectrum of disease, explain the infectious disease process, and illustrate how these affect the surveillance, prevention, and control of infections.

The Infectious Disease Spectrum

By definition, a disease is an illness that is "characterized usually by at least two of these criteria: recognized etiologic agent(s), identifiable group of signs and symptoms, or consistent anatomical alterations."[27]

As illustrated in Figure 1–4, most diseases have a characteristic natural history, or progression, from onset to resolution unless medical intervention occurs. Although this concept applies to both infectious and noninfectious conditions, this discussion will focus on infectious diseases. Conducting an outbreak investigation requires familiarity with the natural history of a disease in order to identify persons who may be infected because not all infections result in disease (i.e., signs and symptoms). If an outbreak is caused by an agent that frequently causes inapparent infection, many infected persons may be missed if an active search for cases is not conducted.

The infectious disease spectrum can be divided into three classes: (1) infection is frequently inapparent, (2) infection results in clinical disease that is rarely fatal, and (3) infection results in severe disease that is usually fatal.

Frequently Inapparent Infection

Agents. Agents that often cause inapparent or subclinical infection include the hepatitis A, B, and C viruses, *M tuberculosis*, polio virus, *N gonorrhea* in females, *Chlamydia trachomatis*, human immunodeficiency virus (HIV), many nontyphoid strains of *Salmonella,* and cytomegalovirus.

Infection control/public health significance. Because they have no signs and symptoms, most persons infected with these agents will not be identified, even though many may be able to spread the infectious agent to others. Since only a small percentage of those infected (the tip of the iceberg) develop clinical disease, only a few will seek medical attention. Therefore, an even smaller percentage is likely to be hospitalized and reported. Statistics on this type of infection are likely to be inaccurate because the number of cases diagnosed and reported will be less than the true number.

If an outbreak is caused by one of these agents, it is necessary to actively search for cases by utilizing the appropriate diagnostic tests, such as serologic tests for the hepatitis viruses, stool cultures for *Salmonella*, and skin tests for *M tuberculosis*, in order to identify infected persons. If diagnostic tests are necessary, the laboratory should be consulted in the early stages of an outbreak investigation to ensure that the correct tests and specimen collection procedures are used, as discussed in Chapter 11.

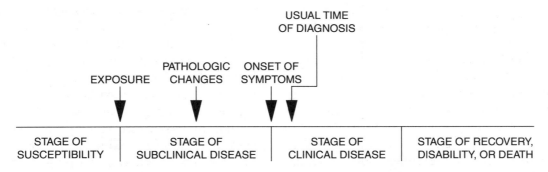

Figure 1–4 The Natural History of Disease. *Source:* Reprinted from Epidemiology Program Office, *Principles of Epidemiology: An Introduction to Applied Epidemiology and Biostatistics,* 2nd ed., p. 43, 1992, Centers for Disease Control and Prevention.

Contact tracing (i.e., finding and treating the contacts of infectious persons) is a public health method used to control the spread of these diseases. Contacts are persons who are exposed to an infectious individual in such a way that infection is likely to occur. For instance, health care workers with prolonged unprotected exposure to a patient subsequently found to be infectious for *M tuberculosis* would be identified as a contact and skin tested to detect infection.

Carriers are persons who have no signs and symptoms but are infectious. These cases are important from an infection control standpoint because they may unwittingly spread their infection to others.

Since patients with inapparent infection may be infectious, health care workers may transfer organisms from one patient to another, or to themselves, if they do not properly follow standard (universal) precautions. It is important to remember that not everyone who has an inapparent infection is infectious (e.g., most people who are infected with *M tuberculosis* become skin test positive, but they are not infectious and cannot spread the infection to others).

Infection Resulting in Rarely Fatal Clinical Disease

Agents. Agents that typically cause clinical disease in those who become infected include the measles and chicken pox viruses and rhinovirus.

Infection control/public health significance. Most persons with measles or chicken pox can be identified clinically. Nevertheless, diagnostic tests should be used to confirm the diagnosis of measles because it is now uncommonly seen in the United States (due to a highly immunized population), and many clinicians are not familiar with its presentation.

Infection Resulting in Usually Fatal Severe Disease

Agents. Agents that cause severe infection that is invariably fatal if not treated include the rabies virus, *Clostridium tetani,* and HIV. Infection with HIV is unique in that it presents with a long subclinical phase in which infection is inapparent and then develops into the acquired immune deficiency syndrome (AIDS), which is invariably fatal. Therefore HIV can be placed into two of the three classes in the infectious disease spectrum.

Infection control/public health significance. Statistics on incidence rates for these diseases are more accurate than the other two classes because these infections are more likely to be reported and can be detected by surveillance systems that compile data from death certificates.

The Infectious Disease Process: The "Chain of Infection"

Certain conditions must be met in order for an infectious disease to be spread from person to person. This process, called the "chain of infection," can occur only when all elements are present (Figure 1–5). In order for the infectious disease process to occur, an infectious agent must leave a reservoir through a portal of exit, be conveyed by an appropriate mode of transmission, and find a suitable portal of entry into a susceptible host. If an outbreak occurs, an investigator must know or determine the likely chain of infection in order to identify effective control measures.

Infectious Agents

When an outbreak of unknown etiology occurs, it is important to remember that a variety of agents can produce similar clinical syndromes. For instance, an outbreak of diarrhea may be caused by a variety of biological agents, such as viruses, parasites, or bacteria; however, it could also be caused by a chemical agent such as a heavy metal or a mushroom toxin. Inherent characteristics of biological agents that affect their ability to cause disease include the following.

Infectious dose. This is the number of organisms needed to cause infection; generally speaking, the larger the dose of infective microorganisms, the greater the chance that infection will result. For example, infection with *Coxiella burnetii*, the rickettsia that causes Q fever, can occur by inhaling only one organism. It is usually necessary to ingest from 100 to 1,000 *Salmonella* organisms to cause infection[28(p.412)]; however, only a few *Shigella* (10–100 organisms) are needed for infection to occur.[28(p.422)] In many foodborne outbreaks, persons who eat a large quantity of a contaminated food are more likely to develop symptoms than those who eat a small quantity because those who eat a greater amount are more likely to have ingested an infectious dose.

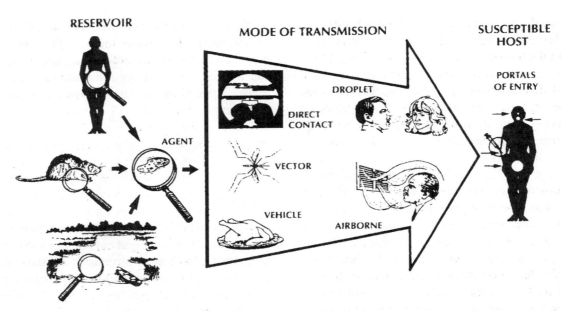

Figure 1–5 The Chain of Infection. *Source:* Reprinted from Epidemiology Program Office, *Principles of Epidemiology: An Introduction to Applied Epidemiology and Biostatistics,* 2nd ed., p. 45, 1992, Centers for Disease Control and Prevention.

Invasiveness. This is the ability of an organism to enter the body and spread through tissue. Examples include the rabies virus, which has a predilection for the brain. Even if it enters the body through the leg, such as from a dog bite, it can spread through tissue to reach the brain.

Infectivity. This is the ability of an agent to initiate and maintain infection. Examples include exposure to chicken pox virus, which generally results in infection in a susceptible host. By contrast, for *Treponema pallidum,* the causative agent of syphilis, only approximately 30 percent of exposures result in infection.[28(p.451)]

Pathogenicity. This is the capacity of an agent to cause disease in a susceptible host. For example, the measles virus is highly pathogenic since almost all persons who become infected will develop a rash, whereas, *Enterococcus faecalis*, which is commonly found in the intestinal tract of humans, rarely causes disease in a normal host and is considered to have low pathogenicity.

Virulence. This is the degree of pathogenicity of an infectious agent: the ability to cause severe disease or death. Virulence is a complex property which combines infectivity, invasiveness, and pathogenicity. For example, although measles is highly pathogenic (it easily causes disease in a susceptible person) it is not very virulent as it rarely causes severe disease. The rabies virus is both highly pathogenic (it causes disease in all who are infected) and extremely deadly, or virulent.

Antigenic variation. This is the ability of an agent to change the antigenic components that are responsible for the specificity of immunity resulting from infection with that agent. For example, influenza A periodically modifies its antigenic structure. This allows the virus to spread more easily through a population that does not have immunity to the new variant. For this reason, the influenza vaccine is modified yearly to protect against those strains of virus which are expected to be prevalent and one must be immunized annually in order to obtain maximum protection.

Viability in the free state. This is the ability of an organism to live outside of a host. For example, the hepatitis B virus (HBV) can survive for at least 7 days on inanimate surfaces at room temperature.[29] For this reason, environmental surfaces and fomites may very well be reservoirs for transmission in an outbreak of hepatitis B. Other organisms, such as human immunodeficiency virus, *Neisseria meningitidis* and *Neisseria gonorrhoeae*, are sensitive to air and will not survive for long on a dry surface, and the tubercle bacillus is quickly killed by sunlight. Therefore, fomites are less important in the transmission of these organisms. (This explains why it is unlikely that one can catch a sexually transmitted disease from the often maligned toilet seat). Some organisms produce spores that may resist heat and drying—spores of *Bacillus anthracis* may remain infective for many years in contaminated soil and articles.

Host specificity. Some agents are species specific and others will infect more than one species. For example, the measles virus, poliovirus, *Neisseria gonorrhoeae,* and *Treponema pallidum* infect only humans; other agents may infect many species. There are numerous serotypes of *Salmonella* that infect humans, other mammals, reptiles, and birds. In some cases, a likely source of an outbreak can be hypothesized if the organism and serotype are known. For instance, since humans are the reservoir for *Salmonella typhi,* an investigator would look for a carrier or for a water or food source contaminated by human feces when investigating an outbreak caused by this organism. An outbreak caused by *Salmonella enteritidis,* however, would suggest a foodborne source because this organism infects both humans and poultry and outbreaks are commonly associated with consumption of raw or undercooked eggs.

Ability to develop resistance to antimicrobials. Some organisms develop resistance to multiple antibiotics, while others remain fairly sensitive; predisposing factors and genetic predilection for developing resistance differs from genus to genus. For example, *Streptococcus pyogenes* (Group A strep) has remained sensitive to penicillin, but *Streptococcus pneumoniae* has become increasingly resistant to penicillin and other antimicrobial agents. *Staphylococcus aureus* developed resistance to penicillin and to methicillin shortly after these antibiotics were introduced. Methicillin-resistant *Staphylococcus aureus* (MRSA), vancomycin-resistant *Enterococcus* (VRE), and antibiotic-resistant strains of Gram-negative organisms, such as *Pseudomonas, Acinetobacter,* and the Enterobacteriaceae (especially *Klebsiella, Serratia and Enterobacter*) are common causes of nosocomial infection in hospitals and long-term care facilities.

Immunogenicity. This is the ability of an agent to stimulate an immunogenic response. For example, infection with some agents will stimulate the production of antibodies that confer immunity. Some organisms, such as the measles, chicken pox, and hepatitis B viruses promote a strong immunogenic response that generally results in long-term immunity to each specific disease. Organisms that stimulate a protective immune response are good candidates for vaccine development. Other agents, such as *Neisseria gonorrhoeae* and *Chlamydia trachomatis*, are poorly immunogenic and reinfection can occur when a person is re-exposed.

Reservoirs

The reservoir is the normal habitat in which an infectious agent lives, multiplies, and grows. Reservoirs for infectious agents exist in humans, animals, and the environment—any of these reservoirs may serve as the source of infection for a susceptible host. Viruses need a living reservoir (human, plant, or animal) to grow and multiply. Gram-positive bacteria such as *Staphylococcus* and *Streptococcus* grow well in a human reservoir but poorly in the environment. Gram-negative bacteria may have a human, animal, or environmental reservoir.

The terms "reservoir" and "source" are frequently used interchangeably; however, they may not be the same. A reservoir is the place where an organism normally lives and reproduces, and the source is the place from which an organism is transmitted to a host through some means of transmission. Sometimes the reservoir and source are the same (e.g., in an outbreak of chicken pox the reservoir and the source of the outbreak may be the same person) and sometimes they are different (e.g., water is a reservoir for *Pseudomonas aeruginosa* that may contaminate a whirlpool bath agitator, which then becomes the source of an outbreak of wound infections). This difference may be important in trying to identify the source of an outbreak so that control measures can be implemented. The inanimate environment, especially fluids, can become contaminated from a reservoir and can serve as the source of an outbreak in the health care setting (e.g., intravenous solutions contaminated with *Enterobacter,* hand lotion contaminated with *Serratia,* eggnog made with unpasteurized eggs harboring *Salmonella*).

Human reservoirs. There are three types of human reservoirs: carriers, colonized persons, and persons who are ill.

1. Carriers are persons who are infected but who have no overt signs and symptoms yet are able to

transmit their infection to others. They are potential sources of infection for others especially because they usually do not know they are infectious and do not take precautions to prevent the spread of their infection to others. There are several types of carrier states:

- Those whose infection is inapparent throughout its course. Also known as subclinical infection, an example of this type of infection is hepatitis A infection, which in children is typically mild or inapparent and jaundice is not a common manifestation. Hepatitis A spreads easily among children in the day care setting and on pediatric units because symptoms, if any, are so slight that little attention is paid to them. Outbreaks in these settings are frequently recognized only after parents or health care providers become infected and develop clinical disease.

- Those who are in the incubatory stage. These are persons who are infected and are infectious but have not yet developed signs and symptoms. For example, a susceptible person who was exposed to chicken pox may have become infected and may be infectious 48 hours before the eruption of chicken pox[28(p.89)]; since he does not know he is infectious, he does not limit contact with others and unwittingly spreads his infection to others.

- Those who are in the convalescent phase. These are persons who continue to be infectious during and after return to health. Those who continue to harbor agents for a prolonged period of time are said to be chronic carriers. For example, approximately 10 percent of untreated persons infected with *Salmonella typhi* will continue to excrete bacilli for three months after onset of symptoms and from 2 to 5 percent will become permanent carriers.[28(p.504)]

2. Those who are colonized. These are persons who harbor an infectious agent but who do not have an infection. A person colonized with an infectious agent is a reservoir and may serve as the source of infection for that organism by transmitting it to another person, either by direct contact or by indirect contact with inanimate objects or environmental surfaces, or by transferring the organism to another site on their own body. For example, approximately 20 to 30 percent of healthy persons carry *Staphylococcus aureus* (coagulase-positive staphylococci) in their anterior nares. These organisms can be transmitted to others or can be inoculated into a break in the colonized person's own skin. Autoinfection is thought to be responsible for at least one-third of staphylococcal infections.[28(p.430)] Many patients in hospitals and residents of long-term care facilities become colonized with antibiotic-resistant organisms, such as methicillin-resistant *Staphylococcus aureus* (MRSA) and vancomycin-resistant *Enterococcus* (VRE), and can serve as the source of infection for others if routine infection control measures such as hand washing and environmental cleanliness are not properly followed.

3. Those who are ill. These are persons who are infected and have signs and symptoms of disease. Because their illness is apparent and precautions can be taken to prevent transmission to others, acute clinical cases are probably less likely to spread infection to others than those who are carriers or who are colonized. For example, if a resident in a long-term care facility develops diarrhea caused by *Clostridium difficile*, precautions such as hand washing and environmental disinfection can be implemented to prevent the transmission of the organism to other residents.

Animal reservoirs. As shown in Table 1–3, animals may serve as reservoirs for many agents that infect humans.[28,30,31] An animal may be a carrier (such as a chicken with *Salmonella*) or may be clinically infected (such as a cat with ringworm). Many foodborne outbreaks in the health care setting have been associated with animal reservoirs—most notably, outbreaks caused by *Salmonella* species from eggs, poultry, and other meats. Infectious agents may be transmitted directly from an animal to human (such as *Pasteurella multocida* transferred from the mouth of a cat to human by a cat bite) or they may be carried by an insect vector (such as *Borrelia burgdorferi*, the causative agent of Lyme disease, which is transmitted by a tick bite).

Although there are no published outbreaks associated with animal-assisted therapy programs, personnel who work in facilities that have such programs need to be aware of the agents that can be transmitted from animals to patients or to residents and need to ensure that appropriate precautions are taken by those in charge of the pets.[30,31] There is one report of an outbreak of *Malassezia pachydermatis* in an intensive care nursery

Table 1–3 Diseases Transmitted from Animal Reservoirs to Humans (Zoonoses)

Disease	Causative Agent	Animal Reservoir(s)	Mode of Transmission
Anthrax	*Bacillus anthracis*	Herbivores, especially sheep and goats	Inhalation of spores from contaminated soil, wool, bones, or hides
Brucellosis	*Brucella* species	Cattle, swine, sheep, goats, dogs	Contact with blood, urine, and tissues (especially placentas and aborted fetuses); ingestion of raw milk and dairy products
Hookworm	*Ancylostoma* species	Cats, dogs	Contact with larva (from feces) in soil
Pasteurellosis	*Pasteurella multocida*, *P haemolytica*	Cats, dogs	Animal bite
Plague	*Yersinia pestis*	Wild rodents (especially ground squirrels)	Bite of infected flea; contact with tissues of infected animals
Psittacosis	*Chlamydia psittaci*	Psittacine birds (parrots, parakeets); poultry	Inhalation of agent from desiccated feces, contaminated dust or feathers
Ringworm	*Trichophyton* species, *Microsporum* species	Cats, dogs, cattle	Direct or indirect contact with infected animals
Rabies	Rabies virus	Skunks, raccoons, bats, dogs, coyotes, foxes, jackals, wolves	Direct contact with saliva of infected animal; corneal transplants from infected person
Salmonellosis	Many *Salmonella* species	Poultry, swine, cattle, rodents, reptiles (especially iguanas, turtles, and snakes), cats, dogs, hedgehogs	Ingestion of organisms in food; fecal-oral transmission
Toxocariasis	*Toxocara canis, T cati*	Dogs, cats	Ingestion of *Toxocara* eggs from the environment
Toxoplasmosis	*Toxoplasma gondii*	Cats and other felines are definitive hosts; sheep, swine, rodents, cattle, and birds may be intermediate hosts	Direct contact with feces; ingestion of raw or undercooked meat
Trichinosis	*Trichinella spiralis*	Swine, dogs, cats, horses, rats, foxes, bears, wolves, boars	Ingestion of viable encysted larvae in raw or undercooked meat
Tularemia	*Francisella tularensis*	Rabbits, hares, muskrats, beavers, hard ticks	Direct contact with infected animal tissue (especially when skinning and processing meat of infected animals); ingestion of undercooked meat or contaminated water; tick bite

that was associated with the colonization of health care workers' pet dogs at home.[32]

Environmental reservoirs. Water and soil are the primary environmental reservoirs for many agents that are pathogenic for humans. *Pseudomonas, Legionellae, Cryptosporidium,* and some *Mycobacterium* species live and multiply in water. Therefore, an aqueous source or reservoir should be considered when investigating an outbreak or cluster of infections caused by one of these organisms. *Aspergillus, Histoplasma, Blastomyces, Cryptococcus,* and *Coccidioides* are fungi that live in the environment in soil or in decaying organic matter; infection with these fungi occurs through inhalation. Outbreaks of *Aspergillus* in health care facilities are frequently associated with disruptions in the physical plant that occur during demolition and renovation.

Portals of Exit

The portal of exit is the path by which an infectious agent leaves its host. The portals of exit and entry for an agent usually correspond to the site in which infection occurs in the body. Agents may leave their human or animal hosts through several portals:

- Respiratory tract. Diseases that are caused by agents that are released through the respiratory tract include the common cold, tuberculosis, influenza, chicken pox, measles, meningococcal disease, pneumococcal disease, infectious mononucleosis, diphtheria, mumps, rubella, and pertussis.
- Genitourinary tract. Diseases of the genital tract that are spread through sexual contact include chlamydia, syphilis, gonorrhea, herpes, lymphogranuloma venereum, and granuloma inguinale. HIV and hepatitis B are bloodborne pathogens that may also be spread through semen and vaginal secretions. Many types of organisms, both gram-positive and gram-negative, can cause urinary tract infections, especially in a catheterized patient, and will be excreted in the urine. Cytomegalovirus is also shed in the urine and in cervical secretions.
- Gastrointestinal tract. Agents that cause gastrointestinal infections and are excreted in feces include *Salmonella, Shigella, Clostridium difficile*, hepatitis A virus, *Vibrio cholerae*, poliovirus, *Campylobacter, Giardia lamblia, Yersinia enterocolitica*, rotavirus, *Escherichia coli*, and the many viral agents that cause acute gastroenteritis.
- Skin and mucous membranes. Organisms that are shed by the skin or mucous membranes include *Herpes simplex* from an oral, skin, or genital lesion; *Treponema pallidum* from a syphilitic lesion or rash; *Staphylococcus aureus* from a skin lesion or wound infection; and the many viral and bacterial agents that cause conjunctivitis.
- Blood. Organisms that are found in blood include HIV, hepatitis B virus, hepatitis C virus, cytomegalovirus, *Treponema pallidum*, and *Plasmodium* species (malaria).
- Transplacental route. Agents that may be transferred from mother to infant across the placenta include the rubella virus, cytomegalovirus, *Treponema pallidum*, hepatitis B virus, HIV, and *Toxoplasma gondii*.

Modes of Transmission

Since microorganisms cannot travel on their own, several modes of transmission facilitate the movement of an agent from its reservoir to a susceptible host. These may be classified as one of three modes of transmission: direct, indirect, and airborne.

Direct transmission. This implies immediate transmission of an infectious agent to an appropriate portal of entry (i.e., one through which infection can occur). Direct transmission can occur through direct contact such as touching, kissing, or sexual intercourse. Many agents that cause nosocomial infections are spread through direct contact and are frequently carried on the hands of health care workers who transfer the organisms from person to person. Direct transmission can also occur through droplet spread. Droplets produced during coughing, talking, sneezing, spitting, or singing may contain infectious agents, which can be carried for a short distance (usually said to be up to 3 feet) to reach the conjunctiva or mucous membranes of the nose or mouth of a susceptible host. Droplet spread is considered direct transmission because two people must be in close proximity for transmission to occur. The meningococcus, pneumococcus, and Group A strep are spread by the droplet route.

Indirect transmission. Transmission by the indirect route involves an intermediate object (inanimate or animate) that carries the agent from the source to a susceptible host. This can be vehicleborne, which occurs when an inanimate object (fomite) serves as a means of transmission for an infectious agent from one host to another. Vehicles in the health care setting include food, water, surgical instruments, medical devices and equipment, intravenous fluids, and blood and blood products. Some agents actively grow and multiply and some can produce toxins in the vehicle (e.g., *Pseudomonas* readily grows and multiplies in fluids; *S aureus* produces an enterotoxin in contaminated foods), while others just passively hitch a ride (e.g., hepatitis A virus in a salad; *M tuberculosis* on a contaminated bronchoscope).

Indirect transmission can also be vectorborne. Vectors are animate intermediaries that carry an infectious agent from host to host. Most vectors are arthropods such as flies, mosquitoes, fleas, lice, and ticks. Insects can transfer organisms by mechanical means (e.g., flies have been shown to carry pathogenic organisms on their feet), or they may be involved in the multiplication or life cycle development of the agent (e.g., *Plasmodium* species multiply in the *Anopheles* mosquito, which injects the organism into humans through a bite).

Airborne transmission. This occurs when microbial aerosols are suspended in air and reach the respiratory tract of a susceptible host. Particles that are between 1 and 5 microns in size are easily inhaled and can bypass the defenses of the upper respiratory tract to be deposited in the alveoli where they grow and multiply. There are two types of aerosols:

- Dust. Particles of dust can carry infective agents such as *Aspergillus* conidia from decaying matter and the Sin Nombre virus (a *Hantavirus*), which is thought to be aerosolized from rodent excreta in soil.
- Droplet nuclei. These are the dried residue of exhaled droplets; they can remain suspended for long periods of time and can be carried on air currents. Droplet nuclei can also be produced by medical procedures such as bronchoscopy and suctioning of the respiratory tract. Chicken pox, measles, influenza, and tuberculosis are spread by the airborne route in droplet nuclei.

Portals of Entry

The portals of entry are similar to the portals of exit described above. Organisms require a specific portal of entry in order to cause infection. If they do not reach this specific portal of entry, they will not be able to establish an infection. For example, enteric pathogens are agents that are transmitted by direct or indirect contact with feces. They are spread by what is commonly called the fecal-oral route (i.e., they are excreted in the feces and enter the body through the mouth). Hepatitis A virus is spread through the fecal-oral route; it is excreted in the feces and is ingested by a host either through direct contact with feces (as may occur by not washing hands after changing a soiled diaper) or indirectly by eating or drinking contaminated food or water.

The skin is an excellent barrier against invasion from infectious agents. Only a few human pathogens, such as the larvae of hookworm and the cercariae of the schistosomes (blood flukes) can effectively penetrate intact skin. Organisms such as *Staphylococcus aureus* and Group A *Streptococcus* can cause infection if they are introduced into a break in the skin; however, they would not be able to initiate infection through intact skin. This is one reason why hand washing is such an important measure for preventing the transmission of infection. If transient organisms such as staphylococci can be washed off the hands before they are introduced into a portal of entry, such as the nose or a wound, then they will not be able to cause an infection.

Salmonella and *Shigella* must be able to reach the intestinal lining in order to cause infection. For this to occur, these organisms generally must be ingested or iatrogenically introduced into the intestine. *Salmonella* has been transmitted in the health care setting by improperly disinfected endoscopes.

Mycobacterium tuberculosis is spread by the airborne route, and the tubercule bacilli must be able to reach the lung in order to initiate a pulmonary infection (i.e., the organism must be able to bypass the hairs, the cilia, and the mucus in the respiratory tract). Generally, a person must inhale the organism for this to occur; however, the tubercule bacilli have also been nosocomially introduced into the lung via contaminated instruments, such as bronchoscopes. Extrapulmonary tuberculosis does occur and can affect any organ or tissue, however, the initial site of infection is almost always the respiratory tract with hematogenous spread to other parts of the body. Although the skin is an excellent barrier against *M tuberculosis*, there are rare reports of primary cutaneous infection caused by direct inoculation.[33]

Susceptible Host

The susceptible host is the final link in the chain of infection. Several factors affect a host's ability to resist infection. These include inherent, or nonspecific, factors; acquired immunity; and secondary resistance factors.

Inherent factors. Inherent, or nonspecific, factors are those that humans are born with, including

- natural barriers such as skin, hairs in the nasal passages, mucous membranes, cilia of the respiratory tract, gastric acidity, and reflexes such as coughing, sneezing, and swallowing
- special mechanisms such as the liver, spleen, and lymph nodes, which can filter organisms from the bloodstream
- hormonal activity such as estrogen, which protects premenopausal females from coronary artery disease

Acquired immunity. Acquired immunity refers to protective antibodies that are directed against a specific agent. There are two types—active immunity and passive immunity. Active immunity occurs when the host develops antibodies in response to an antigen and may be acquired naturally or artificially. It is acquired naturally when the host develops antibodies in response to an infection. For some diseases this immunity persists for the life of the host (e.g., measles and chicken pox). It is acquired artificially in response to a vaccine or toxoid; the duration of protection varies according to disease (e.g., active immunity induced by tetanus toxoid is not permanent and booster doses are recommended every 10 years).[34] Passive immunity results from borrowed antibodies and, like acquired immunity, may be acquired naturally or artificially. Natural immunity is acquired through transfer from mother to fetus; this immunity usually lasts from 6 to 9 months. Immunity is acquired artificially through injection of antiserum (e.g., hepatitis B or varicella-zoster immune globulin) or antitoxin; this protection usually lasts only 4 to 6 weeks.

Secondary resistance factors. Secondary resistance factors are those that affect the host's potential for exposure to an infectious agent. These include extrinsic and intrinsic factors. Extrinsic, or environmental, factors include lack of food, water, or rest; exposure to diagnostic or therapeutic procedures; temperature and humidity; and occupation and socioeconomic status. Examples of extrinsic factors that place the host at risk for nosocomial infection include devices such as ventilators and endotracheal tubes, which compromise the natural defenses in the respiratory tract; surgical procedures and intravascular catheters, which disrupt the skin barrier; urinary catheters, which allow organisms to enter the urinary tract; and chemotherapeutic agents, which are used to suppress the immune system in transplant patients. Intrinsic resistance factors include age, sex, genetic disposition, and diseases that impair the immune response. Examples of diseases that impair the immune response include neoplasias and human immunodeficiency virus infection.

Identifying Effective Measures To Control or Prevent the Spread of Infection

If an agent can be identified—how it enters and exits a host and how it is transmitted—then appropriate prevention and control measures can be determined. These measures are aimed at one of the links in the chain of infection and are usually directed toward the reservoir or source, the mode of transmission, or the susceptibility of the host.

Measures Directed at the Reservoir or Source of an Agent

The nature of the reservoir is of paramount importance in determining the appropriate method of control.

If domestic animals are the reservoir, measures include immunization (e.g., rabies), testing of herds to identify infected animals (e.g., screening cows for bovine tuberculosis), and treatment or destruction of infected animals, such as the destruction of chickens in Japan in 1997 to prevent the spread of avian influenza A (H5N1) to humans. If wild animals are the reservoir, such as rodents for plague and *Hantavirus*, control is more difficult but can be accomplished by limiting the entry of these animals into the living areas of humans. When insects are the reservoir (e.g., mosquitoes for malaria), their entry into dwellings may be limited by screens, or the insects may be eradicated with pesticides or repelled with chemicals. If the reservoir is human, obviously eradication of the host is not a viable option; however, if the infection is recognized, a person can be treated with an antimicrobial to eliminate the agent or can be isolated (i.e., restricted from exposing other persons, such as when a patient with infectious pulmonary tuberculosis is placed in an isolation room or is instructed to stay home until the period of communicability is over).

Measures Directed at Interrupting Transmission

In order to interrupt transmission, measures may be aimed at preventing the organism from entering or exiting the host or at limiting direct contact, indirect contact, or airborne dissemination. Examples include hand washing; standard (universal) precautions; protective barriers, such as gloves, gowns, respirators, and masks used by health care workers; aseptic technique; chemical repellents and window and door screens to protect against insects; isolation and quarantine; and dressings to cover wounds.

Contaminated vehicles can transmit infectious agents from one host to another. Food and water have the potential for affecting large numbers of people from one source and have been the vehicles for many outbreaks in the community and in health care facilities. Measures used to affect this type of transmission include purification of drinking water; pasteurization of milk; irradiation of food; and safe handling and preparation of food, with an emphasis on hand washing, cleanliness of equipment, and proper refrigeration, cooking, and storage. Contaminated medication, equipment, instruments, and devices have served as vehicles in many outbreaks in the health care setting. Measures used to prevent or control these outbreaks include aseptic technique when handling medications and intravenous fluids, and proper cleaning, disinfection, and sterilization of instruments and medical devices.

Measures Directed at the Host

Measures directed at the host focus on reducing host susceptibility and include chemoprophylaxis and immunization. Examples in the health care setting include policies requiring immunity to measles, mumps, rubella, and hepatitis B as a condition of employment (this may be required by law in some areas); bloodborne pathogens exposure management protocols, which include hepatitis B vaccine (active immunization), hepatitis B immune globulin (passive immunization), and chemoprophylaxis for HIV; and tuberculosis control programs, which provide purified protein derivative testing to identify infected persons so that chemoprophylaxis can be given to prevent disease.

Sometimes there may be a shift in emphasis in the primary control measure used to prevent the spread of a disease—such has occurred for tuberculosis and measles. For tuberculosis the change was prompted by the development of effective antimicrobial agents; for measles the change occurred when an effective vaccine was produced. Before the discovery of effective chemotherapy, the primary control measure used to prevent transmission of tuberculosis was placement in a sanitarium or a specialized tuberculosis ward. Now the primary control method is prompt identification and treatment of infectious persons and follow-up of their contacts. Before the measles vaccine was widely implemented, the primary control method was isolation of an infected person; now immunization is the primary control method used.

REFERENCES

1. Roueché B. In the Bughouse. In: *The Medical Detectives*, vol. II. New York: Washington Square Press; 1986:212.

2. Last JM, ed. *A Dictionary of Epidemiology*. 2nd ed. New York: Oxford University Press; 1988:42.

3. Maloney ES. *Chapman's Piloting, Seamanship, and Small Boat Handling*. 62nd ed. New York: Hearst Marine Books; 1996:55.

4. Miller PM. Semmelweis. *Infect Control*. 1982;3:405–409.

5. LaForce FM. The control of infections in hospitals: 1750 to 1950. In: Wenzel RP, ed. *Prevention and Control of Nosocomial Infections*. Baltimore: Williams & Wilkins; 1987:1–12.

6. Snow J. *On the Mode of Communication of Cholera, Second Edition*. London: Churchill; 1885 (reprinted New York: The Commonwealth Fund; 1936).

7. Fredericks DN, Relman DA. Sequence-based identification of microbial pathogens: a reconsideration of Koch's postulates. *Clin Microbiol Rev*. 1996;9:18–33.

8. Lee LA, Gerber AR, Lonsway, DR. *Yersinia enterocolitica* O:3 infections in infants and children associated with the household preparation of chitterlings. *N Engl J Med*. 1990;322:984–987.

9. Christie CDC, Glover AM, Willke MJ, et al. Containment of pertussis in the regional pediatric hospital during the Greater Cincinnati epidemic of 1993. *Infect Control Hosp Epidemiol*. 1995;16:556–563.

10. Faoagali J, Darcy D. Chicken pox outbreak among the staff of a large, urban adult hospital: costs of monitoring and control. *AJIC*. 1995;23:247–250.

11. Raad I, Sheretz R, Russell B, et al. Uncontrolled nosocomial rotavirus transmission during a community outbreak. *AJIC*. 1990;18:24–28.

12. Agerton T et al. Transmission of a highly drug-resistant strain (Strain W1) of *Mycobacterium tuberculosis*: community outbreak and nosocomial transmission via a contaminated bronchoscope. *JAMA*. 1997;278:1073–1077.

13. Centers for Disease Control and Prevention (CDC). Guidelines for preventing the transmission of *Mycobacterium tuberculosis* in health-care facilities, 1994. *MMWR*. 1994;43(RR-13):8–23.

14. CDC. Tuberculosis morbidity—United States, 1996. *MMWR*. 1997;46:695–699.

15. Cantwell MF, Snider DE, Cauthen GM, et al. Epidemiology of tuberculosis in the United States, 1985 through 1992. *JAMA*. 1994;272:535–539.

16. CDC. Tuberculosis morbidity—United States, 1997. *MMWR*. 1998;47:253–257.

17. Centers for Disease Control and Prevention. *Principles of Epidemiology: An Introduction to Applied Epidemiology and Biostatistics*. 2nd ed. Atlanta: US Dept of Health and Human Services, Public Health Service, CDC, Epidemiology Program Office; 1992:32.

18. Last JM, Tyler CW. Epidemiology. In: Last JM, Wallace RB, eds. *Maxcy-Rosenau-Last Public Health and Preventive Medicine*. 13th ed. Stamford, CT: Appleton & Lange; 1992:33.

19. Dwyer DM, Strickler H, Goodman RA, et al. Use of case-control studies in outbreak investigations. *Epidemiol Rev*. 1994;16:109–123.

20. Terdiman JP, Ostroff JW. Gastrointestinal bleeding in the hospitalized patient: a case-control study to assess risk factors, causes, and outcomes. *Am J Med*. 1998;104:349–354.

21. Post WS, Larson MG, Myers RH, et al. Heritability of left ventricular mass: the Framingham Heart Study. *Hypertension*. 1997;30:1025–1028.

22. Research Development Committee, Society for Research and Education in Primary Care Internal Medicine. Clinical research methods: an annotated bibliography. *Ann Intern Med*. 1983;99:419–424.

23. Carpenter LM. Is the study worth doing? *Lancet*. 1993;342:221–223.

24. Glynn JR. A question of attribution. *Lancet*. 1993;342:530–532.

25. Burke JP. Randomized controlled trials in hospital epidemiology. *AJIC*. 1983;11:165–173.

26. Victoria CG. What's the denominator? *Lancet*. 1993;342:345–347.

27. *Stedman's Medical Dictionary*. 25th ed. Baltimore: Williams & Wilkins; 1990: 444.

28. Benenson AS, ed. *Control of Communicable Diseases Manual*. 16th ed. Washington, DC: American Public Health Association; 1995.

29. Bond WW, Favero MS, Petersen NJ, et al. Survival of hepatitis B after drying and storage for one week. *Lancet*. 1981;1:550–551.

30. Goldstein EJC. Household pets and human infections. *Infect Dis Clin North Am*. 1991;5:117–130.

31. Plaut M, Zimmerman EM, Goldstein RA. Health hazards to humans associated with domestic pets. *Annu Rev Public Health*. 1996;17:221–245.

32. Chang HJ, Miller HL, Watkins N, et al. An epidemic of *Malassezia pachydermatis* in an intensive care nursery associated with colonization of health care workers' pet dogs. *N Engl J Med*. 1998;338:706–711.

33. Genne D, Siegrist HH. Tuberculosis of the thumb following a needlestick injury. *Clin Infectious Dis*. 1998;26:210–211.

34. Centers for Disease Control and Prevention. Update on adult immunization. Recommendations of the Immunization Practices Advisory Committee (ACIP). *MMWR*. 1991;40(RR-12):1–94.

SUGGESTED READING

Abramson JH. *Making Sense of Data: A Self-Instruction Manual on the Interpretation of Epidemiological Data*. 2nd ed. New York: Oxford University Press; 1994.

American Academy of Pediatrics. *1997 Red Book: Report of the Committee on Infectious Diseases*. Elk Grove Village, IL: American Academy of Pediatrics; 1997.

Benenson AS, ed. *Control of Communicable Diseases Manual*. 16th ed. Washington, DC: American Public Health Association; 1995.

Bennett JV, Brachman PS, eds. *Hospital Infections*. 4th ed. Boston: Little, Brown and Company; 1997.

Centers for Disease Control and Prevention (CDC). *Principles of Epidemiology: An Introduction to Applied Epidemiology and Biostatistics*. 2nd ed. 1992. (This manual is used in the CDC Self-Study Course 3030-G, Principles of Epidemiology; available from the CDC at 1-800-41-TRAIN.)

Dever GEA. *Epidemiology in Health Services Management*. Gaithersburg, MD: Aspen Publishers; 1984.

Evans AS, Brachman PS, eds. *Bacterial Infections of Humans: Epidemiology and Control*. 3rd ed. New York: Plenum Medical; 1998.

Evans AS, Kaslow RA, eds. *Viral Infections of Humans: Epidemiology and Control*. 4th ed. New York: Plenum Medical; 1997.

Friedman GD. *Primer of Epidemiology*. 4th ed. New York: McGraw Hill; 1994.

Lasker RD. *Medicine and Public Health: The Power of Collaboration*. New York: New York Academy of Medicine, Committee on Medicine and Public Health; 1997.

Last JM. *Public Health and Human Ecology*. 2nd ed. Stamford, CT: Appleton & Lange; 1997.

Lilienfeld DE, Stolley PD. *Foundations of Epidemiology*. 3rd ed. New York: Oxford University Press; 1994.

Mausner JS, Kramer S. *Epidemiology: An Introductory Text*. 2nd ed. Philadelphia: WB Saunders Company; 1985.

Mayhall CG. *Hospital Epidemiology and Infection Control*. Baltimore: Williams & Wilkins; 1996.

Norman GR, Streiner DL. *Biostatistics: The Bare Essentials*. St. Louis, MO: Mosby; 1994.

Olmsted R, ed. *APIC Infection Control and Applied Epidemiology: Principles and Practice*. St. Louis, MO: Mosby; 1996.

Roueché B. *The Medical Detectives* and *The Medical Detectives, Volume II*. New York: Washington Square Press; 1986.

Roueché B. *The Medical Detectives*. Reprint edition. New York: Plume; 1991.

Sackett DL, Haynes RB, Guyatt GH, et al. *Clinical Epidemiology: A Basic Science for Clinical Medicine*. 2nd ed. Boston: Little Brown; 1991.

Wenzel RP, ed. *Prevention and Control of Nosocomial Infections*. 3rd ed. Baltimore: Williams & Wilkins; 1997.

CHAPTER 2

Routine Surveillance Programs
for Health Care Facilities

Kathleen Meehan Arias and Lorraine Messinger Harkavy

INTRODUCTION

In December 1970, the Hospital Infections Section of the Center for Disease Control (now the Centers for Disease Control and Prevention [CDC]) first received reports of episodes of nosocomial bloodstream infections (BSIs) caused by *Enterobacter* species. "Between October 1970 and March 1, 1971, eight United States hospitals in seven states experienced 150 bacteremias caused by *Enterobacter cloacae* or Gram-negative organisms of the *Erwinia* group. There were nine deaths; all were associated with intravenous (IV) fluid therapy. The *Enterobacter* bacteremias in all hospitals were substantially increased as compared to previous time periods. Four hospitals which isolated and identified *Erwinia* had not previously encountered infections with these organisms."[1(p.1227)] The finding that two unusual organisms (*E cloacae* and *Enterobacter agglomerans*) were causing BSIs at multiple hospitals pointed to the likelihood of a common source. The nationwide *Enterobacter* BSI outbreak that affected these hospitals was eventually traced to intrinsic contamination of the plastic cap liners of IV fluids from a single manufacturer. This outbreak of bacteremias associated with contaminated IV infusion fluids may not have been recognized had it not been for the ongoing infection surveillance programs that had been established in these hospitals. This outbreak, which was reported in the March 12, 1971, issue of *Morbidity and Mortality Weekly Report*, "would later be recognized as the largest and most lethal known outbreak of nosocomial infection associated with widespread distribution of a contaminated medical product in the United States.

The report demonstrates the benefit of the emphasis that CDC had placed on nosocomial infection surveillance and control programs starting in the 1960s and illustrated the importance of being able to rapidly assemble data from multiple, widely scattered sites to resolve complex outbreaks."[1(p.1227)] If the nosocomial infection surveillance programs had not existed in these hospitals, the detection of this outbreak would have been more difficult, and the outbreak likely would have resulted in additional deaths. This outbreak resulted in the development of the CDC's Guidelines for Infection Control in Intravenous Therapy,[2] which became the first in a series of guidelines by the CDC on the prevention of nosocomial infections.

Surveillance forms the foundation of an effective infection control program. Personnel in quality management/ quality assurance departments now also recognize that surveillance is a critical component of a performance improvement program in a health care facility. A surveillance system is necessary to identify and recognize nosocomial infections and other adverse events in the health care setting so that prevention and control activities can be identified and implemented to minimize the risk for these events. An effective surveillance program is essential to recognize unusual infections and clusters or outbreaks of disease. In this chapter, the term "disease" is used to describe nosocomial infections and other adverse outcomes and events, such as falls, that are related to health care, and the term "patient" is used to describe residents in long-term care (LTC) facilities and patients in acute, subacute, and ambulatory care facilities.

This chapter explains the reasons for implementing an active surveillance program; discusses the various components of an effective surveillance program for a health care facility; provides definitions for the surveillance of nosocomial infections; outlines the steps in the surveillance process; and discusses how to use surveillance data to recognize problems such as potential outbreaks in order to identify and implement prevention and control measures.

This chapter does not address surveillance in the home care setting. Readers who wish to obtain information on infection surveillance, prevention, and control in home care are referred to the text by Rhinehart and Friedman.[3]

SURVEILLANCE: WHAT IS IT AND WHY DO IT?

Surveillance is "the systematic, active, ongoing observation of the occurrence and distribution of disease within a population, and of the events or conditions that may increase or decrease the risk of such disease occurrence."[4(p.79)] Surveillance systems can be used to collect information about a variety of events. Although infection control professionals use surveillance to focus on nosocomial and community-acquired infections, a surveillance system can also be used to detect medication errors, patient falls, needlesticks in health care workers, and an array of other quality care issues.

Surveillance can be used to measure either outcomes, which are the result of care or performance (such as infections, decubitus ulcers, or patient falls), or processes, which are the actions that are taken to achieve an outcome (such as compliance with an established policy or protocol).[5–8] Two major goals of a surveillance program in a health care facility are:

1. to improve the quality of patient care
2. to identify, implement, and evaluate strategies to prevent and control nosocomial infections and other adverse events

Four objectives of a surveillance program are:

1. to provide baseline, or endemic, rates of disease
2. to identify increases in rates above the baseline, or expected, rates of disease
3. to identify risk factors for disease
4. to evaluate the effectiveness of control measures

Surveillance programs are well-established in acute care hospitals. The Study on the Efficacy of Nosocomial Infection Control, or SENIC project, conducted by the CDC in the mid-1970s, was a landmark study that demonstrated the positive impact that infection control programs had on the reduction of nosocomial infection rates in hospitals.[9,10] SENIC found that hospitals could reduce their nosocomial infection rates by approximately 32 percent if they implemented an infection surveillance and control program that included certain critical components, such as appropriate surveillance activities, vigorous control efforts, and proper staffing.[9]

In 1970, the CDC established the National Nosocomial Infections Study, now the National Nosocomial Infections Surveillance (NNIS) system, to create a national database of nosocomial infections and to improve surveillance methods in hospitals.[11] The hospitals that participate in NNIS use the CDC's surveillance protocol, which includes standardized data collection forms and criteria.[11] These hospitals submit their data to the CDC, and then the CDC compiles it, analyzes it separately for each hospital, pools it into an aggregate database, and then reports it back to each hospital. The aggregate NNIS reports are periodically published in the *American Journal of Infection Control*[12] and are also available on the CDC's Web site (http://www.cdc.gov/ncidod/hip). Data from NNIS has been used to identify risk factors for nosocomial infection and measures that can be used to reduce these risks.[13] Some hospitals have used NNIS data to support the implementation of infection prevention and control measures and have been able to document a subsequent reduction in nosocomial infection rates.[14]

Many LTC facilities have surveillance programs for nosocomial infections. However, these are generally not as well-established as those in the acute care setting[15,16] and there is no national database for nosocomial surveillance in LTC facilities. Little has been published about surveillance methods in the ambulatory care setting.[17,18]

SURVEILLANCE METHODS

Each facility must develop a surveillance program that will meet the organizational objectives and fulfill the needs of its performance improvement initiatives. There is no one surveillance system that is appropriate for all institutions. The Surveillance Initiative Working Group of the Association for Professionals in Infection Control and Epidemiology (APIC) noted that "[a]lthough there is no single or 'right' method of surveillance design or implementation, sound epidemiologic principles must form the foundation of effective systems and must be understood by key participants in the surveillance program and supported by senior management."[5(p.277)]

A variety of surveillance methods have been used in health care facilities. These methods can be separated into four major categories:

1. total prospective (or house-wide) surveillance, in which all patients are monitored for nosocomial infections at all body sites[19]
2. targeted (or focused) surveillance, in which selected infections, infection sites, or organisms are surveyed[11,13]
3. prevalence surveys, in which the number of active infections during a specified period of time is counted, and a prevalence rate is calculated[20,21]
4. periodic surveillance, which may be conducted in several ways; using this method, hospital-wide surveillance may be conducted for a specified time period (such as one month in each quarter of a calendar year), or total surveillance may be conducted for a specified period of time on selected units and then shifted to other units so that the entire hospital can be surveyed over the course of the year[21,22]

Because prevalence surveys and periodic surveillance are not ideal for detecting clusters and outbreaks, they will not be discussed in this chapter.

Total (House-Wide) Surveillance

Total house-wide surveillance was recommended by the CDC in the early 1970s and was the most common type of surveillance conducted in hospitals throughout the 1970s.[19] In this type of surveillance, all nosocomial infections are identified prospectively by reviewing daily microbiology reports, patient records, patients on isolation precautions, and patients who are receiving antibiotics and by making rounds on patient care units. At the end of each month, an overall infection rate is calculated using the total number of infections detected in that month as the numerator and the total number of patients discharged during that month as the denominator. In addition, infection rates may be calculated by service and by patient care unit.[11,19]

Two of the drawbacks of total surveillance is that it is labor intensive and the data "are of limited value since they are not able to measure the influence of exposure to significant risk factors for nosocomial infections, such as urinary catheterization, ventilators, and types of surgical operations."[11(p.29)] Many infection control professionals have long questioned the value of total surveillance because it has limited utility in providing facilities with the data needed to improve infection prevention and control efforts. Although house-wide surveillance is no longer recommended by most authorities,[23–27] 58 percent of the respondents in a survey conducted in 1995 by the APIC education committee reported that they conducted facility-wide surveillance for all infections.[28]

Targeted (Focused) Surveillance

A targeted surveillance program may focus on selected patient care units (such as intensive care, hemodialysis, or bone marrow transplant units), specific procedures (such as surgery), infections associated with specific devices (such as ventilator-associated pneumonia [VAP]), or organisms of epidemiologic importance (such as methicillin-resistant *Staphylococcus aureus* [MRSA], *Clostridium difficile*, or *Mycobacterium tuberculosis*). Targeted surveillance programs generally focus on high-risk, high-volume, or high-cost nosocomial infections that are potentially preventable. In 1986, the CDC introduced targeted surveillance into the NNIS system when it eliminated the requirement for participating hospitals to conduct hospital-wide surveillance and offered several options called surveillance components.[11,13] The four NNIS surveillance components are hospital-wide, adult and pediatric intensive care unit (ICU), high-risk nursery, and surgical patient.

For additional information on surveillance methodologies, refer to one of several infection control reference texts that are listed in the Suggested Reading section at the end of this chapter (Olmsted, Mayhall, Bennett and Brachman, or Wenzel).

GUIDELINES FOR DEVELOPING AND EVALUATING A SURVEILLANCE PROGRAM

Developing a Surveillance Program

A well-designed surveillance program should provide for the ongoing collection, management, analysis, and dissemination of data to control and prevent disease.

Regardless of the setting, those who are designing a surveillance program for a health care facility should establish a system that can prevent the most infections and other adverse events with the resources available.

In 1984, Robert Haley, MD, recommended a priority-directed approach to surveillance that he termed "surveillance by objective."[29] Building on Dr. Haley's recommendations, the following list can be used when designing a surveillance program today.

1. Target those outcomes that will be prevented (e.g., influenza, urinary tract infections, respiratory tract infections, decubitus ulcers, medication errors, specific injuries) and those processes that will be improved (e.g., influenza immunization rates in long-term care facility residents or personnel compliance with hand washing) and develop specific indicators with objectives.
2. "Assign priorities to these objectives. Since there is never enough time or resources to do everything, one must rank the objectives."[29(p.88)]
3. "Allocate time and resources commensurate with the assigned priorities."[29(p.88)]
4. After completing the first three steps, design the surveillance, prevention, and control strategies so they can support the objectives.
5. After a defined period, evaluate the surveillance, prevention, and control program and revise it as needed.

Guidelines for developing and evaluating surveillance programs have been published by the CDC[30] and APIC.[5] Based on these references, a review of the literature,[4,7,8,11,15–19,21,25,26,31] and personal experience, the following steps should be taken (although not necessarily all in the order listed) when designing a surveillance system for a health care facility.

- Identify the surveillance method(s) to be used.
- Assess and define the population and select the indicators to be studied.
- Determine the period of time of the data collection.
- Select surveillance criteria.
- Determine the data gathering process.
- Identify how to analyze the data.
- Design an interpretive surveillance report(s).
- Identify who will receive the report(s).
- Develop a written surveillance plan.

Identify the Surveillance Method(s) To Be Used

Before designing a surveillance program, the facility must decide whether to conduct total (whole-house) or targeted surveillance. Some accrediting agencies and states may require total surveillance in an LTC facility, so health care facilities should check accrediting requirements and local regulations before designing a program. The authors recommend a priority-directed, targeted (or focused) approach to surveillance if there are no regulatory requirements for total surveillance.

Assess and Define the Population and Select the Indicators To Be Studied

Each facility must assess its patient (or resident) population and identify those who are at greatest risk for adverse health outcomes. The facility must then choose the indicators or events (outcomes, processes, and organisms) to be studied. Surveillance indicators should be selected based on the characteristics of the population(s) to be studied, identified risk factors for infection, types of treatment provided and procedures performed, the level of care provided, relevant regulations, accrediting agency requirements, available resources, and risk, performance/quality improvement, and cost reduction initiatives. Surveillance indicators may measure outcomes, processes, or the occurrence of organisms of epidemiologic significance (as defined by the facility). An effective surveillance program will have a mixture of outcome and process monitors and will target organisms and diseases that have been demonstrated to cause health care-associated problems in the population being studied (or in similar populations as identified by a review of the literature). Some surveillance indicators should focus on personnel.

Acute care facilities. In the acute care setting, the highest rates of nosocomial infections occur in ICUs. ICU patients have been shown to be at high risk of infection due to their underlying disease and conditions, their compromised host status, and the invasive diagnostic and therapeutic treatments that they receive.[32] Thus it is not surprising that many outbreaks reported in the literature occur in critical care unit patients (see Chapter 3). Those responsible for designing a surveillance program in a hospital should target their surveillance to defined populations (such as patients in a specific ICU or patients undergoing a specific surgical procedure) so that the number of patients in the population under study (i.e., the population at risk) can be identified. This is necessary if infection rates are to be calculated.[11]

Many infection control programs monitor device-associated infections, such as central line-associated BSI and VAP in ICU patients, because these devices place a patient at risk for developing a nosocomial infection. Reports have shown that hospitals that have used device-related nosocomial infection rates to monitor trends over time have been able to identify potential problem areas and to implement changes that have reduced the risk of infection and that have improved specific nosocomial infection rates.[14] In addition, if a hospital uses NNIS system methodology to define infections, collect data, and calculate rates, then it can use the published NNIS rates for comparison with other hospitals.[12] Many hospital outbreaks have been associated with the improper use and care of ventilators, as discussed in Chapter 3. Because VAP can result in significant morbidity and mortality and increased patient costs and length of stay, many facilities conduct surveillance for VAP and use their surveillance data to identify and implement infection prevention and control measures.[14]

Patients who have surgery are at risk for developing surgical site infections (SSIs), and this risk is influenced by characteristics of the patient, operation, personnel, and hospital.[33] Because it is neither necessary nor an efficient use of resources to monitor all surgical procedures all of the time, most facilities select several high-risk, high-volume, or high-cost procedures that are performed at the facility. CDC has published the list of operative procedures that are included in the NNIS system.[34] Personnel who are responsible for developing a surveillance program in a hospital should consider monitoring one or more of these procedures, using the NNIS system methodology, so that external comparative rates (see caveats below) are available. Much has been written about surveillance methods for SSIs. Because a complete discussion of this topic is beyond the scope of this chapter, the reader is referred to several references.[11,17,18,33-40]

Health care facilities should routinely conduct surveillance for organisms that are epidemiologically significant, such as MRSA,[41] multiply-resistant gram-negative rods such as *Pseudomonas aeruginosa*, *E cloacae* or *Klebsiella pneumoniae*, vancomycin-resistant *Enterococcus*,[42] *C difficile*,[43] respiratory syncytial virus (RSV),[44] rotavirus,[45] and *M tuberculosis*[46] so that isolation precautions can be implemented as soon as possible to prevent transmission to other patients. In addition, all health care facilities should routinely monitor laboratory reports for organisms of public health importance, such as *Salmonella* or *Staphylococ-*

cus aureus with reduced susceptibility to vancomycin (VISA). All cases of *Salmonella* should be reported to the local health department, and all cases of confirmed or presumptive VISA should be reported immediately through local and state health departments to the CDC's Hospital Infections Program. Isolates of suspected VISA should be saved and sent to the CDC, and patients from whom VISA is isolated should be placed on isolation precautions as specified by the CDC.[47] Institutions must choose which organisms to monitor based on the ages and the characteristics of the population served, the incidence or presence of an organism in the facility and in the community, and the facility's public health responsibilities (e.g., reporting reportable diseases). For example, pediatric units should monitor organisms that frequently cause nosocomial infections in children, such as RSV and rotavirus.

Health care facilities play an integral role in recognizing community outbreaks. For instance, in 1994 the staff of a community hospital detected a cluster of community-acquired Legionnaires' disease and reported this to the health department. This led to the recognition of an outbreak of legionellosis among the passengers of a cruise ship.[48]

Infection control personnel should also work with the employee health service department to monitor and identify communicable infections in personnel, such as tuberculosis, chickenpox, and conjunctivitis, so that appropriate work restrictions can be implemented.

In addition to nosocomial infection surveillance in patients and in personnel, those responsible for risk and quality management programs in hospitals should have a surveillance system for detecting noninfectious outcomes of care in patients (such as medication errors) and adverse events in personnel (such as sharps injuries). Both quality management and infection control programs should select some surveillance indicators that assess the processes or activities that affect patient outcomes (such as biological monitoring of steam sterilizers and use of aseptic technique and barriers when inserting central lines) and employee health (such as employee practices that result in sharps injuries).

Ambulatory care facilities. Few studies have been done on the risk factors for infection in the ambulatory care setting.[18,49] This is not surprising because the term "ambulatory care" encompasses a variety of settings. "Ambulatory care facility" as used in this chapter refers to a hospital-based or free-standing facility or office in which health care is provided and in which patients reside for less than 24 hours. Examples include emergency rooms, dialysis centers, physician's offices, urgent care centers, ambulatory surgery centers, and clinics.

With the exception of ambulatory surgery and dialysis center patients, it is often difficult to identify specific populations at risk of developing a nosocomial infection that is related to health care provided in the ambulatory setting.[18] When compared to the acute care and LTC settings, ambulatory care facilities have a greater challenge regarding the surveillance of health care-associated infections. Patients cared for in these locations are frequently seen for relatively brief periods, often over a few hours. The patients may not be well-known to the provider, may be seen for only one encounter, and are frequently lost to follow-up once they leave the facility. Follow-up of these patients is usually left to the primary care provider, who may have a limited working relationship with other care providers.

Persons who are responsible for managing infection control programs in ambulatory care settings should be familiar with the numerous outbreaks that have occurred in these settings[49,50] (see Chapter 5). Examples of frequently reported outbreaks in ambulatory care facilities are[49,50]

- BSIs and hepatitis B infections associated with improper infection control practices in hemodialysis centers
- tuberculosis associated with unrecognized cases of pulmonary disease or improper isolation precautions used for patients with known pulmonary tuberculosis
- keratoconjunctivitis in ophthalmology clinics associated with poor infection control practices, such as lack of hand washing or improper disinfection of instruments

In addition, bronchoscopy and gastrointestinal endoscopy procedures have been associated with many outbreaks in outpatient health care facilities.[50] Infections associated with these procedures are difficult to detect unless they occur in clusters or are caused by an unusual or uncommon pathogen.

There is little published about effective surveillance methods for ambulatory care settings, with the exception of SSI surveillance in ambulatory surgery centers. Ambulatory surgery centers should identify the procedures that are most commonly performed at the facility and should use facility-specific data and literature reviews to identify those that have the highest risk for infectious and noninfectious complications.[17,33] If SSI surveillance is performed, high-volume and/or high-risk procedures should be monitored.

The CDC is developing a national surveillance system to study the incidence of bloodstream and vascular access-site infections, hospitalizations, and antimicrobial use in hemodialysis patients.[51] Hemodialysis centers should consider participating in this program. Information on the dialysis surveillance system can be obtained from the CDC's Web site at http://www.cdc.gov/ncidod/hip/dialysis. Hemodialysis centers should routinely perform quality assurance tests on hemodialysis water. Documentation of this testing and any actions taken based on the test results can serve as a process monitor.

Ophthalmology offices and clinics should conduct surveillance for patients who develop conjunctivitis following care in the office or clinic (an outcomes indicator). These settings could also implement a performance improvement monitor on the proper use of hand washing, multidose medications, or disinfection of equipment (process indicators).

Personnel who are responsible for developing an infection surveillance, prevention, and control program in the ambulatory care setting should focus on both risk reduction and infection prevention activities (i.e., process indicators) and on outcomes measurements, such as infections, whenever possible. Process-oriented surveillance indicators for an ambulatory care setting such as a physician's office or a clinic could include compliance with reporting reportable diseases, compliance with a sterility assurance protocol (i.e., biological, physical, and chemical monitoring) for all sterilizers used in the facility, and immunization rates for patients. Many studies have revealed glaring deficiencies in the processing of endoscopes, despite the fact that numerous outbreaks have been associated with the use of contaminated bronchoscopes and gastrointestinal endoscopes.[52] Therefore, those who are designing a surveillance program for an endoscopy suite should develop process monitors, such as personnel compliance with specific cleaning and disinfection/sterilization protocols for endoscopes. In this setting, monitoring the processes used (i.e., attention to proper cleaning and disinfection practices) will more likely lead to improved patient care than monitoring an outcome (such as infection), which is difficult to detect, especially in an ambulatory population that is frequently lost to follow-up. Ambulatory care facilities should also conduct surveillance for the occurrence of diseases of epidemiologic importance (such as salmonellosis, tuberculosis, and Legionnaires' disease) in their patient population and should report these diseases to the health department.

LTC facilities. Much has been published about endemic and epidemic nosocomial infections and risk factors for infection in the LTC setting.[16,53–63] However, infection surveillance methodology for the LTC setting has not been as well defined as it has been for the acute care setting, and many facilities probably lack an effective, ongoing surveillance program.[62] Surveillance programs in the LTC setting should be designed and implemented to promote the ongoing collection, analysis, and dissemination of information on infections in the facility. Surveillance data should be used to plan infection prevention and control activities, including educational programs.[61] Surveillance indicators should be based on those infections that commonly occur in the facility—especially on those that are potentially preventable—and on those processes shown to reduce the risk of nosocomial infections in LTC facilities (e.g., annual influenza vaccination).[16] Guidelines for developing infection surveillance programs in LTC facilities have been published by APIC and the Society for Healthcare Epidemiology of America (SHEA),[16] Smith,[15,58] the Canadian Ministry of National Health and Welfare,[64] and Rusnak.[65] As in the acute care setting, targeted or focused surveillance programs are recommended because they are a more efficient use of scarce infection control resources and they permit the calculation of site-specific rates (such as urinary tract infections).[16]

The most commonly occurring outbreaks in the LTC setting are respiratory diseases (influenza and tuberculosis), gastrointestinal diseases, and scabies.[16] Colonization and infection with MRSA occurs frequently in many LTC facilities. Therefore, surveillance programs must be capable of detecting these infections. Ahlbrecht et al were able to demonstrate positive outcomes in a pilot study that involved infection surveillance and a team approach to infection prevention and control in a 220-bed community-based nursing home.[66] They also suggested some data elements in the minimum data set from the Health Care Financing Admin-

istration that may be useful in targeting surveillance in nursing home residents.[66]

In addition to infection surveillance, LTC facilities should have a program for monitoring noninfectious outcomes of care, such as falls and decubiti, and processes such as influenza rates in residents and personnel.[8]

Selecting surveillance indicators. Table 2–1 lists suggested indicators for surveillance programs in a variety of health care settings and provides references (when available) that either explain or illustrate the use of these indicators or can provide criteria for developing an indicator.[67–94]

Determine the Period of Time of the Data Collection

Surveillance data should be collected on an ongoing basis in order to identify trends, detect organisms and diseases of epidemiologic importance, and recognize clusters and outbreaks. There is no defined time period or number of events that must be measured; however, it is difficult to interpret rates for events that occur infrequently and for procedures that are rarely performed. In practice, many infection control professionals collect data on each indicator for a defined period, such as a year, and then analyze and assess the information obtained to determine if it is useful for identifying potential problems and methods for improvement. If the indicator does not appear to be useful, its use should be discontinued. For example, if a facility selects central line-related BSI rates as a nosocomial infection surveillance indicator on a cardiac care unit and discovers that these infections rarely occur, then consideration should be given to discontinuing this particular indicator.

Select Surveillance Criteria

Criteria, or case definitions, are a key element of any surveillance system. To be able to accurately analyze surveillance data over time, consistent definitions must be used to determine the presence of a nosocomial infection, the occurrence of an adverse health-related event, or compliance to a policy. Criteria must be used the same way and applied consistently by all persons who collect or evaluate surveillance data to ensure the accuracy and reproducibility of the results. If data elements are not defined consistently, then it will not be possible to determine the presence and the true incidence of a disease or to determine if control measures implemented to control a disease are effective.

Table 2–1 Suggested Indicators for Surveillance Programs in Health Care Facilities

Indicator	Type(s) of Setting	Indicator	Selected Reference(s)
BSIs associated with central lines	Acute	Outcome	11, 12, 34, 67, 68
BSIs in selected populations	Acute	Outcome	69
Local site infections and/or phlebitis associated with peripheral intravascular therapy	Acute, LTC	Outcome	70
VAP	Acute, LTC	Outcome	11, 12, 14, 67, 71
Catheter-associated urinary tract infections	Acute, LTC	Outcome	11, 12, 34, 71
SSI	Acute, Amb	Outcome	33–35
Decubitus ulcers	LTC, Acute	Outcome	57, 72, 73
Conjunctivitis	Ophthalmology offices and clinics	Outcome	74
Influenza in residents and personnel	LTC	Outcome	75
Sharps injuries in personnel	Acute, LTC, Ambulatory surgery centers	Outcome	76
PPD conversions in personnel	Acute, LTC, Amb	Outcome	46
PPD conversions in residents	LTC	Outcome	58, 77
Newly diagnosed tuberculosis cases	Acute, LTC, Amb	Outcome	46
Infection/colonization with MRSA or VRE	Acute, LTC	Outcome	41, 78, 79
Respiratory syncytial virus infection	Pediatric	Outcome	44, 80
Rotavirus infection	Pediatric	Outcome	45
Clostridium difficile diarrhea	LTC, Acute	Outcome	43, 81
BSIs, pyrogenic reactions, vascular access infections, MRSA, or VRE in hemodialysis patients	Hemodialysis centers	Outcome	51
Resident or patient falls	LTC, Acute	Outcome	82, 83
Medication errors	Acute, LTC	Outcome	84, 85
Occurrence of reportable diseases	Acute, LTC, Amb	Outcome	Local/state regulations, 86
Influenza vaccination rates in personnel, patients, and residents	LTC, Acute, Amb	Process	87
Personnel adherence to standard precautions or isolation precautions	Acute, LTC, Amb	Process	50, 88
Personnel adherence to cleaning, disinfection, or sterilization protocols	Acute, LTC, Amb	Process	89, 90
Adherence to performance testing/quality assurance program for sterilizers (e.g., appropriate use of biological indicator)	Wherever sterilizers are used	Process	90, 91
Proper functioning of isolation rooms used for tuberculosis	Acute, LTC, Amb	Process	46
Proper use of activated gluteraldehyde solutions	Acute, LTC, Amb	Process	See instructions on product label
Hepatitis B vaccination rates in personnel	Acute, LTC, Amb	Process	92
Hepatitis B vaccination rates in patients	Hemodialysis centers	Process	51
Adherence to reportable disease regulations	Acute, LTC, Amb	Process	86
Use of appropriate hand-washing practices by personnel	Acute, LTC, Amb	Process	93, 94

Note: BSI, bloodstream infection; LTC, long-term care; VAP, ventilator-associated pneumonia; SSI, surgical site infection; PPD, purified protein derivative; Amb, ambulatory care; MRSA, methicillin-resistant *Staphylococcus aureus*; VRE, vancomycin-resistant *Enterococcus*.

Criteria allow all persons involved in the surveillance process (all those who collect, analyze, evaluate, and use the data) to have a common understanding of the events that are being monitored. To be acceptable to all of the users of the data, the criteria used in a surveillance program should reflect generally accepted definitions of the specific disease or event being studied. For example, if SSI surveillance is going to be performed, then the infection control department and the surgery department must agree upon the criteria for defining the presence of an SSI.

Criteria frequently combine specific clinical findings with the results of laboratory and other diagnostic tests. The most widely used sets of definitions for nosocomial infection are those developed by the CDC for acute care hospitals in the NNIS system[34,35,67] and those developed by McGeer et al for LTC.[95] The McGeer definitions were intended "for use in facilities that provide homes for elderly residents who require 24-hour personal care under professional nursing supervision."[95(p.1)] Copies of the CDC definitions appear in Exhibits 2–1 and 2–2. The McGeer definitions focus on the clinical presentations of infections and minimize the need for confirmatory diagnostic or laboratory tests that are infrequently performed in the LTC setting.

Whenever possible, previously published, standardized definitions should be used. Definitions may be obtained from professional organizations and federal and state agencies. Case definitions for many infectious diseases can be found in Appendixes C, H, I, and J.

Exhibit 2–1 CDC Definitions for Nosocomial Infections, 1988

The Hospital Infections Program, Centers for Infectious Diseases (CDC) developed a set of definitions for surveillance of nosocomial infections. The definitions were introduced into hospitals participating in the National Nosocomial Infections Study (NNIS) in 1987 and were modified based on comments from infection control personnel in NNIS hospitals and others involved in surveillance, prevention, and control of nosocomial infections. The definitions were implemented in NNIS hospitals in January 1988 and are the current CDC definitions for nosocomial infections.

PRINCIPLES USED IN DEFINITIONS

The definitions are based on several important principles. First, information used to determine the presence and classification of an infection involves various combinations of clinical findings and results of laboratory and other diagnostic tests. Clinical evidence is derived from direct observation of the patient or review of information in the patient's chart or other ward or unit records, for example, temperature sheet or Kardex. Laboratory evidence consists of results of cultures, antigen- or antibody-detection tests, and microscopic visualization methods. Supportive data are derived from other diagnostic studies, such as results of X-ray studies, ultrasound examination, computed tomography (CT) scan, magnetic resonance imaging, radiolabel scans, endoscopic procedures, biopsies, and needle aspiration. For infections in which clinical manifestations are different in neonates and infants than in older persons, specific criteria are included.

Second, a physician's or surgeon's diagnosis of infection derived from direct observation during surgery, endoscopic examination, or other diagnostic study, or based on clinical judgment, is an acceptable criterion for an infection, unless there is compelling evidence to the contrary (e.g., information written on the wrong patient's record or a presumptive diagnosis that was not substantiated by subsequent studies). For infections at some sites, however, a physician's clinical diagnosis in the absence of supportive data must be accompanied by initiation of appropriate antimicrobial therapy to satisfy the criterion.

Third, for an infection to be defined as nosocomial, there must be no evidence that the infection was present or incubating at the time of hospital admission. An infection that occurs in the following special situations is considered nosocomial: (1) infection that is acquired in the hospital and becomes evident after hospital discharge and (2) newborn infection that is the result of passage through the birth canal.

Fourth, infection that occurs as the result of the following special situations is not considered nosocomial: (1) infection that is associated with a complication or extension of infection(s) already present on admission, unless a change in pathogen or symptoms strongly suggests the acquisition of a new infection and (2) infection in an infant that is known or proved to have been acquired transplacentally (e.g., herpes simplex, toxoplasmosis, rubella, cytomegalovirus, or syphilis) and becomes evident shortly after birth.

Fifth, except for a few situations that are referred to in the definitions, no specific time during or after hospitalization is given to determine whether an infection is nosocomial or community acquired. Thus each infection must be assessed for evidence that links it to hospitalization.

DEFINITIONS FOR NOSOCOMIAL INFECTIONS

Definitions for primary bloodstream infection, pneumonia, and urinary tract infection are presented first and are followed by other sites of infection listed alphabetically.

continues

Exhibit 2–1 continued

PRIMARY BLOODSTREAM INFECTION

Primary bloodstream infection includes laboratory-confirmed bloodstream infection and clinical sepsis. The definition of clinical sepsis is intended primarily for infants and neonates.

Laboratory-confirmed bloodstream infection must meet one of the following criteria:

1. Recognized pathogen isolated from blood culture, AND pathogen is not related to infection at another site.[1]
2. One of the following: fever (>38° C), chills, or hypotension AND any of the following:
    a. Common skin contaminant[2] isolated from two blood cultures drawn on separate occasions, AND organism is not related to infection at another site[1]
    b. Common skin contaminant isolated from blood culture from patient with intravascular access device, AND physician institutes appropriate antimicrobial therapy
    c. Positive antigen test on blood[3] AND organism is not related to infection at another site
3. Patient ≤12 months of age[4] has one of the following: fever (>38° C), hypothermia (<37° C), apnea, or bradycardia AND any of the following:
    a. Common skin contaminant isolated from two blood cultures drawn on separate occasions AND organism is not related to infection at another site[1]
    b. Common skin contaminant isolated from blood culture from patient with intravascular access device AND physician institutes appropriate antimicrobial therapy
    c. Positive antigen test on blood AND pathogen is not related to infection at another site

Clinical sepsis must meet either of the following criteria:

1. One of the following clinical signs or symptoms with no other recognized cause: fever (>38° C), hypotension (systolic pressure: ≤90 mm Hg), or oliguria (>20 mL/hr) AND all of the following:
    a. Blood culture not done or no organism or antigen detected in blood
    b. No apparent infection at another site
    c. Physician institutes appropriate antimicrobial therapy for sepsis
2. Patient ≤12 months of age has one of the following clinical signs or symptoms with no other recognized cause: fever (>38° C, hypothermia (<37° C), apnea, or bradycardia, AND all of the following:
    a. Blood culture not done or no organism or antigen detected in blood
    b. No apparent infection at another site
    c. Physician institutes appropriate antimicrobial therapy for sepsis

PNEUMONIA

Pneumonia is defined separately from other infections of the lower respiratory tract. The criteria for pneumonia involve various combinations of clinical, radiographic, and laboratory evidence of infection. In general, expectorated sputum cultures are not useful in diagnosing pneumonia but may help identify the etiologic agent and provide useful antimicrobial susceptibility data. Findings from serial chest X-ray studies may be more helpful than those from a single X-ray film.

Pneumonia must meet one of the following criteria:

1. Rales or dullness to percussion on physical examination of chest AND any of the following:
    a. New onset of purulent sputum or change in character of sputum
    b. Organism isolated from blood culture
    c. Isolation of pathogen from specimen obtained by transtracheal aspirate, bronchial brushing, or biopsy
2. Chest radiographic examination shows new or progressive infiltrate, consolidation, cavitation, or pleural effusion AND any of the following:
    a. New onset of purulent sputum or change in character of sputum
    b. Organism isolated from blood culture
    c. Isolation of pathogen from specimen obtained by transtracheal aspirate, bronchial brushing, or biopsy
    d. Isolation of virus or detection of viral antigen in respiratory secretions
    e. Diagnostic single antibody titer (IgM) or fourfold increase in paired serum samples (IgG) for pathogen
    f. Histopathologic evidence of pneumonia
3. Patient ≤12 months of age has two of the following: apnea, tachypnea, bradycardia, wheezing, rhonchi, or cough AND any of the following:
    a. Increased production of respiratory secretions
    b. New onset of purulent sputum or change in character of sputum
    c. Organism isolated from blood culture
    d. Isolation of pathogen from specimen obtained by transtracheal aspirate, bronchial brushing, or biopsy
    e. Isolation of virus or detection of viral antigen in respiratory secretions
    f. Diagnostic single antibody titer (IgM) or fourfold increase in paired serum samples (IgG) for pathogen
    g. Histopathologic evidence of pneumonia
4. Patient ≤12 months of age has chest radiologic examination that shows new or progressive infiltrate, cavitation, consolidation, or pleural effusion AND any of the following:
    a. Increased production of respiratory secretions
    b. New onset of purulent sputum or change in character of sputum

continues

Exhibit 2–1 continued

c. Organism isolated from blood culture
d. Isolation of pathogen from specimen obtained by trans-tracheal aspirate, bronchial brushing, or biopsy
e. Isolation of virus or detection of viral antigen in respiratory secretions
f. Diagnostic single antibody titer (IgM) or fourfold increase in paired serum samples (IgG) for pathogen
g. Histopathologic evidence of pneumonia

URINARY TRACT INFECTION

Urinary tract infection includes symptomatic urinary tract infection, asymptomatic bacteriuria, and other infections of the urinary tract.

Symptomatic urinary tract infection must meet one of the following criteria:

1. One of the following: fever (>38° C), urgency, frequency, dysuria, or suprapubic tenderness AND a urine culture[5] of $\geq 10^5$ colonies/mL urine with no more than two species of organisms
2. Two of the following: fever (>38° C), urgency, frequency, dysuria, or suprapubic tenderness AND any of the following:
    a. Dipstick test positive for leukocyte esterase and/or nitrate
    b. Pyuria (≥ 10 white blood cells [WBC]/mL[3] or ≥ 3 WBC/high-power field of unspun urine)
    c. Organisms seen on Gram stain of unspun urine
    d. Two urine cultures with repeated isolation of the same uropathogen[6] with $\geq 10^2$ colonies/mL urine in nonvoided specimens
    e. Urine culture with $\leq 10^5$ colonies/mL urine of single uropathogen in patient being treated with appropriate antimicrobial therapy
    f. Physician's diagnosis
    g. Physician institutes appropriate antimicrobial therapy
3. Patient ≤ 12 months of age has one of the following: fever (>38° C), hypothermia (<37° C), apnea, bradycardia, dysuria, lethargy, or vomiting AND urine culture of $\geq 10^5$ colonies/mL urine with no more than two species of organisms
4. Patient ≤ 12 months of age has one of the following: fever (>38° C), hypothermia (<37° C), apnea, bradycardia, dysuria, lethargy, or vomiting AND any of the following:
    a. Dipstick test positive for leukocyte esterase and/or nitrate
    b. Pyuria
    c. Organisms seen on Gram stain of unspun urine
    d. Two urine cultures with repeated isolation of same uropathogen with $\geq 10^2$ organisms/mL urine in nonvoided specimens
    e. Urine culture with $\leq 10^5$ colonies/mL urine of a single uropathogen in patient being treated with appropriate antimicrobial therapy
    f. Physician's diagnosis
    g. Physician institutes appropriate antimicrobial therapy

Asymptomatic bacteriuria must meet either of the following criteria:

1. An indwelling urinary catheter is present within seven days before urine is cultured AND patient has no fever (>38° C), urgency, frequency, dysuria, or suprapubic tenderness AND has urine culture of $\geq 10^5$ organisms/mL urine with no more than two species of organisms.
2. No indwelling urinary catheter is present within seven days before the first of two urine cultures with $\geq 10^5$ organisms/mL urine of the same organism with no more than two species of organisms AND patient has no fever (>38° C), urgency, frequency, dysuria, or suprapubic tenderness.

Other infections of the urinary tract (kidney, ureter, bladder, urethra, or tissues surrounding the retroperitoneal or perinephric spaces) must meet one of the following criteria:

1. Organism isolated from culture of fluid (other than urine) or tissue from affected site
2. An abscess or other evidence of infection seen on direct examination, during surgery, or by histopathologic examination
3. Two of the following: fever (>38° C), localized pain, or tenderness at involved site AND any of the following:
    a. Purulent drainage from affected site
    b. Organism isolated from blood culture
    c. Radiographic evidence of infection[7]
    d. Physician's diagnosis
    e. Physician institutes appropriate antimicrobial therapy
4. Patient ≤ 12 months of age has one of the following: fever (>38° C), hypothermia (<37° C), apnea, bradycardia, lethargy, or vomiting AND any of the following:
    a. Purulent drainage from affected site
    b. Organism isolated from blood culture
    c. Radiographic evidence of infection
    d. Physician's diagnosis
    e. Physician institutes appropriate therapy

BONE AND JOINT INFECTION

Bone and joint infection includes osteomyelitis, joint or bursa infection, and vertebral disk infection.

Osteomyelitis must meet one of the following criteria:

1. Organism cultured from bone
2. Evidence of osteomyelitis seen during surgery or by histopathologic examination
3. Two of the following with no other recognized cause: fever (>38° C), localized swelling, tenderness, heat, or drainage at suspected site of infection AND any of the following:
    a. Organism isolated from blood culture
    b. Positive antigen test on blood
    c. Radiographic evidence of infection

continues

Exhibit 2–1 continued

Joint or bursa infection must meet one of the following criteria:

1. Organism isolated from culture of joint fluid or synovial biopsy
2. Evidence of joint or bursa infection seen during surgery or by histopathologic examination
3. Two of the following with no other recognized cause: joint pain, swelling, tenderness, heat, evidence of effusion or limitation of motion AND any of the following:
   a. Organisms and white blood cells seen on Gram stain of joint fluid
   b. Positive antigen test on blood, urine, or joint fluid
   c. Cellular profile and chemistries of joint fluid compatible with infection and not explained by underlying rheumatologic disorder
   d. Radiographic evidence of infection

Vertebral disk space infection must meet one of the following criteria:

1. Organism isolated from culture of involved site tissue obtained during surgery or needle aspiration
2. Evidence of infection at involved site seen during surgery or by histopathologic examination
3. Fever (>38° C) with no other recognized cause or pain at involved site AND radiographic evidence of infection
4. Fever (>38° C) with no other recognized cause AND pain at involved site AND positive antigen test on blood or urine

CARDIOVASCULAR SYSTEM INFECTION

Cardiovascular system infection includes arterial or venous infection, endocarditis, myocarditis or pericarditis, and mediastinitis. Mediastinitis is grouped with cardiovascular system infections because it most often occurs after cardiac surgery.

Arterial or venous infection must meet one of the following criteria:

1. Organism isolated from culture of arteries or veins removed during surgery AND blood culture not done or no organism isolated from blood culture
2. Evidence of infection at involved vascular site seen during surgery or by histopathologic examination
3. One of the following: fever (>38° C), pain, erythema, or heat at involved vascular site AND both of the following:
   a. More than 15 colonies cultured from intravascular cannula tip using semiquantitative culture method
   b. Blood culture not done or no organism isolated from blood culture
4. Purulent drainage at involved vascular site AND blood culture not done or no organism isolated from blood culture
5. Patient ≤12 months of age has one of the following: fever (>38° C), hypothermia (<37° C), apnea, bradycardia, lethargy, pain, erythema, or heat at involved vascular site AND both of the following:

a. More than 15 colonies cultured from intravascular-cannula tip using semiquantitative culture method
b. Blood culture not done or no organism isolated from blood culture

Endocarditis of natural or prosthetic heart valve must meet one of the following criteria:

1. Organism isolated from culture of valve or vegetation
2. Two of the following with no other recognized cause: fever (>38° C), new or changing murmur; embolic phenomena, skin manifestations (i.e., petechiae, splinter hemorrhages, painful subcutaneous nodules), congestive heart failure, or cardiac conduction abnormality AND physician institutes appropriate antimicrobial therapy if diagnosis is made antemortem AND any of the following:
   a. Organism isolated from two blood cultures
   b. Organisms seen on Gram stain of valve when culture is negative or not done
   c. Valvular vegetation seen during surgery or autopsy
   d. Positive antigen test on blood or urine
   e. Evidence of new vegetation seen on echocardiogram
3. Patient ≤12 months of age has two or more of the following with no other recognized cause: fever (>38° C), hypothermia (<37° C), apnea, bradycardia, new or changing murmur, embolic phenomena, skin manifestations, congestive heart failure, or cardiac conduction abnormality AND physician institutes appropriate antimicrobial therapy if diagnosis is made antemortem AND any of the following:
   a. Organism isolated from two blood cultures
   b. Organisms seen on Gram stain of valve when culture is negative or not done
   c. Valvular vegetation seen during surgery or autopsy
   d. Positive antigen test on blood or urine
   e. Evidence of new vegetation seen on echocardiogram

Myocarditis or pericarditis must meet one of the following criteria:

1. Organism isolated from culture of pericardial tissue or fluid obtained by needle aspiration or during surgery
2. Two of the following with no other recognized cause: fever (>38° C), chest pain, paradoxical pulse, or increased heart size AND any of the following:
   a. Abnormal electrocardiogram (ECG) consistent with myocarditis or pericarditis
   b. Positive antigen test on blood
   c. Evidence of myocarditis or pericarditis on histologic examination of heart tissue
   d. Fourfold rise in type-specific antibody with or without isolation of virus from pharynx or feces
   e. Pericardial effusion identified by echocardiogram, CT scan, magnetic resonance imaging, angiography, or other radiographic evidence of infection

continues

Exhibit 2–1 continued

3. Patient ≤12 months of age has two of the following with no other recognized cause: fever (>38° C), hypothermia (<37° C), apnea, bradycardia, paradoxical pulse, or increased heart size AND any of the following:
   a. Abnormal ECG consistent with myocarditis or pericarditis
   b. Positive antigen test on blood
   c. Histologic examination of heart tissue shows evidence of myocarditis or pericarditis
   d. Fourfold rise in type-specific antibody with or without isolation of virus from pharynx or feces
   e. Pericardial effusion identified by echocardiogram, CT scan, magnetic resonance imaging, angiography, or other radiographic evidence of infection

Mediastinitis must meet one of the following criteria:

1. Organism isolated from culture of mediastinal tissue or fluid obtained during surgery or needle aspiration
2. Evidence of mediastinitis that is seen during surgery or by histopathologic examination
3. One of the following: fever (>38° C), chest pain, or sternal instability AND any of the following:
   a. Purulent drainage from mediastinal area
   b. Organism isolated from blood culture or culture of drainage from mediastinal area
   c. Mediastinal widening on X-ray examination
4. Patient ≤12 months of age has one of the following: fever (>38° C), hypothermia (<37° C), apnea, bradycardia, or sternal instability AND any of the following:
   a. Purulent drainage from mediastinal area
   b. Organism isolated from blood culture or culture of drainage from mediastinal area
   c. Mediastinal widening on X-ray examination

CENTRAL NERVOUS SYSTEM INFECTION

Central nervous system infection includes intracranial infection, meningitis or ventriculitis, and spinal abscess without meningitis.

Intracranial infection (brain abscess, subdural or epidural infection, and encephalitis) must meet one of the following criteria:

1. Organism isolated from culture of brain tissue or dura
2. Abscess or evidence of intracranial infection seen during surgery or by histopathologic examination
3. Two of the following with no other recognized cause: headache, dizziness, fever (>38° C), localizing neurologic signs, changing level of consciousness, or confusion AND physician institutes appropriate antimicrobial therapy if diagnosis is made antemortem AND any of the following:
   a. Organism seen on microscopic examination of brain or abscess tissue obtained by needle aspiration or by biopsy during surgery or autopsy
   b. Positive antigen test on blood or urine

   c. Radiographic evidence of infection
   d. Diagnostic single antibody titer (IgM) or fourfold increase in paired serum samples (IgG) for pathogen
4. Patient ≤12 months of age has two of the following with no other recognized cause: fever (>38° C), hypothermia (<37° C), apnea, bradycardia, localizing neurologic signs, or changing level of consciousness AND physician institutes appropriate antimicrobial therapy if diagnosis is made antemortem AND any of the following:
   a. Organisms seen on microscopic examination of brain or abscess tissue obtained by needle aspiration or by biopsy during surgery or autopsy
   b. Positive antigen test on blood or urine specimen
   c. Radiographic evidence of infection
   d. Diagnostic single antibody titer (IgM) or fourfold increase in paired serum samples (IgG) for pathogen

Meningitis or ventriculitis must meet one of the following criteria:

1. Organism isolated from culture of cerebrospinal fluid (CSF)
2. One of the following with no other recognized cause: fever (>38° C), headache, stiff neck, meningeal signs, cranial nerve signs, or irritability, AND physician institutes appropriate antimicrobial therapy if diagnosis is made antemortem AND any of the following:
   a. Increased white cells, elevated protein, and/or decreased glucose in CSF
   b. Organisms seen on Gram stain of CSF
   c. Organism isolated from blood culture
   d. Positive antigen test on CSF, blood, or urine
   e. Diagnostic single antibody titer (IgM) or fourfold increase in paired serum samples (IgG) for pathogen
3. Patient ≤12 months of age has one of the following with no other recognized cause: fever (>38° C), hypothermia (<37° C), apnea, bradycardia, stiff neck, meningeal signs, cranial nerve signs, or irritability AND physician institutes appropriate antimicrobial therapy if diagnosis is made antemortem AND any of the following:
   a. Increased white cells, elevated protein, and/or decreased glucose in CSF
   b. Organisms seen on Gram stain of CSF
   c. Organism isolated from blood culture
   d. Positive antigen test on CSF, blood, or urine
   e. Diagnostic single antibody titer (IgM) or fourfold increase in paired serum samples (IgG) for pathogen

Spinal abscess without meningitis (an abscess of the spinal epidural or subdural space, without involvement of the CSF or adjacent bone structures) must meet one of the following criteria:

1. Organism isolated from culture of abscess in spinal epidural or subdural space
2. Abscess in spinal epidural or subdural space seen during surgery or autopsy or by histopathologic examination

continues

Exhibit 2–1 continued

3. One of the following with no other recognized cause: fever (>38° C), back pain, focal tenderness, radiculitis, paraparesis, or paraplegia AND physician institutes appropriate antimicrobial therapy if diagnosis is made antemortem AND either of the following:
   a. Organism isolated from blood culture
   b. Radiographic evidence of spinal abscess

EYE, EAR, NOSE, THROAT, AND MOUTH INFECTION

Eye infection includes conjunctivitis and other eye infections. Ear infections include otitis externa, otitis media, otitis interna and mastoiditis. Nose, throat, and mouth infections include oral cavity infections, upper respiratory infections, and sinusitis.

Conjunctivitis must meet either of the following criteria:

1. Pathogen isolated from culture of purulent exudate obtained from conjunctiva or contiguous tissues, such as eyelid, cornea, meibomian glands, or lacrimal glands
2. Pain or redness of conjunctiva or around eye AND any of the following:
   a. WBCs and organisms seen on Gram stain of exudate
   b. Purulent exudate
   c. Positive antigen test on exudate or conjunctival scraping
   d. Multinucleated giant cells seen on microscopic examination of conjunctival exudate or scrapings
   e. Positive viral culture on conjunctival exudate
   f. Diagnostic single antibody titer (IgM) or fourfold increase in paired serum samples (IgG) for pathogen

Eye infections other than conjunctivitis must meet either of the following criteria:

1. Organism isolated from culture of anterior or posterior chamber or vitreous fluid
2. Two of the following with no other recognized cause: eye pain, visual disturbance, or hypopyon AND any of the following:
   a. Physician's diagnosis
   b. Positive antigen test on blood
   c. Organism isolated from blood culture

Otitis externa must meet either of the following criteria:

1. Pathogen isolated from culture of purulent drainage from ear canal
2. One of the following: fever (>38° C), pain, redness, or drainage from ear canal AND organisms seen on Gram stain of purulent drainage

Otitis media must meet either of the following criteria:

1. Organism isolated from culture of fluid from middle ear obtained by tympanocentesis or surgery

2. Two of the following: fever (>38° C), pain in eardrum, inflammation, retraction or decreased mobility of eardrum, or fluid behind eardrum

Otitis interna must meet either of the following criteria:

1. Organism isolated from culture of fluid from inner ear obtained at surgery
2. Physician's diagnosis

Mastoiditis must meet either of the following criteria:

1. Organism isolated from culture of purulent drainage from mastoid
2. Two of the following with no other recognized cause: fever (>38° C), pain, tenderness, erythema, headache, or facial paralysis AND either of the following:
   a. Organisms seen on Gram stain of purulent material from mastoid
   b. Positive antigen test on blood

Oral cavity infection (mouth, tongue, or gums) must meet one of the following criteria:

1. Organism isolated from culture of purulent material from tissues or oral cavity
2. Abscess or other evidence of oral cavity infection seen on direct examination, during surgery, or by histopathologic examination
3. One of the following: abscess, ulceration, or raised white patches on inflamed mucosa, or plaques on oral mucosa AND any of the following:
   a. Organisms seen on Gram stain
   b. Positive potassium hydroxide (KOH) stain
   c. Multinucleated giant cells seen on microscopic examination of mucosal scrapings
   d. Positive antigen test on oral secretions
   e. Diagnostic single antibody titer (IgM) or fourfold increase in paired serum samples (IgG) for pathogen
   f. Physician's diagnosis and treatment with topical or oral antifungal therapy

Sinusitis must meet either of the following criteria:

1. Organism isolated from culture of purulent material obtained from sinus cavity
2. One of the following: fever (>38° C), pain or tenderness over the involved sinus, headache, purulent exudate, or nasal obstruction AND either of the following:
   a. Positive transillumination
   b. Radiographic evidence of infection

Upper respiratory tract infection (pharyngitis, laryngitis, epiglottis) must meet one of the following criteria:

continues

Exhibit 2–1 continued

1. Two of the following: fever(>38° C), erythema of pharynx, sore throat, cough, hoarseness, or purulent exudate in throat AND any of the following:
   a. Organism isolated from culture of specific site
   b. Organism isolated from blood culture
   c. Positive antigen test on blood or respiratory secretions
   d. Diagnostic single antibody titer (IgM) or fourfold increase in paired serum samples (IgG) for pathogen
   e. Physician's diagnosis
2. Abscess seen on direct examination, during surgery, or by histopathologic examination
3. Patient ≤12 months of age has two of the following: fever (>38° C), hypothermia (<37° C), apnea, bradycardia, nasal discharge, or purulent exudate in throat AND any of the following:
   a. Organism isolated from culture of specific site
   b. Organism isolated from blood culture
   c. Positive antigen test on blood or respiratory secretions
   d. Diagnostic single antibody titer (IgM) or fourfold increase in paired serum samples (IgG) for pathogen
   e. Physician's diagnosis

GASTROINTESTINAL SYSTEM INFECTION

Gastrointestinal system infections include gastroenteritis, hepatitis, necrotizing enterocolitis, gastrointestinal tract infections, and intra-abdominal infections not specified elsewhere.

Gastroenteritis must meet either of the following criteria:

1. Acute onset of diarrhea (liquid stools for more than 12 hours) with or without vomiting or fever (>38° C) AND no likely noninfectious cause (e.g., diagnostic tests, therapeutic regimen, acute exacerbation of a chronic condition, psychologic stress)
2. Two of the following with no other recognized cause: nausea, vomiting, abdominal pain, or headache AND any of the following:
   a. Enteric pathogen isolated from stool culture or rectal swab
   b. Enteric pathogen detected by routine or electron microscopy examination
   c. Enteric pathogen detected by antigen or antibody assay on feces or blood
   d. Evidence of enteric pathogen detected by cytopathic changes in tissue culture (toxin assay)
   e. Diagnostic single antibody titer (IgM) or fourfold increase in paired serum samples (IgG) for pathogen

Hepatitis must meet the following criterion: Two of the following with no other recognized cause: fever (>38° C), anorexia, nausea, vomiting, abdominal pain, jaundice, or history of transfusion within the previous three months AND any of the following:

1. Positive antigen or antibody test for hepatitis A, hepatitis B, or delta hepatitis
2. Abnormal liver function tests (e.g., elevated alanine/aspartate aminotransferase [ALT/AST] and bilirubin)
3. Cytomegalovirus (CMV) detected in urine or oropharyngeal secretions

Infant necrotizing enterocolitis must meet the following criterion: Two of the following with no other recognized cause: vomiting, abdominal distention, or prefeeding residuals AND persistent microscopic or gross blood in stools AND any of the following abdominal radiographic abnormalities:

1. Pneumoperitoneum
2. Pneumotosis intestinalis
3. Unchanging "rigid" loops of small bowel

Gastrointestinal (GI) tract infection (esophagus, stomach, small bowel, large bowel, and rectum), excluding gastroenteritis and appendicitis, must meet either of the following criteria:

1. Abscess or other evidence of infection seen during surgery or by histopathologic examination
2. Two of the following with no other recognized cause and compatible with infection of the organ or tissue involved: fever (>38° C), nausea, vomiting, abdominal pain, or tenderness AND any of the following:
   a. Organism isolated from culture of drainage or tissue obtained during surgery or endoscopy or from surgically placed drain
   b. Organisms seen on Gram or KOH stain or multinucleated giant cells seen on microscopic examination of drainage or tissue obtained during surgery or endoscopy or from surgically placed drain
   c. Organism isolated from blood culture
   d. Radiographic evidence of infection
   e. Pathologic findings on endoscopic examination (e.g., *Candida* esophagitis or proctitis)

Intra-abdominal infection (including gallbladder, bile ducts, liver [other than viral hepatitis], spleen, pancreas, peritoneum, subphrenic or subdiaphragmatic space, or other intra-abdominal tissue or area not specified elsewhere) must meet one of the following criteria:

1. Organism isolated from culture of purulent material from intra-abdominal space obtained during surgery or needle aspiration
2. Abscess or other evidence of intra-abdominal infection seen during surgery or by histopathologic examination
3. Two of the following with no other recognized cause: fever (>38° C), nausea, vomiting, abdominal pain, or jaundice AND any of the following:

continues

Exhibit 2–1 continued

a. Organism isolated from culture of drainage from surgically placed drain (e.g., closed suction drainage system, open drain, or T-tube drain)
b. Organisms seen on Gram stain of drainage or tissue obtained during surgery or needle aspiration
c. Organism isolated from blood culture and radiographic evidence of infection

LOWER RESPIRATORY TRACT INFECTION (EXCLUDING PNEUMONIA)

Lower respiratory tract infection (excluding pneumonia) includes infections such as bronchitis, tracheobronchitis, bronchiolitis, tracheitis, lung abscess, and empyema.

Bronchitis, tracheobronchitis, bronchiolitis, tracheitis, without evidence of pneumonia, must meet either of the following criteria:

1. Patient has no clinical or radiographic evidence of pneumonia AND has two of the following: fever (>38° C), cough, new or increased sputum production, rhonchi, wheezing, AND either of the following:
   a. Organism isolated from culture obtained by deep tracheal aspirate or bronchoscopy
   b. Positive antigen test on respiratory secretions
2. Patient ≤12 months of age has no clinical or radiographic evidence of pneumonia AND has two of the following with no other recognized cause: fever (>38° C), cough, new or increased sputum production, rhonchi, wheezing, respiratory distress, apnea, or bradycardia AND any of the following:
   a. Organism isolated from culture of material obtained by deep tracheal aspirate or bronchoscopy
   b. Positive antigen test on respiratory secretions
   c. Diagnostic single antibody titer (IgM) or fourfold increase in paired serum samples (IgG) for pathogen

Other infections of the lower respiratory tract must meet one of the following criteria:

1. Organisms seen on smear or isolated from culture of lung tissue or fluid, including pleural fluid
2. Lung abscess or empyema seen during surgery or by histopathologic examination
3. Abscess cavity seen on radiographic examination of lung

REPRODUCTIVE TRACT INFECTION

A group of infections that occur in obstetric and gynecology patients and in male urology patients is defined as reproductive tract infection. Such infections include endometritis, episiotomy infection, vaginal cuff infection, and other infections of the male or female reproductive tract.

Endometritis must meet either of the following criteria:

1. Organism isolated from culture of fluid or tissue from endometrium obtained during surgery, by needle aspiration, or by brush biopsy
2. Purulent drainage from uterus AND two of the following: fever (>38° C), abdominal pain, or uterine tenderness

Episiotomy site infection must meet either of the following criteria:

1. Purulent drainage from episiotomy
2. Episiotomy abscess

Vaginal cuff infection must meet one of the following criteria:

1. Purulent drainage from vaginal cuff
2. Abscess at vaginal cuff
3. Pathogen isolated from culture of fluid or tissue obtained from vaginal cuff

Other infections of the male or female reproductive tract (epididymis, testes, prostate, vagina, ovaries, uterus, or other deep pelvic tissues, excluding endometritis or vaginal cuff infection) must meet one of the following criteria:

1. Organism isolated from culture of tissue or fluid from affected site
2. Abscess or other evidence of infection seen during surgery or by histopathologic examination
3. Two of the following: fever (>38° C), nausea, vomiting, pain, tenderness, or dysuria AND either of the following:
   a. Organism isolated from blood culture
   b. Physician's diagnosis

SKIN AND SOFT TISSUE INFECTION

Skin and soft tissue infection includes skin infection (other than incisional wound infection), soft tissue infection, decubitus ulcer infection, burn infection, breast abscess or mastitis, omphalitis, infant pustulosis, and newborn circumcision infection. Separate criteria are presented for each infection.

Skin infection must meet either of the following criteria:

1. Purulent drainage, pustules, vesicles, or boils
2. Two of the following at affected site: localized pain or tenderness, swelling, redness, or heat AND any of the following:
   a. Organism isolated from culture of aspirate or drainage from affected site; if organism is normal skin flora, must be pure culture of single organism
   b. Organism isolated from blood culture
   c. Positive antigen test on infected tissue or blood

continues

Exhibit 2–1 continued

d. Multinucleated giant cells seen on microscopic examination of affected tissue
e. Diagnostic single antibody titer (IgM) or fourfold increase in paired serum samples (IgG) for pathogen

Soft tissue infection (necrotizing fasciitis, infectious gangrene, necrotizing cellulitis, infectious myositis, lymphadenitis, or lymphangitis) must meet one of the following criteria:

1. Organism isolated from culture of tissue or drainage from affected site
2. Purulent drainage from affected site
3. Abscess or other evidence of infection seen during surgery or by histopathologic examination
4. Two of the following at affected site: localized pain or tenderness, redness, swelling, or heat AND any of the following:
   a. Organism isolated from blood culture
   b. Positive antigen test on blood or urine
   c. Diagnostic single antibody titer (IgM) or fourfold increase in paired serum samples (IgG) for pathogen

Decubitus ulcer infection, including both superficial and deep infection, must meet the following criterion: Two of the following: redness, tenderness, or swelling of wound edges AND either of the following:

1. Organism isolated from culture of fluid obtained by needle aspiration or biopsy of tissue obtained from ulcer margin
2. Organism isolated from blood culture

Burn infection must meet one of the following criteria:

1. Change in burn wound appearance or character, such as rapid eschar separation, or dark brown, black, or violaceous discoloration of the eschar, or edema at wound margin AND histologic examination of burn biopsy specimen that shows invasion of organisms into adjacent viable tissue
2. Change in burn wound appearance or character, such as rapid eschar separation, or dark brown, black, or violaceous discoloration of the eschar, or edema at wound margin AND either of the following:
   a. Organism isolated from blood culture in absence of other identifiable infection
   b. Isolation of herpes simplex virus, histologic identification of inclusions by light or electron microscopy, or visualization of viral particles by electron microscopy in biopsy specimens or lesion scrapings
3. Burn patient has two of the following: fever (>38° C) or hypothermia (<36° C), hypotension (systolic pressure ≤90 mm Hg), oliguria (<20 mL/hr), hyperglycemia at previously tolerated level of dietary carbohydrate, or mental confusion AND any of the following:
   a. Histologic examination of burn biopsy specimen that shows invasion of organisms into adjacent viable tissue

b. Organism isolated from blood culture
c. Isolation of herpes simplex virus, histologic identification of inclusions by light or electron microscopy, or visualization of viral particles by electron microscopy in biopsy specimens or lesion scrapings

Breast abscess or mastitis must meet one of the following criteria:

1. Organism isolated from culture of affected breast tissue or fluid obtained by incision and drainage or needle aspiration
2. Breast abscess or other evidence of infection seen during surgery or by histopathologic examination
3. Fever (>38° C), local inflammation of the breast, and physician's diagnosis

Omphalitis in newborn (≤30 days of age) must meet either of the following criteria:

1. Erythema and/or serous drainage from umbilicus and either of the following:
   a. Organism isolated from culture of drainage or needle aspirate
   b. Organism isolated from blood culture
2. Erythema and purulent drainage at umbilicus

Pustulosis in infant (≤12 months of age) must meet the following criterion:

1. Infant has pustules AND physician's diagnosis or
2. Infant has pustules AND physician institutes appropriate antimicrobial therapy

Circumcision infection in newborn (≤30 days of age) must meet one of the following criteria:

1. Newborn has purulent drainage from circumcision site
2. Newborn has one of the following: erythema, swelling, or tenderness at circumcision site AND pathogen isolated from culture of site
3. Newborn has one of the following: erythema, swelling, or tenderness at circumcision site, and skin contaminant isolated from culture of site AND physician's diagnosis or physician institutes appropriate antimicrobial therapy

SYSTEMIC INFECTION

Systemic infection is defined as infection that involves multiple organs or systems, without an apparent single site of infection. Such infections are usually of viral origin and can usually be identified by clinical criteria alone (e.g., measles, mumps, rubella, and varicella); they occur infrequently as nosocomial infections.

continues

Exhibit 2–1 continued

COMMENTS

Although the definitions presented here were developed for use in hospitals participating in NNIS to standardize and improve the quality of nosocomial infection data reported to CDC, other hospitals may wish to adopt these definitions for use in their surveillance programs. By doing so and by using similar surveillance methods, comparisons may be made with NNIS data. In addition to use in routine surveillance programs for endemic nosocomial infections, these definitions can be used for prevalence surveys, special studies, and outbreak investigations.

[1]When an organism isolated from blood culture is compatible with a related nosocomial infection at another site, the bloodstream infection is classified as a secondary bloodstream infection. Exceptions to this are intravascular device–associated bloodstream infections, all of which are classified as primary even if localized signs of infection are present at the access site.

[2]Organisms that are normal skin flora (e.g., diphtheroids, *Bacillus* sp., *Propionibacterium* sp., coagulase-negative staphylococci, or micrococci).

[3]Detection of bacterial, fungal, or viral antigen (e.g., *Candida* sp., herpes simplex, varicella zoster, *Haemophilus influenzae, Streptococcus pneumoniae, Neisseria meningitidis,* group B streptococci) by rapid diagnostic test (e.g., counterimmunoelectrophoresis, coagulation, or latex agglutination).

[4]These criteria apply specifically to infants ≤12 months of age; they may infrequently apply to older infants and children.

[5]For urine specimens to be of value in determining whether a nosocomial infection exists, they must be obtained aseptically using an appropriate technique, such as clean catch collection, bladder catheterization, or suprapubic aspiration.

[6]Gram-negative bacteria or *Staphylococcus saprophyticus.*

[7]Radiographic evidence of infection includes abnormal results of ultrasound examination, CT scan, magnetic resonance imaging, or radiolabel scan (e.g., gallium or technetium).

Source: Reprinted from CDC definitions for Nosocomial Infections, 1988, The Hospital Infections Program, Center for Infectious Diseases, Centers for Disease Control, Public Health Service, U.S. Department of Health and Human Services.

Exhibit 2–2 CDC Definitions of Nosocomial Surgical Site Infections, 1992: A Modification of CDC Definitions of Surgical Wound Infections

In 1988, the Centers for Disease Control (CDC) published definitions of nosocomial infections. However, because of journalistic style and space constraints, these definitions lacked some of the detail provided to National Nosocomial Infections Surveillance (NNIS) System hospitals in the *NNIS Manual* (unpublished). After the NNIS System hospitals had had considerable experience with the definitions and in response to a request for review by The Surgical Wound Infection Task Force, a group composed of members of The Society for Hospital Epidemiology of America, the Association for Practitioners in Infection Control, the Surgical Infection Society, and the CDC, we slightly modified the definition of surgical wound infection and changed the name to surgical site infection (SSI).

The changes were made for two reasons. First, in the 1988 definitions, it was not clear that for deep surgical wound infections, specifying the anatomic location of the deep infection was necessary. For example, NNIS System hospitals would report osteomyelitis as the specific site of a deep surgical wound infection if it followed an orthopedic operative procedure. Hospitals unfamiliar with this two-level designation might not have gleaned this information from the 1988 definitions. In this revision, we have included a Table listing specific sites. Second, we have removed the term "wound," because in surgical terminology, "wound" connotes only the incision from skin to deep soft tissues. We introduce the term "organ/space" to define any part of the anatomy (e.g., organs or spaces), other than the incision, opened or manipulated during the operative procedure. The distinction between this component of the surgical site and the incision is important in the pathogenesis of SSI following certain operative procedures.

The following revised definitions should be used for surveillance of SSI by hospitals wishing to compare their SSI data with NNIS System SSI data. This article includes some additional considerations when comparing hospital data to NNIS System data.

GENERAL CRITERIA

The American College of Surgeons, in the *Manual on Control of Infection in Surgical Patients,* classified surgical infections into the following groups according to anatomical location and pathophysiologic changes: wound infection, regional extension, organ or visceral infection, systemic infection, and remote coexisting or complicating infections. The first three groups are covered in the following definitions of SSI and involve the skin, subcutaneous tissue, deep soft tissues (e.g., fascial and muscle layers) of the incision, and organs or spaces opened or manipulated during an operative procedure. Systemic and remote or complicating infections that follow an operative procedure (e.g., postoperative pneumonia following cholecystectomy) are considered surgical patient infections but are not classified as SSI because they are not associated with the surgical site. The exception is a bloodstream infection secondary to an incisional or organ/space SSI.

As with all CDC definitions of nosocomial infections, a physician's or surgeon's diagnosis of infection is an acceptable criterion for an SSI unless there is compelling evidence to the contrary (e.g., information written on the wrong patient's record or presumptive diagnosis not substantiated by subsequent studies).

continues

Exhibit 2–2 continued

DEFINITIONS OF SSI

For surveillance classification purposes, SSI are divided into incisional SSI and organ/space SSI. Incisional SSI are further classified into those involving only the skin and subcutaneous tissue (called superficial incisional SSI) and those involving deep soft tissues of the incision (called deep incisional SSI [e.g., fascial and muscle layers]). Organ/space SSI involve any part of the anatomy (e.g., organs or spaces), other than the incision, opened or manipulated during the operative procedure.

Superficial Incisional SSI

Superficial incisional SSI must meet the following criteria: the infection occurs within 30 days after the operative procedure and involves only skin or subcutaneous tissue of the incision. In addition, it must meet at least one of the following: purulent drainage from the superficial incision; organisms isolated from an aseptically obtained culture of fluid or tissue from the superficial incision; at least one of the following signs or symptoms of infection—pain or tenderness, localized swelling, redness or heat, and the superficial incision is deliberately opened by a surgeon unless the incision is culture-negative; or diagnosis of superficial incisional SSI by the surgeon or attending physician.

The following are not reported as superficial incisional SSI: stitch abscess (minimal inflammation and discharge confined to the points of suture penetration); infection of an episiotomy or newborn circumcision site (episiotomy and circumcision are not considered NNIS System operative procedures); infected burn wound; and incisional SSI that extends into the fascial and muscle layers (see deep incisional SSI). (Note: specific criteria are used for infected episiotomy and circumcision sites and burn wounds.)

Deep Incisional SSI

Deep incisional SSI must meet the following criteria: the infection occurs within 30 days after the operative procedure if no implant (i.e., a nonhuman-derived implantable foreign body [e.g., prosthetic heart valve, nonhuman vascular graft, mechanical heart, or hip prosthesis] that is permanently placed in a patient during surgery) is left in place or within one year if an implant is in place and the infection appears to be related to the operative procedure and the infection involves deep soft tissues (e.g., fascial and muscle layers) of the incision. In addition, it must meet at least one of the following: purulent drainage from the deep incision but not from the organ/space component of the surgical site; a deep incision that spontaneously dehisces or is deliberately opened by a surgeon when the patient has at least one of the following signs or symptoms—fever (>38° C), localized pain, or tenderness, unless the incision is culture-negative; an abscess or other evidence of infection involving the deep incision is found on direct examination, during reoperation, or by histopathologic or radiologic examination; or diagnosis of a deep incisional SSI by a surgeon or attending physician.

Organ/Space SSI

An organ/space SSI involves any part of the anatomy (e.g., organs or spaces), other than the incision, opened or manipulated during the operative procedure. Specific sites are assigned to organ/space SSI to further identify the location of the infection. The Table lists the specific sites that must be used to differentiate organ/space SSI. An example is appendectomy with subsequent subdiaphragmatic abscess, which would be reported as an organ/space SSI at the intra-abdominal specific site.

Organ/space SSI must meet the following criteria: the infection occurs within 30 days after the operative procedure if no implant is left in place or within one year if implant is in place and the infection appears to be related to the operative procedure and the infection involves any part of the anatomy (e.g., organs or spaces), other than the incision, opened or manipulated during the operative procedure. In addition, it must meet at least one of the following: purulent drainage from a drain that is placed through a stab wound into the organ/space (if the area around a stab wound becomes infected, it is not an SSI—it is considered a skin or soft tissue infection, depending on its depth); organisms isolated from an aseptically obtained culture of fluid or tissue in the organ/space; an abscess or other evidence of infection involving the organ/space that is found on direct examination, during reoperation, or by histopathologic or radiologic examination; or diagnosis of an organ/space SSI by a surgeon or attending physician.

SSI Involving More Than One Specific Site

An infection that involves *both* superficial and deep incision sites is classified as deep incisional SSI.

Occasionally, an organ/space infection drains through the incision. Such infection generally does not involve reoperation and is considered a complication of the incision. Therefore, it is classified as a deep incisional SSI.

TABLE
Specific Sites of Organ/Space SSI

Arterial or venous infection	Myocarditis or pericarditis
Breast abscess or mastitis	Oral cavity (mouth, tongue, or
Disc space	gums)
Ear, mastoid	Osteomyelitis
Endometritis	Other infections of the lower
Endocarditis	respiratory tract
Eye, other than conjunctivitis	Other infections of the urinary
Gastrointestinal tract	tract
Intra-abdominal, not specified	Other male or female
elsewhere	reproductive tract
Intracranial, brain abscess or	Sinusitis
dura	Spinal abscess without meningitis
Joint or bursa	Upper respiratory tract,
Mediastinitis	pharyngitis
Meningitis or ventriculitis	Vaginal cuff

Source: From the Hospital Infections Program, National Center for Infectious Diseases, Centers for Disease Control, Public Health Service, U.S. Department of Health and Human Services, Atlanta, Georgia.

Each facility must evaluate its case mix of patients and the availability of diagnostic and laboratory facilities in order to determine which definitions are both appropriate and applicable to its setting. Factors that should be considered when evaluating surveillance criteria include the sophistication of the data collector, the applicability of the particular set of definitions to the population being surveyed, the availability and accuracy of laboratory and other diagnostic tests performed on the population, and the availability of laboratories that can provide needed feedback regarding specimen collection and analysis. Many facilities adapt currently available definitions for their use. This makes it impossible for the facility to compare its performance to that of other institutions.

Some problems with current definitions. Many definitions of infections have serious drawbacks. Infection control professionals have long recognized the difficulty of classifying some diseases, especially pneumonia and BSIs, when doing surveillance. Many investigators have proposed different definitions for classifying pneumonia but there is no consensus on a practical definition for this disease.[96] The CDC NNIS definitions for pneumonia and BSIs are rather nonspecific and difficult to use consistently. When evaluating a potential BSI, it is often difficult to determine if an organism isolated from a blood culture is a true infection or a contaminant. The CDC has recognized this problem and is currently revising the BSI and the pneumonia definitions in the NNIS system. Those using these definitions must realize that incidence rates may change when a definition is changed and this must be recognized when analyzing surveillance data and must be noted when writing a surveillance report.

The characteristics of patients residing in licensed LTC facilities dramatically changed in the 1990s. The McGeer et al[95] definitions were written in 1989, before the widespread use of IV therapy and mechanical ventilators and the presence of patients with acquired immune deficiency syndrome in many LTC facilities. Some LTC facilities—especially those that care for residents with significant acuity, such as those who are ventilator dependent or who have a central venous catheter—have adopted some of the CDC NNIS definitions for use in the LTC setting.

Ambulatory surgery facilities should use the CDC NNIS system criteria when conducting SSI surveillance.[34,35] Unfortunately, standardized surveillance criteria for other ambulatory care settings, such as dialysis centers, have not been established.

Determine the Data Gathering Process

The data gathering process will depend on the surveillance indicators that are chosen.[5,8,24]

Identify what data will be collected. Data collection should be limited to the essential information needed to determine if the criteria for the disease or event being monitored is met. Although the variables to be collected will depend on the particular event being surveyed, when monitoring patient outcomes the following data points should be considered:

1. for nosocomial infections:
   * patient name, medical record or identification number, age, sex, location in the facility (unit, room number, bed number), physician name and service, date of admission, date of infection onset, type of infection, date of discharge, transfer, or death
   * information needed to classify the specific nosocomial infection being monitored: relevant laboratory/diagnostic tests, date(s) done/results, cultures done/date collected/site of culture/result, antibiotic susceptibility pattern of significant isolates, signs/symptoms specific for the disease criteria
   * risk factors for infection: host factors (such as underlying disease), surgical procedures (name of procedure, surgeon, ASA [American Society of Anesthesiologists] score, duration of procedure), presence of invasive devices (date of insertion, duration, location and types of vascular access devices; use and duration of urinary catheter or mechanical ventilator)
2. for noninfectious events:[8]
   * patient name, medical record or identification number, age, sex, location in the facility (unit, room number, bed number), physician name and service, date of admission, date, time and location of the occurrence, outcome of event, personnel involved (when relevant), date of discharge, transfer, or death, and risk factors for event (e.g., identified risk factors for falls include poor vision, preexisting neurological deficits, and medications such as psychotropic drugs)

Identify when data will be collected. The approach to collecting surveillance data (concurrent and/or retrospective) depends on the event being studied and the available resources. The advantages of conducting concurrent surveillance (i.e., collecting data while the patient is still under the care of the facility) include the ability to observe findings that are not always recorded in the patient's record (such as the presence of drainage at a surgical incision site), to interview those caring for the patient (direct caregivers frequently provide insight into circumstances and factors that may influence patient outcomes), to detect clusters or potential outbreaks in a timely manner, to institute immediate control measures (such as isolation precautions), and to provide informal education about infection control to caregivers, patients, or family members (this is especially important in LTC facilities that have high staff turnover rates). Some data, such as information on falls and other accidents, should be recorded at the time of the incident so that important information is not overlooked or forgotten. If data is collected concurrently, then patient length of stay will affect the frequency of data collection. Some experts recommend that routine infection surveillance be performed at least once a week in the LTC setting.[53]

The disadvantages of concurrent surveillance are the time involved in locating and reviewing charts on a busy unit and the incompleteness of the patient's medical record if test results are not yet available when the chart is reviewed. In some circumstances it may be more efficient to conduct retrospective or closed-record surveillance, especially if there is little or no opportunity for intervention. Retrospective chart review allows the surveyor to review laboratory and other diagnostic reports that may not be completed or placed in the medical record until after discharge.

Identify sources of data. After deciding what data elements are needed, the sources of the data should be identified. Sources may include[24]

- patient or resident records
- daily microbiology reports provided by the laboratory
- daily list of patients or residents admitted (including diagnosis) provided by the admissions department
- monthly report of the number of patients admitted and discharged and the number of patient-days for each unit in the facility, as provided by the facility's administrative or financial department
- interviews with caregivers
- verbal and written reports from caregivers
- Kardex on the patient units
- lists of patients on isolation precautions (this can sometimes be generated through the facility's computer information system)
- reports of antibiotic orders generated by the pharmacy
- chest radiograph results from the radiology department (these are often available through the hospital information system or through an audio system by telephone)
- incident reports from the risk management department
- observations of health care worker's practices
- activity/procedure logs from the emergency room, operating room, respiratory therapy department, or outpatient offices or clinics
- other personnel who regularly review records (such as quality management and utilization review)
- employee health reports for needlesticks and other personnel injuries or exposures
- the medical records department for lists of patients who were coded with the same disease or condition

Infection control personnel should work with the facility's information services department to identify any other sources of information.[97]

Identify who will collect the data. The persons who are responsible for collecting nosocomial infection surveillance data must be capable of interpreting clinical notes, collecting the data elements needed to evaluate the presence of nosocomial infection, and using a standardized data collection tool. The availability of surveillance personnel may affect the frequency and accuracy of data collection. If the person who is responsible for data collection leaves the position or is on an extended leave of absence, then someone else should be trained and assigned responsibility for the data collection process. If data is not collected for short periods, it may not be of major consequence; however, if data collection is interrupted for long periods, significant events such as outbreaks or clusters may be missed.

For some nosocomial infection indicators, personnel in several departments may be given the responsibility for collecting data. For example, respiratory therapy personnel can often provide the number of ventilator-days in a specific patient care unit and ICU personnel can collect and record each day the number of patients with a urinary catheter or a central line. (Note: "central line" must be defined[34] so that data can be consistently collected each day regardless of who collects it.)

Design data collection tools. Standardized data collection tools must be designed and used to collect the necessary data elements for the surveillance indicators. Several types of data collection forms may be needed.

1. A case report form can be used to collect surveillance data on each patient reviewed.
   - If a manual data collection and management system is used, this case report form should be designed so it is consistent with the order in the patient medical record so that information can be collected and recorded efficiently. This should minimize the need to search back and forth through the chart.
   - If a computer database is used, the case report form should be designed so the order is the same as the data entry screen on the computer. Whenever possible, both the computer database and the case report form should be set up so the information is consistent with the order in the patient medical record.
   - A one-page data collection form should be used as much as possible.
2. A line-listing form can be used to record all cases who have a particular disease (such as all patients from whom MRSA has been isolated or all patients with an SSI following total hip arthroplasty) and to visualize factors that may be common to these patients (if the group is small).
3. A form can be used to record the number of patients on a specified unit who have a central line or urinary catheter or who are on mechanical ventilation.[11]

Examples of data collection forms can be found in Appendixes B, H, I, and J and in several of the references.[8,11,58,64,65] The forms used in the NNIS system were published in 1991.[11] Any of these forms can be used as prototypes from which a facility-specific form can be modeled.

Using technology to store, manage, and analyze surveillance data. Before data can be analyzed, it must be organized. Data collection and consolidation can be accomplished using either a manual or computerized system. The basic premises are the same; however, the data can be more easily manipulated when a computer is used, so computers and computerized databases should be used whenever possible. Unfortunately, manual systems are frequently used even when computers may be readily available.

When manual systems are used, the user should be able to take information from the individual or case forms in an orderly manner and transcribe it easily onto a line-listing form (a manual database) that is organized to correspond to the case form. Line listings can then be used to display data in a variety of ways (e.g., by organism, infection site, procedure, date of event, or service).

Those responsible for coordinating infection surveillance, prevention, and control programs should learn how to use computers to store, manage, and analyze surveillance data, if they are not yet doing so. Basic software packages, such as Microsoft Office, contain word processing, spreadsheet, database, and graphics programs that are useful for infection control surveillance. Data collection forms can be designed using a word processing program, and corresponding line listings can be developed using either a word processing, spreadsheet, or database (the most useful method) program. There are several commercially available software programs designed to manage nosocomial infection surveillance.[97] The use of computers to manage infection control and quality management data is beyond the scope of this chapter, so refer to a review article by Reagan for further information.[97]

Much data is collected at the bedside or in clinical areas. Therefore, unless portable computers or bedside terminals are used to collect the information, a paper form must still be used to record the data on site. The information then must be entered into a computer. Smyth et al described the use of an automated data entry system employing optical scanning of a specially designed form to enter surveillance data into a computer database.[98] This method reduced both the time and errors associated with manual data entry. Although widely used for other purposes (such as grading examinations), optical scanning technology has rarely been used for entering surveillance data in health care facilities.

Some facilities have developed comprehensive, hospital-wide software systems. These "expert" systems can merge and/or evaluate existing patient information databases to identify patients with a high probability of having a nosocomial infection. These patients can then be targeted for chart review, antibiotic management, or infection control intervention.[97,99]

Identify How To Analyze the Data

When designing a surveillance program, the types of measurements desired (usually rates and proportions) must be determined prior to conducting surveillance so that the appropriate data can be identified and consistently collected. Ratios, rates, and proportions are explained in detail in Chapter 10. The basic formula used to calculate rates, ratios, and proportions is:

$$\text{rate, ratio, or proportion} = (x \,/\, y) \times 10^n$$

where x (the numerator) is compared to y (the denominator) and 10^n is used to transform the result of the division into a uniform quantity. The value of n depends on the type of frequency measure being computed.

A rate is used in health care epidemiology to measure the frequency or occurrence of a disease or event in a specified population over time. The formula is:

$$\text{rate} = \frac{\text{the number of cases or events in a specified time period}}{\text{the number of persons in the population at risk during the same time period}} \times 10^n$$

To calculate accurate rates of disease frequency, the appropriate numerators and denominators must be used. For instance, when calculating an incidence rate, persons who have the disease or condition being studied are called the "cases," and these become the numerator. The persons who are at risk of developing the disease or condition being studied are called the "population at risk," and these become the denominator.

Criteria or case definitions must be used to identify cases, as discussed above. During the course of an outbreak investigation, the case definition may be expanded in order to identify all the persons who may be affected and later narrowed to include only those who have been diagnosed with the disease being studied, as explained in Chapter 8. However, when conducting routine surveillance, it is imperative that a single case definition for each disease or event be applied at all times, so that the surveyors can accurately track trends (rates) over time.

The selection of an appropriate denominator is one of the most important aspects of measuring disease fre-

quency.[100] It is important to ensure that the number used closely represents the true population at risk. For example, incidence rates measure the frequency with which new cases or events occur in a defined population at risk during a specified period. The formula for calculating an incidence rate is:

$$\text{incidence rate} = \frac{\text{number of cases or events that occur in a defined time period}}{\text{number of persons in population at risk during the same period}} \times 10^n$$

If one wishes to measure the incidence of primary bloodstream infections (PBSIs) in an ICU, the numerator would be the number of new PBSIs in the ICU during a defined period, and the denominator would be the number of patients discharged from the ICU during that period (because the number discharged would be a close approximation of the population at risk). However, because a patient's risk of developing a PBSI is known to increase as the time spent in the ICU increases, a more accurate measure of a patient's risk of developing a PBSI would be an incidence density rate. The incidence density is a type of incidence rate that incorporates time, such as patient-days, in the denominator. The formula is:

$$\text{incidence density} = \frac{\text{number of new cases that occur in a defined time period}}{\text{the time each person in population at risk is observed, totaled for all persons}} \times 10^n$$

Using the above formula, one could calculate the incidence density rate of PBSIs in the ICU as follows:

$$\frac{\text{ICU PBSI rate}}{\text{per 1,000 patient-days}} = \frac{\text{number of new cases PBSI in the ICU in a defined period}}{\text{total number of patient-days in the ICU in the defined period}} \times 1,000$$

where the denominator is the total number of days spent in the ICU by *all* of the patients who were in the ICU during the defined period, and $n = 3$ to show the rate per 1,000 patient-days.

One can also calculate device-associated infection rates. One could calculate the number of PBSIs that are associated with a central line in the above ICU population by using the steps shown in Exhibit 2–3.

There are also many methods for calculating SSI rates.[36] One can calculate service-specific, surgeon-

Exhibit 2–3 How To Calculate a Device-Associated Infection Rate

Step 1:	Decide on the time period for your analysis. It may be a month, a quarter, six months, a year, or some other period.
Step 2:	Select the patient population for analysis, i.e., the type of intensive care unit or a birthweight category in the high-risk nursery.
Step 3:	Select the infections to be used in the numerator. They must be site specific and must have occurred in the selected patient population. Their date of onset must be during the selected time period.
Step 4:	Determine the number of device-days which is used as the denominator of the rate. Device-days are the total number of days of exposure to the device (central line, ventilator, or urinary catether) by all of the patients in the selected population during the selected time period.

Example: Five patients on the first day of the month had one or more central lines in place: five on day 2, two on day 3, five on day 4, three on day 5, four on day 6, and four on day 7. Adding the number of patients with central lines on days 1 through 7, we would have $5 + 5 + 2 + 5 + 3 + 4 + 4 = 28$ central line-days for the first week. If we continued for the entire month, the number of central line-days for the month is simply the sum of the daily counts.

Step 5:	Calculate the device-associated infection rate (per 1,000 device-days) using the following formula:

$$\frac{\text{Number of device-associated infections for a specified site}}{\text{Number of device-days}} \times 1,000$$

Example: **Central line-associated BSI rate per 1,000 central line-days =**

$$\frac{\text{Number of central line-associated BSI}}{\text{Number of central line-days}} \times 1,000$$

Source: Reprinted from National Nosocomial Infections Surveillance (NNIS) System Report, Data Summary from October 1986–April 1998, Issued June, 1998. Hospital Infectious Program, National Center for Infectious Diseases, Centers for Disease Control and Prevention, Public Health Service, US Department of Health and Human Services, Atlanta, Georgia.

specific, or procedure-specific rates. Examples are shown below (in these cases, $n = 2$, and the rate is expressed as a percentage).

$$\text{Cardiology service-specific rate (\%)} = \frac{\text{number SSIs in patients on cardiology service}}{\text{number patients operated on by cardiology service}} \times 100$$

$$\text{Surgeon-specific rate (\%)} = \frac{\text{number SSIs in patients operated on by Dr. A}}{\text{number patients operated on by Dr. A}} \times 100$$

$$\text{Procedure-specific rate (\%)} = \frac{\text{number SSIs after coronary artery bypass graft (CABG) surgery}}{\text{number CABG procedures done}} \times 100$$

Prevalence is a measure of the frequency of the occurrence of active (new and old) cases of a disease in a specified population during a defined time period. A prevalence rate is calculated using the formula:

$$\text{Prevalence rate} = \frac{\text{all new and existing cases during a specific time period}}{\text{population at risk during same time period}} \times 10^n$$

Incidence versus prevalence rates. A prevalence rate differs from an incidence rate in that a prevalence rate measures the occurrence of both new and existing cases of a disease and an incidence rate measures new cases only. For this reason, prevalence rates are generally higher than incidence rates. Some published studies report prevalence (not incidence) rates of infection. Therefore, one must be careful that the same types of rates are being compared when comparing rates in a facility to those in the literature.

When developing a surveillance program one must first identify which rates will be calculated and then identify which numerator and denominator will be used before any data is collected.

Comparing rates: risk stratification, data collection, and benchmarking. Different populations have different risks for disease or injury. For instance, a new mother in a mother-baby unit is less likely to develop a nosocomial infection than a critically ill patient in an ICU. A health care worker who uses needles to give injections is more likely to sustain a needlestick than a clerk in the same facility. For this reason, a risk stratification method (a system of adjusting rates based on risk) must be incorporated into the surveillance program.[5,11,12,24,33,36]

Calculating incidence rates based on patient-days or device-days is one method of risk stratification, and this is used in the NNIS system.[11,12] Surgical wound infection rates have long been calculated using a risk assessment system,[36,101–103] and the NNIS system uses a risk index based on wound classification, duration of the operation (time of incision to time of closure), and ASA score.[12,103]

Because a thorough discussion of risk stratification methods is beyond the scope of this chapter, refer to the references noted above and to the review article by Gross.[104] It should be noted that risk assessment systems must be used for measuring all outcomes of care, not only for nosocomial infections.[105,106]

Data analysis should be limited to those personnel who are trained to consistently apply specific criteria for the event being monitored. Studies have shown that even when personnel are trained to identify the presence, type, and site of nosocomial infections, there is variation in their ability to do so.[107,108] In addition, surveillance that is conducted prospectively (at least in part) has been shown to be more accurate than surveillance conducted by retrospective chart review.[109]

Factors that affect variations in data collection and analysis must be kept in mind when comparing rates over time in a health care facility and especially when comparing rates with other institutions.[110–113] Surveillance indicators that are used for comparing rates with external databases (benchmarking) should meet the criteria delineated by SHEA and APIC.[110]

Many hospitals use the NNIS system data for benchmarking nosocomial infection rates. In order to benchmark rates, a facility must use the NNIS system methodology for collecting data and for calculating and analyzing rates.[11,12] There is currently no similar national database for comparing or benchmarking nosocomial infection rates in the LTC setting. However, there is a published report of a regional data set of infection rates for LTC facilities that demonstrates the potential for developing a pooled data set for interfacility (among different facilities) comparison.[114] There are few national databases for comparing other types of events relating to health care. Although the use of benchmarking is

attractive and comparing rates to others can lead to improvement in the quality of care,[14,71] health care facilities must be aware of the problems inherent in comparing rates among facilities and the need for risk stratification, validation of the data collection process, and standardization of the methods used for analysis and interpretation of the findings.[110,112,115–118]

Develop an Interpretive Report

"Measurement, or surveillance, is an essential step in enabling an organization to learn about what it produces (outcomes) and how it produces it (process)."[119(p.137)] Surveillance reports should be designed to provide accurate, interpretable information and to stimulate improvement of the process or the outcomes being measured.[5] Methods for using visual displays (charts, graphs, and tables) to present the findings are discussed in Chapter 12.

The content, format, and level of detail of each report will depend on the intended audience. Reports should be designed to contain the following information: time frame of the study, numbers of cases or events detected, number in the population studied, the rates, the methodology that was used to collect the data and calculate the rates, the criteria that was used to define the numerator and denominator, any actions taken, the likely risk factors that influenced the occurrence of the events, and any recommendations for prevention and control measures.

Determine Who Should Receive the Report

Reports should be given to those persons in the facility who can alter the outcomes or processes (i.e., those who can develop and implement strategies to reduce the risk factors). Those who produce the reports should periodically meet with those who receive the reports to discuss the findings, rates, any clusters detected, and any recommendations for improvement.

Develop a Written Surveillance Plan

A written surveillance plan should be developed and reviewed periodically (usually annually) to assess the usefulness of the program. The written plan should contain the following information:

- a brief description of the facility
- the types of services provided
- the objectives of the surveillance program
- a brief description of the surveillance indicators (both outcome and process)

- the methodology for data collection (total or targeted)
- the methodology for calculating and analyzing rates
- a description of the surveillance criteria used (e.g., NNIS[34,35,67] or McGeer et al[95])
- the types of reports provided and persons to whom they are sent
- the process for evaluating the program

Evaluating a Surveillance Program

Each surveillance program should be periodically assessed to evaluate its usefulness. Guidelines for evaluating surveillance systems were published by the CDC in 1988.[30] A surveillance system is considered useful if it contributes to the prevention and control of adverse health events.

When assessing the usefulness of the program, one should begin with a review of the program's objectives. "Depending on the objectives of a particular surveillance system, the system may be considered useful if it satisfactorily addresses at least one of the following questions. Does the system:

a. Detect trends signaling changes in the occurrence of disease?
b. Detect epidemics?
c. Provide estimates of the magnitude of morbidity and mortality related to the health problem under surveillance?
d. Stimulate epidemiologic research likely to lead to control or prevention?
e. Identify risk factors associated with disease occurrence?
f. Permit assessment of the effects of control measures?
g. Lead to improved clinical practice by the healthcare providers who are the constituents of the surveillance system?"[30(p.5)]

REGULATIONS AND ACCREDITING REQUIREMENTS AFFECTING SURVEILLANCE PROGRAMS

Federal and state regulations require hospitals and LTC facilities to have infection control programs.[16,65,120–123] The federal Health Care Financing Administration (HCFA) mandates the collection and analysis of data on outcomes and adverse events in facilities that accept Medicare or Medicaid patients. For example, the HCFA's Long Term Care Conditions of Participation requires a facility to develop a program to investigate, control, and prevent infections in the facility and to maintain a record of incidents and corrective actions related to infections.[123]

In addition to legal requirements, health care facilities are also subject to guidelines or recommendations that are recognized as standards of care (such as CDC guidelines[46,77]) and to accrediting agency requirements (such as the Joint Commission on Accreditation of Healthcare Organizations [Joint Commission] or the Rehabilitation Accreditation Commission [CARF]).

The Joint Commission requires hospitals, LTC facilities, and ambulatory care facilities to have infection surveillance, prevention, and control programs that include the ongoing review and analysis of nosocomial infection data.[124–126] The Joint Commission specifies that a health care facility must design and implement a surveillance program that is appropriate to the environment. Organizations that are accredited by CARF must have an infection control program that addresses infections acquired in the community, infections acquired in the facility, and trends.[127] Although the expectations of the various agencies regarding the methodology and type of data collected varies, there is general agreement that a health care facility must collect nosocomial infection data, analyze the data to determine the significance of the findings, and implement programs or activities that will reduce the risk of nosocomial infections.

All states in the United States and many municipalities have "notifiable disease" requirements. The CDC publishes a recommended list of diseases that should be reported to the National Notifiable Disease Surveillance System (NNDSS);[86] however, state and local laws governing reporting vary somewhat for the diseases or conditions that must be reported by health care providers to the local health department. The list of the CDC notifiable diseases is shown in Exhibit 2–4.

PUBLIC HEATLH SERVICE

Health care facilities play an important role in the identification, surveillance, and reporting of communicable diseases and in the early recognition of community outbreaks.[48] Even though it may not seem important to report one case of a reportable disease, that case

Exhibit 2–4 The 52 Infectious Diseases That Were Designated as Notifiable at the National Level During 1996

Acquired immune deficiency syndrome	Gonorrhea	Psittacosis
Anthrax	*Haemophilus influenzae,* invasive disease	Rabies, animal
Botulism*	Hansen disease (leprosy)	Rabies, human
Brucellosis	Hantavirus pulmonary syndrome	Rocky Mountain spotted fever
Chancroid*	Hemolytic uremic syndrome, post-diarrheal	Rubella
Chlamydia trachomatic, genital infection	Hepatitis A	Salmonellosis*
	Hepatitis B	Shigellosis*
Cholera	Hepatitis C/non-A, non-B	Streptococcal disease, invasive, group A
Coccidioidomycosis*	HIV infection, pediatric	*Streptococcus pneumoniae,* drug-resistant*
Congenital rubella syndrome	Legionellosis	
Congenital syphilis	Lyme disease	Streptococcal toxic-shock syndrome
Cryptosporidiosis	Malaria	Syphilis
Diphtheria	Measles (Rubeola)	Tetanus
Encephalitis, California	Meningococcal disease	Toxic-shock syndrome
Encephalitis, eastern equine	Mumps	Trichinosis
Encephalitis, St. Louis	Pertussis	Tuberculosis
Encephalitis, western equine	Plague	Typhoid fever
Escherichia coli O157:H7	Poliomyelitis, paralytic	Yellow fever

Note: Although varicella is not a nationally notifiable disease, the Council of State and Territorial Epidemiologists recommends reporting of cases of this disease to CDC.

*Not currently published in the *MMWR* weekly tables.

Source: Reprinted from Summary of Notifiable Diseases, United States, 1996, *MMWR* 1997, 45(53): iv, Centers for Disease Control and Prevention.

may be part of a larger outbreak that would not be recognized unless each health care provider reported each case that they diagnosed.

Community outbreaks are frequently detected by health care providers when several patients present with the same symptoms within a short period of time. Health care facilities should have a mechanism for routinely reporting suspected community outbreaks of infectious and noninfectious diseases. For example, several years ago a patient was admitted to a local hospital with dehydration and gastroenteritis. The patient told her attending physician that several of her friends, all of whom had attended the same wedding reception, were also ill and another had just been admitted to the same hospital with similar symptoms. The physician reported this to the infection control staff who interviewed both patients, confirmed the report, and called the local health department. The health department investigated the cases and uncovered an outbreak of *Salmonella enteritidis* food poisoning among the attendees of the wedding. The source of the *Salmonella* was found to be a contaminated commercially packaged meat product. Contamination of the meat product may not have been recognized if this cluster of cases had not been promptly reported.

CONCLUSION

Routine surveillance programs in health care facilities should be implemented to measure outcomes and processes related to health care. An effective surveillance program should be able to detect and quantify the occurrence of adverse events, such as nosocomial infections, and of diseases of public health importance. A major objective of the program is to identify clusters and outbreaks of disease so that control measures can be implemented to prevent new cases from occurring.

REFERENCES

1. Centers for Disease Control and Prevention. Nosocomial bacteremias associated with intravenous fluid therapy—USA. *MMWR.* 1997;46: 1227–1233.

2. Goldmann DA, Maki DG, Rhame FS, Kaiser AB, Tenney JH, Bennett JV. Guidelines for infection control in intravenous therapy. *Ann Intern Med.* 1973;79:848–850.

3. Rhinehart E, Friedman MM. *Infection Control in Home Care*. Gaithersburg, MD: Aspen Publishers, Inc; 1999.

4. Haley RW, Gaynes RP, Aber RC, et al. Surveillance of nosocomial infections. In: Bennett JV, Brachman PS, eds. Hospital Infections. 3rd ed. Boston: Little Brown and Co.; 1992.

5. Lee TB, Baker OG, Lee JT, et al. Recommended practices for surveillance. *Am J Infect Control*. 1998;26:277–288.

6. Baker OG. Process surveillance: an epidemiologic challenge for all health care organizations. *Am J Infect Control*. 1997;25:96–101.

7. Lee TB. Surveillance in acute care and nonacute care settings: current issues and concepts. *Am J Infect Control*. 1997;25:121–124.

8. Massanari RM, Wilkerson K, Swartzendruber S. Designing surveillance for noninfectious outcomes of medical care. *Infect Control Hosp Epidemiol*. 1995;16:419–426.

9. Haley RW, Culver DH, White JW, et al. The efficacy of infection surveillance and control programs in preventing nosocomial infections in U.S. hospitals. *Am J Epidemiol*. 1985;121:182–205.

10. Centers for Disease Control and Prevention. Public health focus: surveillance, prevention and control of nosocomial infections. *MMWR*. 1992;41:783–787.

11. Emori TG, Culver DH, Horan TC, et al. National nosocomial infections surveillance system (NNIS): description of surveillance methods. *Am J Infect Control*. 1991;19:19–35.

12. Centers for Disease Control and Prevention. National Nosocomial Infections Surveillance (NNIS) report, data summary from October 1986—April 1998, issued June 1998. *Am J Infect Control*. 1998;26:522–533.

13. Gaynes RP, Culver DH, Emori TG, et al. The national nosocomial infections surveillance system: plans for the 1990s and beyond. *Am J Med*. 1991;91(Suppl 3B):3B-116S—3B-120S.

14. Gaynes RP, Solomon S. Improving hospital-acquired infection rates: the CDC experience. *J Qual Improvement*. 1996;22:457–467.

15. Smith PW. Infection surveillance in long-term care facilities. *Infect Control Hosp Epidemiol*. 1991;12:55–58.

16. Smith P, Rusnack P. Infection prevention and control in the long-term-care facility. *Am J Infect Control*. 1997;25:488–512.

17. Manian FA. Surveillance of surgical site infections in alternative settings: exploring the current options. *Am J Infect Control*. 1997;25:102–105.

18. Nafziger DA, Lundstrom T, Chandra S, Massanari RM. Infection control in ambulatory care. *Infect Dis Clin North Amer*. 1997;11:279–296.

19. Centers for Disease Control. *Outline for Surveillance and Control of Nosocomial Infections*. Atlanta, GA: Centers for Disease Control; 1970.

20. US Dept of Health and Human Services. *Prevalence Survey for Nosocomial Infections: Revised*. Atlanta, GA: Hospital Infections Program, Centers for Disease Control and Prevention; 1992.

21. Pottinger JM, Herwaldt LA, Perl TM. Basics of surveillance—an overview. *Infect Control Hosp Epidemiol*. 1997;18:513–527.

22. Chelgren G, La Force FM. Limited, periodic surveillance proves practical and effective. *Hospitals*. 1978;52:151–152,154.

23. Tousey PM. Epidemiologic methods for selective surveillance. *Am J Infect Control*. 1987;15:148–158.

24. Lee TB, Baker OG. Surveillance. In: Olmsted RN, ed. *APIC Infection Control and Applied Epidemiology: Principles and Practice*. St. Louis, MO: Mosby–Year Book; 1996:5-1—5-18.

25. Haley RW. *Managing Hospital Infection Control for Cost Effectiveness*. Chicago: American Hospital Association; 1986.

26. Perl TM. Surveillance, reporting, and the use of computers. In: Wenzel RP, ed. *Prevention and Control of Nosocomial Infections*. 2nd ed. Baltimore: Williams & Wilkins; 1993:139–176.

27. Scheckler WE. Surveillance, foundation for the future: a historical overview and evolution of methodologies. *Am J Infect Control*. 1997;25:106–111.

28. Pirwitz S, Manian F. Prevalence of use of infection control rituals and outdated practices: Education Committee survey results. *Am J Infect Control*. 1997;25:28–33.

29. Haley RW. Surveillance by objective: a new priority-directed approach to the control of nosocomial infections. *Am J Infect Control*. 1985;13:78–89.

30. Centers for Disease Control. Guidelines for evaluating surveillance systems. *MMWR*. 1988;37(S-5):1–18.

31. Gaynes RP, Horan TC. Surveillance of nosocomial infections. In: Mayhall CG, ed. *Hospital Epidemiology and Infection Control*. Baltimore: Williams & Wilkins; 1996:1017–1031, App-A–App-C.

32. Wenzel RP, Thompson RL, Landry SM, et al. Hospital-acquired infections in intensive care unit patients: an overview with emphasis on epidemics. *Infect Control Hosp Epidemiol*. 1983;4:371–375.

33. Mangram AJ, Horan TC, Pearson ML, Silver LC, Jarvis WR, and the Hospital Infection Control Practices Advisory Committee. Guideline for the prevention of surgical site infection, 1999. *Infect Control Hosp Epidemiol*. 1999;20:247–280.

34. Horan TC, Emori TG. Definitions of key terms used in the NNIS system. *Am J Infect Control*. 1997;25:112–116.

35. Horan, TC, Gaynes RP, Martone WJ, Jarvis WR, Emori TG. CDC definitions of nosocomial surgical site infections, 1992: a modification of CDC definitions of surgical wound infections. *Infect Control Hosp Epidemiol*. 1992;13;606–608.

36. Roy MC, Perl TM. Basics of surgical-site surveillance. *Infect Control Hosp Epidemiol*. 1997;18:659–668.

37. Roberts FJ, Walsh A, Wing P, Dvorek M, Schweigel J. The influence of surveillance methods on surgical wound infection rates in a tertiary care spinal surgery service. *Spine*. 1998;23:366–370.

38. Fields CL. Outcomes of a postdischarge surveillance system for surgical site infections at a Midwestern regional referral center hospital. *Am J Infect Control*. 1999;27:158–164.

39. Lee JT. Wound infection surveillance. *Infect Dis Clin North Am*. 1992;6:643–656.

40. Cardo DM, Falk PS, Mayhall CG. Validation of surgical wound surveillance. *Infect Control Hosp Epidemiol*. 1993;14:22–215.

41. Boyce JM, Jackson MM, Pugliese G, et al. Methicillin-resistant *Staphylococcus aureus* (MRSA): a briefing for acute care hospitals and nursing facilities. *Infect Control Hosp Epidemiol*. 1994;15:105–115.

42. The Hospital Practices Advisory Committee. Recommendations for preventing the spread of vancomycin resistance: recommendations of the Hospital Practices Advisory Committee (HICPAC). *Am J Infect Control*. 1995;23:87–94.

43. Mylotte JM. Laboratory surveillance method for nosocomial *Clostridium difficile* diarrhea. *Am J Infect Control*. 1998;26:16–23.

44. Filippel MB, Rearick T. Respiratory syncytial virus. *Nurs Clin North Am*. 1993;28:651–671.

45. Bernstein DI, Ward RL. Rotaviruses. In: Feigin RD, Cherry JD, eds. *Textbook of Pediatric Infectious Diseases*. 4th ed. Philadelphia: WB Saunders Company; 1998:1901–1922.

46. Centers for Disease Control and Prevention. Guidelines for preventing the transmission of *Mycobacterium tuberculosis* in health-care facilities. *MMWR*. 1994;43(RR-13):1–132.

47. Centers for Disease Control and Prevention. Interim guidelines for prevention and control of staphylococcal infection associated with reduced susceptibility to vancomycin. *MMWR.* 1997;46:626–635.

48. Guerrero JC, Filippone C. A cluster of Legionnaire's disease in a community hospital—a clue to a larger epidemic. *Infect Control Hosp Epidemiol.* 1996;17:177–178.

49. Goodman RA, Solomon SL. Transmission of infectious diseases in outpatient health care settings. *JAMA.* 1991;265:2377–2380.

50. Herwaldt LA, Smith SD, Carter CD. Infection control in the outpatient setting. *Infect Control Hosp Epidemiol.* 1998;19:41–74.

51. Tokars JI, Miller ER, Alter MJ, Arduino MJ. *National Surveillance of Dialysis-Associated Diseases in the United States, 1997.* Atlanta, GA: National Center for Infectious Diseases, Centers for Disease Control and Prevention, Public Health Service, Department of Health and Human Services; 1999.

52. Kaczmarek RG, Moore RM, McCrohan J, et al. Multi-state investigation of the actual disinfection/sterilization of endoscopes in health care facilities. *Am. J. Med.* 1992;92:257–261.

53. Smith PW. Consensus conference on nosocomial infections in long-term care facilities. *Am J Infect Control.* 1987;15:97–100.

54. Jackson MM, Fierer J. Infections and infection risk in residents of long-term care facilities: a review of the literature, 1970–1984. *Am J Infect Control.* 1985;13:63–77.

55. Jacobson C, Strausbaugh LJ. Incidence and impact of infection in nursing home care unit. *Am J Infect Control.* 1990;18:151–159.

56. Vermaat JH, Rosebrugh E, Ford-Jones EL, Ciano J, Kobayashi J, Miller G. An epidemiologic study of nosocomial infections in a pediatric long-term care facility. *Am J Infect Control.* 1993;21:183–188.

57. Garibaldi RA, Brodine S, Matsumiya S. Infections among patients in nursing homes: policies, prevalence and problems. *N Engl J Med.* 1981;305:731–735.

58. Smith PW, ed. *Infection Control in Long-Term Care Facilities.* 2nd ed. Albany, NY: Delmar Publishers, Inc; 1994.

59. Jackson MM, Fierer J, Barrett-Connor E, et al. Intensive surveillance for infections in a three-year study of nursing home patients. *Am J Epidemiol.* 1992;135:685–696.

60. Darnowski SB, Gordon M, Simor AE. Two years of infection surveillance in a geriatric long-term care facility. *Am J Infect Control.* 1991;19:185–190.

61. Vlahov D, Tenney JH, Cervino KW, Shamer DK. Routine surveillance for infections in nursing homes: experience at two facilities. *Am J Infect Control.* 1987;15:47–53.

62. Goldrick BA. Infection control programs in skilled nursing long-term care facilities: an assessment, 1995. *Am J Infect Control.* 1999;27:4–9.

63. Nicolle LE, Garibaldi RA. Infection control in long-term care facilities. *Infect Control Hosp Epidemiol.* 1995;16:348–353.

64. Ministry of National Health and Welfare. *Canadian Infection Control Guidelines for Long Term Care Facilities.* Ottawa, Ontario, Canada: Ministry of National Health and Welfare; 1994.

65. Rusnak PG. Long term care. In: Olmsted RN, ed. *APIC Infection Control and Applied Epidemiology: Principles and Practice.* St. Louis, MO: Mosby–Year Book; 1996.

66. Ahlbrecht H, Shearen C, Degelau J, Guay DRP. Team approach to infection prevention and control in the nursing home setting. *Am. J. Infect Control.* 1999;27:64–70.

67. Garner JS, Jarvis WR, Emori TG, et al. CDC definitions for nosocomial infections. *Am J Infect Control.* 1988;16:128–140.

68. Sheretz RJ. Surveillance for infections associated with vascular catheters. *Infect Control Hosp Epidemiol.* 1996;17:746–752.

69. Yokoe DS, Anderson J, Chambers R, et al. Simplified surveillance for nosocomial bloodstream infections. *Infect Control Hosp Epidemiol.* 1998;19:657–660.

70. Intravenous Nurses Society. *The Intravenous Nursing Standards of Practice.* Cambridge, MA: Intravenous Nurses Society; 1998.

71. Richards C, Gaynes R, and the National Nosocomial Surveillance (NNIS) System. Improving nosocomial infection rates: institutional interventions needed for success [abstract]. *Am J Infect Control.* 1999;27:221.

72. Berlowitz DR, Halpern J. Evaluating and improving pressure ulcer care: the VA experience with administrative data. *Joint Comm J Qual Improv.* 1997;23:424–433.

73. Panel for the Prediction and Prevention of Pressure Ulcers in Adults. *Pressure Ulcers in Adults: Prediction and Prevention.* Clinical Practice Guideline, Number 3, AHCPR Publication No. 92–0047. Rockville, MD: AHCPR; 1992.

74. Gottsch JD. Surveillance and control of epidemic keratoconjunctivitis. *Trans Amer Ophthalmology Soc.* 1996;94:539–587.

75. Maryland Department of Health and Mental Hygiene (DHMH). *Guidelines for the Prevention and Control of Upper and Lower Acute Respiratory Illness (Including Influenza and Pneumonia) in Long Term Care Facilities.* 1997. Baltimore, MD: Maryland DHMH, Epidemiology and Disease Control Program; 1997. [Reprinted in Appendix H.]

76. Patel N, Tignor GH. Device-specific sharps injury and usage rates: an analysis by hospital department. *Am J Infect Control.* 1997;25:77–84.

77. Centers for Disease Control. Prevention and control of tuberculosis in facilities providing long-term care to the elderly: recommendations of the Advisory Committee for the Elimination of Tuberculosis. *MMWR.* 1990;39(RR-10).

78. Wenzel RP, Reagan DR, Bertino JS Jr, Baron EJ, Arias K. Methicillin-resistant *Staphylococcus aureus* outbreak: a consensus panel's definition and management guidelines. *Am J Infect Control.* 1998;26:102–110.

79. Pittet D, Safran E, Harbarth S, et al. Automatic alerts for methicillin-resistant *Staphylococcus aureus* surveillance and control: role of a hospital information system. *Infect Control Hosp Epidemiol.* 1996;17:496–502.

80. Kirkland T, Taylor G. Respiratory syncytial virus surveillance in an acute tertiary care facility [abstract]. *Am J Infect Control.* 1999;27:221.

81. Agnes K, Tan A, Chacko A, Roghmann M. Use of electronic surveillance for *C. difficile* infections [abstract]. *Am J Infect Control.* 1999;27:220.

82. Mitchell A, Jones N. Striving to prevent falls in an acute care setting—action to enhance quality. *J Clin Nurs.* 1996;5:213–220.

83. Welton JM, Jarr S. Automating and improving the data quality of a nursing department quality management program at a university hospital. *Joint Comm J Qual Improv.* 1997;23:623–635.

84. Lesar TS, Briceland L, Stein DS. Factors related to errors in medication prescribing. *JAMA.* 1997;277:312–317.

85. Mohseni IE, Wong DH. Medication errors analysis is an opportunity to improve practice. *Am J Surg.* 1998;175:4–9.

86. Centers for Disease Control and Prevention. Summary of notifiable diseases, United States, 1996. *MMWR.* 1997;45(53):1–83.

87. Centers for Disease Control and Prevention. Prevention and control of influenza: recommendations of the Advisory Committee on Immunization Practices (ACIP). *MMWR.* 1999;48(RR-04):1–28.

88. Garner JS, and the Hospital Infection Control Practices Advisory Committee. Guideline for isolation precautions in hospitals. *Am J Infect Control.* 1996;24:24–52.

89. Rutala WA, and the APIC Guidelines Committee. APIC guideline for selection and use of disinfectants. *Am J Infect Control.* 1996;24:313–342.

90. Association of Operating Room Nurses. *1999 Standards and Recommended Practices.* Denver, CO: Association of Operating Room Nurses, Inc; 1999.

91. Association for the Advancement of Medical Instrumentation. *Sterilization, Part 1: Sterilization in Health Care Facilities.* Arlington, VA: Association for the Advancement of Medical Instrumentation; 1998.

92. Doebbling BN, Ferguson KJ, Kohout FJ. Predictors of hepatitis B vaccine acceptance in health care workers. *Med Care.* 1996;34:58–72.

93. Larson E, Kretzer EK. Compliance with handwashing and barrier precautions. *J Hosp Infect.* 1995;30(Suppl):88–106.

94. Centers for Disease Control and Prevention. Handwashing and glove use in a long-term care facility—Maryland, 1992. *MMWR.* 1993;42:672–675.

95. McGeer A, Campbell B, Emori TG, et al. Definitions of infection for surveillance in long-term care facilities. *Am J Infect Control.* 1991;19:1–7.

96. Goldmann D. Contemporary challenges for hospital epidemiology. *Am J Med.* 1991;91(Suppl 3B):8S–15S.

97. Reagan DR. Microcomputers in hospital epidemiology. *Infect Control Hosp Epidemiol.* 1997;18:440–448.

98. Smyth ET, McIlvenny G, Barr JG, Dickson LM, Thompson IM. Automated entry of hospital infection surveillance data. *Infect Control Hosp Epidemiol.* 1997;18:486–491.

99. Carr JR, Fitzpatrick P, Izzo JL, et al. Changing the infection control paradigm from off-line to real time: the experience at Millard Fillmore Health System. *Infect Control Hosp Epidemiol.* 1997;18:255–259.

100. Victora CG. What's the denominator? *Lancet.* 1993;342:97–99.

101. Haley RW, Culver DH, Morgan WM, White JW, Emori TG, Hooton TM. Identifying patients at high risk of surgical wound infection: a simple multivariate index of patient susceptibility and wound contamination. *Am J Epidemiol.* 1985;121:206–215.

102. Haley RW. Nosocomial infections in surgical patients: developing valid measures of intrinsic patient risk. *Am J Med.* 1991;91(Suppl 3B):145S–151S.

103. Culver DH, Horan TC, Gaynes RP, et al. Surgical wound infection rates by wound class, operative procedure, and patient risk index. *Am J Med.* 1991;91(Suppl 3B):152S–157S.

104. Gross PA. Basics of stratifying for severity of illness. *Infect Control Hosp Epidemiol.* 1996;17:675–686.

105. Bailit JL, Dooley SL, Peaceman AN. Risk adjustment for interhospital comparison of primary cesarean rates. *Obstet Gynecol.* 1999;93:1025–1030.

106. Zinn JS, Aaronson WE, Rosko MD. The use of standardized indicators as quality improvement tools: an application in Pennsylvania nursing homes. *Am J Med Qual.* 1993;8:72–78.

107. Simonds DN, Horan TC, Kelley R, Jarvis WR. Detecting pediatric nosocomial infections: how do infection control and quality assurance personnel compare? *Am J Infect Control.* 1997;25:202–208.

108. Larson E, Horan T, Cooper B, et al. Study of the definition of nosocomial infections (SDNI). *Am J Infect Control.* 1991;19:259–267.

109. Haley RW, Schaberg DR, McClish DK, et al. The accuracy of retrospective chart review in measuring nosocomial infection rates. *Am J Epidemiol.* 1980;111:516–533.

110. Scheckler WE, Brimhall D, Buck AS, et al. Requirements for infrastructure and essential activities of infection control and epidemiology in hospitals: a consensus panel report. *Am J Infect Control.* 1998;26:47–60.

111. National Nosocomial Infection Surveillance System. Nosocomial infection rates for interhospital comparison: limitations and possible solutions. *Infect Control Hosp Epidemiol.* 1991;12:609–621.

112. The Quality Indicator Study Group. An approach to the evaluation of quality indicators of outcome of care in hospitalized patients, with a focus on nosocomial infection indicators. *Infect Control Hosp Epidemiol.* 1995;16:308–316.

113. Keita-Perse O, Gaynes RP. Severity of illness scoring systems to adjust nosocomial infection rates: a review and commentary. *Am J Infect Control.* 1996;24:429–434.

114. Stevenson KB. Regional data set of infection rates for long-term care facilities: description of a valuable benchmarking tool. *Am J Infect Control.* 1999;27:20–26.

115. Cleves MA, Weiner JP, Cohen W, et al. Assessing HCFA's Health Care Quality Improvement Program. *Joint Comm J Qual Improv.* 1997;23:550–560.

116. Hofer TP, Bernstein SJ, Hayward RA, DeMonner S. Validating quality indicators for hospital care. *Joint Comm J Qual Improv.* 1997;23:455–467.

117. Phillips CD, Zimmerman D, Bernabei R, Jonsson PV. Using the Resident Assessment Instrument for quality enhancement in nursing homes. *Age Ageing.* 1997;26(Suppl 2):77–81.

118. Morris JN, Hawes C, Fries BE, et al. Designing the national resident assessment instrument for nursing homes. *Gerontologist.* 1990;30:293–307.

119. Lovett LL, Massanari MM. Role of surveillance in emerging health systems: measurement is essential but not sufficient. *Am J Infect Control.* 1999;27:135–140.

120. Bobinski MA. Legal issues in hospital epidemiology and infection control. In: Mayhall CG, ed. *Hospital Epidemiology and Infection Control.* Baltimore: Williams & Wilkins; 1996:1138–1145.

121. Occupational Safety and Health Administration. Directive—CPL 2.106—Enforcement Procedures and Scheduling for Occupational Exposure to Tuberculosis. U.S. Department of Labor, Occupational Safety and Health Administration; 1996. [Can be downloaded from the OSHA Web site at http://www.osha.gov.]

122. Department of Labor, Occupational Safety and Health Administration. Occupational exposure to bloodborne pathogens: final rule. *Federal Register.* December 6, 1991;56(235):64004–64182.

123. US Dept of Health and Human Services, Health Care Financing Administration. Medicare and Medicaid requirements for long term care. *Federal Register.* September 26, 1991;56:48826–48879.

124. The Joint Commission on Accreditation of Healthcare Organizations. Surveillance, prevention, and control of infection. In: *Comprehensive Accreditation Manual for Hospitals.* Chicago, IL: Joint Commission on Accreditation of Healthcare Organizations; 1999.

125. The Joint Commission on Accreditation of Healthcare Organizations. Surveillance, prevention, and control of infection. In: *1998–1999 Comprehensive Accreditation Manual for Long Term Care.* Chicago, IL: Joint Commission on Accreditation of Healthcare Organizations; 1999:609–629.

126. The Joint Commission on Accreditation of Healthcare Organizations. Surveillance, prevention, and control of infection. In: *1998–1999 Comprehensive Accreditation Manual for Ambulatory Care.* Chicago, IL: Joint Commission on Accreditation of Healthcare Organizations; 1999:501–518.

127. CARF . . . The Rehabilitation Commission. *1999 Medical Rehabilitation Standards Manual.* Tucson, AZ: CARF . . . The Rehabilitation Commission; 1999:1.L-31—1.L-41.

SUGGESTED READING

Bennett JV, Brachman PS, eds. *Hospital Infections*. 4th ed. Boston: Little, Brown; 1998.

CDC. Public health focus: surveillance, prevention, and control of nosocomial infections. *MMWR*. 1992;41:783–787.

Haley RW, Culver DH, White JW, et al. The efficacy of infection surveillance and control programs in preventing nosocomial infections in U.S. hospitals. *Am J Epidemiol*. 1985;121:182–205.

Lee TB, Baker OG, Lee JT, et al. Recommended practices for surveillance. *Am J Infect Control*. 1998;26:277–288.

Massanari RM, Wilkerson K, Swartzendruber S. Designing surveillance for noninfectious outcomes of medical care. *Infect Control Hosp Epidemiol*. 1995;16:419–426.

Mayhall CG, ed. *Hospital Epidemiology and Infection Control*. 2nd ed. Baltimore: Williams & Wilkins; 1999.

Olmsted R, ed. *APIC Infection Control and Applied Epidemiology: Principles and Practice*. St. Louis: Mosby; 1996.

Roy MC, Perl TM. Basics of surgical-site infection surveillance. *Infect Control Hosp Epidemiol*. 1997;18:659–668.

Smith PW, ed. *Infection Control in Long-Term Care Facilities*. 2nd ed. Albany, NY: Delmar Publishers, Inc; 1994.

Smith P, Rusnack P. Infection prevention and control in the long-term-care facility. *Am J Infect Control*. 1997;25:488–512.

Wenzel RP, ed. *Prevention and Control of Nosocomial Infections*. 3rd ed. Baltimore: Williams & Wilkins; 1997.

CHAPTER 3

Outbreaks Reported in Acute Care Facilities

Kathleen Meehan Arias

An ounce of prevention is worth a pound of cure.
—Anonymous

INTRODUCTION

Outbreaks of infectious diseases in hospitals have long been recognized. A study of the nosocomial transmission of epidemic louse-borne typhus fever was published in England in 1864[1] and "hospital fever" is one of the many names given to this disease. In the mid-1800s, Ignaz Semmelweis recommended hand washing to prevent the spread of puerperal fever, and Florence Nightingale promoted isolation of infected patients, a clean environment, and hygienic handling of food and water to prevent the spread of disease. Despite the advances of modern medicine, outbreaks continue to occur as a result of health care provided in a variety of settings.[2–9] The hospital outbreaks of typhus and puerperal fevers that occurred in the 1800s have been replaced in the late 1900s by outbreaks of methicillin-resistant *Staphylococcus aureus* (MRSA) and vancomycin-resistant *Enterococcus* (VRE). However, the primary control measures used to prevent the spread of infectious agents remain the same: hand washing, isolation of infected persons, environmental cleanliness, and safe handling of food and water.

Personnel responsible for managing infection control and quality management programs in health care facilities should study reports of outbreak investigations to expand their knowledge of the epidemiology of nosocomial infections and other iatrogenic events. By reviewing the findings of these investigations, it is possible to identify

- factors contributing to outbreaks (e.g., agents, common sources and reservoirs, and modes of transmission; devices, products, and other vehicles; procedures, practices, and technical errors)
- measures for controlling or preventing a similar outbreak

If an outbreak is suspected in a health care facility, a literature search should be conducted to identify relevant articles, as discussed in Chapter 9.

The purpose of this chapter is to identify outbreaks that have been reported in acute care facilities. It is not intended to be an exhaustive review of outbreaks that have occurred in hospitals. Rather, its purpose is to provide an overview of the wide variety of organisms, diseases, and conditions that have been responsible for epidemics in the acute care setting. Information on the agents, reservoirs, and modes of transmission is included, along with the control measures that were used to interrupt the outbreak. The reports discussed in this chapter were identified by performing electronic literature searches of the MEDLINE and CINHAL databases, by reviewing the tables of contents of selected journals and the references in the bibliographies of relevant articles, and by accessing information through the Centers for Disease Control and Prevention's (CDC—formerly Centers for Disease Control until October 27, 1992, Center for Disease Control between 1970 and 1980, and Communicable Disease Center from 1946 to 1970) home page via the Internet. The reports of these investigations highlight the importance of maintaining an active surveillance program in all health care settings in order to identify an outbreak or a cluster of events.

Most of the outbreaks discussed in this text have been grouped into the settings in which they occurred. But personnel responsible for managing infection control and quality management programs should be familiar with outbreaks that have been reported in all types of health care settings because procedures, practices, products, and devices may be used in more than one setting. The organisms discussed in this chapter are associated with outbreaks that are generally reported in acute care facilities, although transmission may occur in other settings. Organisms such as methicillin-resistant *S aureus*, vancomycin-resistant *Enterococcus*, *Mycobacterium tuberculosis*, *Sarcoptes scabiei*, and *Clostridium difficile*, which have been reported to cause outbreaks in both acute care and long-term care facilities, are discussed in Chapter 7. Although the terms "outbreak" and "epidemic" are most commonly used in reference to infectious diseases, they are also used to describe the sudden occurrence or increase of noninfectious diseases and conditions; therefore, examples of outbreaks caused by noninfectious agents are also included.

ENDEMIC VERSUS EPIDEMIC INFECTIONS

Most hospital-acquired infections are endemic and are generally considered endogenous in origin.[2] Because the majority of these infections originate from the patient's own flora, only a third are believed to be preventable.[10] Only a small proportion of nosocomial infections occur as part of an epidemic. Results of one study showed that patients involved in epidemics accounted for 3.7 percent of all nosocomial infections detected over a 5-year period.[11] In another study it was estimated that true outbreaks involved approximately 2 percent of all patients who contracted a nosocomial infection.[3] Among infections reported to the National Nosocomial Infections Surveillance system, approximately 5 percent occurred in epidemics.[5] Although these numbers are small, they are important because these infections (1) result in significant morbidity and mortality, (2) may cause disruption of services, (3) may be costly to investigate and control, and (4) are potentially preventable.

The organisms responsible for causing the majority of endemic and epidemic infections in hospitals change over time. In the 1950s and 1960s, a pandemic of *S aureus* caused major outbreaks in communities and hospitals. In the 1970s, gram-negative organisms, such as the Enterobacteriaceae and *Pseudomonas aerugi-*

nosa, emerged as major nosocomial pathogens. Throughout the 1980s, methicillin-resistant *S aureus* became established in many hospitals, and in the late 1980s and early 1990s multidrug-resistant *Mycobacterium tuberculosis* (MDR-TB) caused multiple outbreaks in health care facilities, affecting both patients and personnel. A major concern in the 1990s has been the nosocomial spread of antibiotic-resistant organisms such as MDR-TB and VRE and the anticipated emergence of vancomycin-resistant *S aureus*.

Infection control personnel and health care providers need to be aware of both newly recognized infectious agents and reemerging pathogens that have the potential for causing endemic and epidemic nosocomial infections[12–15] such as those listed in Table 3–1.

ORGANISMS RESPONSIBLE FOR HOSPITAL-ASSOCIATED OUTBREAKS

Organisms that have frequently been associated with outbreaks in the acute care setting include *Enterococcus*, *Pseudomonas*, *Serratia*, *Enterobacter*, *Salmonella*, *Mycobacterium*, and *Candida* species; *S aureus*; and group A streptococcus. When the site of infection and the organism causing a suspected outbreak is known, it is possible to use the knowledge gained from published reports of outbreaks to develop hypotheses on the likely modes of transmission and potential sources and reservoirs.

There are four major modes of transmission of microorganisms that are commonly involved in nosocomial outbreaks: contact, vehicle (common source), droplet spread, and airborne. Outbreaks caused by *S aureus* are associated with human reservoirs because this organism is transmitted directly by person-to-person contact, indirectly from patient to patient on the hands of personnel, or by a human disseminator, such as a nasal carrier. Organisms such as *Pseudomonas*, *Flavobacterium*, *Mycobacterium gordonae* and *chelonae*, and gram-negative bacteria such as *Klebsiella*, *Enterobacter*, and *Serratia* readily grow in fluids and are frequently associated with common source outbreaks involving contaminated solutions. *Aspergillus* and *Legionella* are spread by airborne transmission. Epidemics caused by these two organisms usually involve environmental sources, such as cooling towers or contaminated potable water for *Legionella,* and construction or some disruption in the physical plant for *Aspergillus.* Many organisms have more than one mode of transmis-

Table 3–1 Emerging Infectious Diseases with a Significant Link to the Hospital Setting, 1976 to 1996

Disease/Agent	Hospital Link
Legionnaires' disease	Repeated outbreaks in the hospital setting since its recognition in 1976.
Ebola virus	Each of the major African outbreaks (Zaire 1976, Sudan 1976, Sudan 1979, Zaire 1995) have been propagated in the hospital setting and have affected health care workers.
Clostridium difficile	Predominantly a complication of hospital care and frequently disseminated in the hospital environment. First recognized as the cause of pseudomembranous colitis in 1977.
HIV/AIDS*	Transmission to health care workers was reported shortly after the disease was recognized in 1981 and produced a revolution in infection control approaches, leading to universal precautions.
Toxic shock syndrome	Detected when unusual disease manifestations were recognized in hospitalized women.
Escherichia coli O157:H7	Since its recognition in 1982, many major outbreaks have been detected due to clusters of patients hospitalized with hemolytic-uremic syndrome, the major complication of this infection; rare transmission to health care workers also has been documented.
Hepatitis C	A transfusion-associated and bloodborne agent that has been tied closely to the hospital setting and has produced nosocomial outbreaks.
Hantavirus pulmonary syndrome (Sin Nombre virus)	First recognized in 1993, when unusual illnesses and deaths were detected among previously healthy persons with unexplained adult respiratory distress syndrome.
Variant Creutzfeldt-Jakob disease	Hospital-based surveillance in Britain for Creutzfeldt-Jakob disease led to the recognition of a variant form of illness possibly linked to bovine spongiform encephalopathy.
Methicillin-resistant *Staphylococcus aureus*	The most common nosocomial pathogen. Acquires resistance to methicillin and rapidly spreads from hospital to hospital; is more frequent in the intensive care setting, where antimicrobial use is high.
Vancomycin-resistant *Enterococcus*	A less common nosocomial pathogen; has acquired resistance to the last antimicrobial widely available to treat it.
Nosocomial gram-negative rods	Increasing acquisition of resistance among an array of gram-negative rods such as *Pseudomonas, Klebsiella, Enterobacter, and Serratia* species.
Multidrug-resistant tuberculosis	Beginning in 1989, a series of outbreaks of multidrug-resistant tuberculosis occurred in the hospital setting, mostly involving HIV-infected patients, but also spreading to health care workers.

*HIV = human immunodeficiency virus; AIDS = acquired immune deficiency syndrome.

Source: Reprinted with permission from S.M. Ostroff, Emerging Infectious Diseases in the Institutional Setting: Another Hot Zone, *Infection Control and Hospital Epidemiology,* Vol. 17, No. 8, p. 486, © 1996, SLACK Incorporated.

---

sion[16–19] and may have several potential sources or reservoirs in the health care setting, as shown in Table 3–2.

OUTBREAKS ASSOCIATED WITH PRODUCTS, DEVICES, AND PROCEDURES (COMMON SOURCE OUTBREAKS)

Since some products, devices, and procedures are repeatedly associated with hospital epidemics, it is useful to study published reports of these outbreaks so that preventive measures can be identified and implemented. The Hospital Infections Program of the Centers for Disease Control and Prevention conducted investigations of 125

nosocomial outbreaks occurring from January 1980 to July 1990 and reported the following.[4]

1. Products, procedures, or devices were involved in 46 percent of the outbreaks: 22 percent were product related, 13 percent were procedure related, and 11 percent were device related.
2. Bacterial pathogens caused 62 percent of the outbreaks, fungi caused 9 percent, viruses caused 8 percent, mycobacteria caused 4 percent, and toxins or other organisms caused 18 percent.
3. The proportion of outbreaks caused by products, devices, and procedures increased from 47 per-

Table 3–2 Organisms Associated with Outbreaks in the Health Care Setting, Their Likely Modes of Transmission, and Potential Sources

Organism	Site of Infection	Likely Mode(s) of Transmission	Potential Sources/Reservoirs
Clostridium difficile	Gastrointestinal	Contact; cross-infection via hands	Infected patients
		Vehicle/common source	Contaminated equipment
Enterococcus species	Genitourinary, surgical wound	Contact; cross-infection via hands	Infected or colonized patients
		Vehicle/common source	Contaminated equipment
Group A streptococcus	Surgical wound	Contact	Infected personnel
	Pharyngeal	Vehicle/common source	Food contaminated by infected personnel
Hepatitis A	Liver	Vehicle/common source	Food contaminated by infected personnel
		Contact; cross-infection via hands	Infected patients and personnel
Influenza	Respiratory	Droplet	Infected patients or personnel
Legionella	Respiratory	Airborne	Contaminated water
Mycobacterium species, not tuberculosis	Respiratory	Vehicle/common source	Contaminated bronchoscope
Mycobacterium tuberculosis	Respiratory	Airborne	Infected patients or personnel
		Vehicle/common source	Contaminated bronchoscope
Pseudomonas species	Blood, respiratory	Vehicle/common source	Contaminated fluids, devices, and equipment
		Contact; cross-infection via hands	Infected and colonized patients
Salmonella species	Gastrointestinal	Vehicle/common source	Food contaminated by improper handling or by personnel carrier
		Contact; cross-infection via hands	Infected patients
Staphylococcus aureus	Surgical wound	Contact	Personnel carrier
	Skin, respiratory, blood	Contact; cross-infection via hands	Infected and colonized patients
	Gastrointestinal	Vehicle/common source	Food contaminated by infected personnel

cent in the first half of the decade to 67 percent between 1986 and July 1990.

Outbreaks Associated with Products

Multiple outbreaks of infections, illnesses, or adverse reactions associated with the use of products have been reported.[20–59] Many of these outbreaks involved products that were intrinsically or extrinsically contaminated by microbial agents or their toxins; however, several outbreaks did not have an infectious etiology. Infection control personnel in all health care set-tings should be familiar with the types of products associated with epidemics because these products may be used not only in acute care facilities, but also in the long-term care and ambulatory care settings.[30,32,33,58,60]

Intrinsic Contamination of Products

As used here, the term intrinsic refers to contamination that occurs before a product's arrival at a health care facility, such as a product contaminated during manufacture. These products may cause widespread outbreaks in multiple facilities before they are recognized.[22,54] A variety of intrinsically contaminated products have been associated with outbreaks: intravenous fluid, povidone-iodine solution, packed red blood cells, fresh-frozen plasma, polygeline plasma extender, human albumin, mouthwash, saline solution, and peritoneal dialysis fluid, as shown in Table 3–3.

Hospital personnel should notify the manufacturer, the local health department, and the appropriate government agency (e.g., in the case of antiseptics or drugs, the Food and Drug Administration [FDA] Medical Products Reporting Program at 800-332-1088) if a product that is associated with a cluster of infections is believed to be intrinsically contaminated. In addition, health care providers using the item should be notified of the suspected contamination and should be instructed to remove all of the implicated product from stock and save it for further study. Although health care facilities may not be able to prevent infections associated with an intrinsically contaminated product, infection control personnel should be alert to clusters or increasing numbers of isolates of unusual organisms, as these may possibly be associated with intrinsically or extrinsically contaminated products. Active surveillance programs are necessary to recognize promptly any product-associated outbreaks so that measures can be taken to identify the implicated product and to prevent its continued use.[22]

Extrinsic Contamination of Products

Extrinsic contamination occurs during the use of a product. Extrinsically contaminated products associated with outbreaks include antimicrobial soap, antiseptics and disinfectant solutions, saline solution, gauze dressings, gentian violet and other dyes, albuterol, infant formula, and dextrose solution (Table 3–4). Some products, such as benzalkonium chloride solution, have been associated with multiple outbreaks and are no longer recommended for use in the health care setting because of the ease with which they can become contaminated.[60–64] In 1976 the Center for Disease Control recommended the elimination of benzalkonium chloride solution as an antiseptic; however, a study reported in 1991 that many health care facilities were still using this product.[64] Personnel who are using benzalkonium chloride for skin antisepsis should be instructed to use an alternative product.[65] Other products, such as the anesthetic agent propofol, have been associated with multiple outbreaks but are still widely used.[37–39] Health care personnel who use propofol should be made aware of the hazards associated with it

and should be instructed to adhere to the manufacturer's instructions for preventing contamination.

Since many types of solutions have the potential to become contaminated during use, health care personnel should be educated on the proper handling of fluids and the use of aseptic technique. Even hand care products, such as lotions[66–68] and plain and antimicrobial soap,[52,69] can become contaminated during use and can serve as reservoirs for infectious agents.

Noninfectious Adverse Events Related to Products

Clinicians also need to maintain surveillance for noninfectious adverse reactions due to therapeutic agents. Products that have resulted in clusters of illness, deaths, and injury in hospitals include disinfectants, intravenous additives, and infectious waste containers (Table 3–5). Health care providers should notify the facility's pharmacy, the manufacturer, and the Food and Drug Administration (FDA MedWatch at 800-332-1088) if a therapeutic agent is associated with a cluster of adverse reactions.

Outbreaks Associated with Devices

Devices used for therapeutic and diagnostic procedures have long been associated with epidemics in the acute care and ambulatory care areas.[70–93] As invasive devices are used more frequently, especially in the intensive care setting, the risk of infection and of epidemics increases. Outbreaks have been traced to contaminated endoscopes used for endoscopic retrograde cholangiopancreatography (ERCP)[70–72] and upper gastrointestinal procedures,[70,72–76] bronchoscopes,[70,77–81] automated endoscope washers,[72,76,79,80] respiratory therapy equipment,[82,83] hemodynamic monitoring systems,[84–87] jet gun injectors,[88] reusable fingerstick blood-sampling devices,[89,90] urologic apparatus,[91,92] electronic thermometers,[93] and hemodialysis equipment.[94] In addition, adverse reactions in patients have resulted from residual gluteraldehyde on devices that were not thoroughly rinsed after soaking in a gluteraldehyde solution.[95,96]

Table 3–6 lists selected device-related outbreaks and the infection control and technical errors associated with their occurrence. The major reasons for these epidemics were (1) improper cleaning and disinfection procedures, (2) contamination of endoscopes by automatic washers/disinfectors, and (3) improper handling of sterile equipment.

Table 3–3 Outbreaks Involving Intrinsically Contaminated Products

Outbreak	Year(s) Reported (Reference No.)	Product	Comments
Enterobacter cloacae and *Enterobacter agglomerans* septicemia	1976[20,21] 1978[22]	Intravenous fluid	1971—nationwide outbreak of septicemia (reference 21 is reprint of original report with a discussion of the outbreak)
Pseudomonas (currently *Burkholderia*) *cepacia* peritonitis and pseudobacteremia	1981[25] 1992[26]	Povidone-iodine	1981—first report of nosocomial infections caused by intrinsically contaminated povidone-iodine
Pseudomonas aeruginosa peritonitis and wound infection	1982[30]	Poloxamer-iodine solution	Outbreak in outpatients on chronic peritoneal dialysis
Yersinia enterocolitica bacteremia, endotoxin shock, and deaths	1988[34] 1997[35]	Packed red blood cells	Not true outbreak as cases occurred sporadically—donors likely bacteremic when they donated blood (however, transfused blood products should be considered as potential sources when patients develop sepsis of unknown etiology shortly after transfusion)
Hepatitis A in a neonatal intensive care unit	1990[36]	Fresh-frozen plasma	Outbreak in 9 nurses, 1 infant, and infant's mother (the index case was the infant who became infected from a transfusion of fresh-frozen plasma)
Hepatitis C	1994[41]	Intravenous immuno-globulin	Worldwide outbreak; first recognized outbreak of bloodborne pathogens associated with immune globulin product licensed in the United States
Fever and hypotension after cardiac surgery	1995[44]	Polygeline plasma extender	Product intrinsically contaminated by cell wall products of *Bacillus stearothermophilus*
Primary cutaneous aspergillosis	1996[47]	Contaminated gauze (one case prompted an investigation)	Evidence of water exposure in gauze (contamination probably occurred prior to arrival at hospital)
Cutaneous lesions caused by *Paecilomyces lilacinus*	1996[48]	Skin lotion	Lesions in immunocompromised patients (2 patients died; product recalled)
Enterobacter cloacae bacteremia	1997[50]	Human albumin	Intrinsic contamination resulted in worldwide recall of Albuminar
Burkholderia (currently *Ralstonia*) *pickettii* bacteremia	1997[53]	Saline solution	Saline used to flush indwelling intravascular devices
Sterile peritonitis following continuous cycling peritoneal dialysis	1997[54]	Peritoneal dialysis fluid	Nationwide outbreak resulted in recall of product; contaminated by endotoxin
Ralstonia pickettii respiratory tract colonization	1998[56]	0.9% saline solution used for respiratory therapy	*R pickettii* isolated from several products marketed as sterile
Endotoxin-like reactions	1998[57]	Intravenous gentamicin	Reactions associated with once-daily dosing of gentamicin received from one manufacturer
Enterobacter cloacae bloodstream infections	1998[58]	Prefilled saline syringes	Outbreak in outpatient hematology/oncology service at a hospital
Burkholderia cepacia respiratory tract infection and colonization in an intensive care unit	1998[59]	Alcohol-free mouthwash	Product used for routine oral care of ventilated patients

Table 3–4 Outbreaks Involving Extrinsically Contaminated Products

Outbreak	Year(s) Reported (Reference No.)	Product	Comments (Reason for Extrinsic Contamination, When Applicable)
Pseudobacteremia due to *Pseudomonas* (currently *Burkholderia*) *cepacia* and/ or *Enterobacter* species	1976[23]	Contaminated benzalkonium chloride antiseptic	Antiseptic used to prepare skin prior to venipuncture (several patients may have become bacteremic)
Endotoxemia following computerized axial tomography	1980[27]	Possible contamination of radiopaque contrast medium and glucagon	Source not determined but contaminated hot water bath had been used to warm contrast medium prior to infusion
Serratia marcescens bacteremia	1981[28]	Heparinized saline irrigation fluid likely	Saline possibly contaminated when first mixed
Cutaneous aspergillosis	1981[29]	Outside packaging of dressing supplies	Outside of packages contaminated by spores and dust during construction in central inventory supply area
Mycobacterium chelonae surgical wound infections	1987[32]	Gentian violet skin-marking solution	Gentian violet—used to mark incision site prior to plastic surgery in a surgeon's office—contaminated with *M chelonae*
Serratia marcescens septic arthritis	1987[33]	Benzalkonium chloride antiseptic solution	Patients who had received injections of methylprednisolone in orthopaedic surgeons' office (likely reservoir was canister of cotton balls soaking in benzalkonium chloride solution; *S marcescens* was isolated from canister and used multidose vials)
Postoperative febrile episodes, and bloodstream and surgical site infections	1990[37] 1995[38] 1997[39]	Propofol	Multiple outbreaks resulting from lack of aseptic technique (this lipid-based medication is easily contaminated)
Pseudomonas (currently *Ralstonia*) *pickettii* bacteremia	1991[40]	Fentanyl citrate	Narcotic theft by employee who replaced fentanyl with contaminated distilled water
Burkholderia cepacia respiratory tract infection and colonization in mechanically ventilated patients	1995[42] 1996[43]	Albuterol multidose vial	Lack of aseptic technique by respiratory therapy and intensive care unit personnel (respiratory therapy personnel carried multidose vials in their pockets)
Pseudomonas aeruginosa ventilator-associated respiratory tract infections and colonization	1995[45]	Food coloring dye added to nasogastric tube feedings	*P aeruginosa* isolated from 32-oz bottles of food coloring dye; multiple-use bottles were replaced by single-use vials
Gram-negative rod colonization and infection in a neonatal intensive care unit	1997[49]	Infant formula	Formula contaminated during preparation; contamination associated with use of blender
Neonatal infection and colonization with *Serratia marcescens*	1997[52]	1% chloroxylenol antiseptic hand soap	Nursing staff used personal bottles of soap, which became contaminated during use
Burkholderia cepacia septicemia in cardiac patients	1998[55]	5% dextrose solution used to dilute heparin	One-liter bag of solution used to dilute heparin for multiple patients on cardiology ward

Table 3–5 Products Associated with Clusters of Noninfectious Adverse Events

Outbreak	Year(s) Reported (Reference No.)	Product	Comments
Neonatal hyperbilirubinemia	1978[24]	Phenolic disinfectant detergent	Infants exposed to a phenol solution used for disinfecting nursery surfaces
Cluster of unusual illness and deaths in neonates	1986[31]	Commercially available intravenous vitamin E preparation	Product newly marketed; precise constituents in E-ferol that caused illness and death unable to be determined
Increase in needlestick injuries in hospital employees	1995[46]	Fiberboard infectious waste containers	Product replaced in hospital and injuries occurred when needles pierced walls of new container
Illness and sudden deaths in adult patients	1997[51]	Commercially available amino acid additive used for peripheral parenteral nutrition (PPN)	Additive caused precipitate in the PPN

Measures used to prevent these types of outbreaks include

- careful attention to cleaning and disinfection protocols for endoscopes and bronchoscopes
- careful maintenance and quality control of automated endoscope washing and disinfection machines
- careful attention to cleaning and disinfection protocols for respiratory therapy equipment
- proper use and dilution of disinfectant solutions
- consistent use of disposable single-patient use equipment for hemodynamic monitoring and urodynamic testing
- strict adherence to sterile technique when handling sterile supplies
- correct use and cleaning of devices in accordance with manufacturers' instructions

Outbreaks Associated with Procedures

Many diagnostic and therapeutic procedures place a patient at risk for developing a nosocomial infection or other iatrogenic event, such as injury or allergic reaction. Most procedure-related infections are not associated with outbreaks and are usually thought to be a result of host factors such as impaired or disrupted host defenses, immunosuppression, colonization with hospital-acquired organisms, and underlying diseases. However, outbreaks have been associated with procedures such as gastrointestinal endoscopy,[70,72–76] bronchoscopy,[70,77–81] hemodialysis,[94,97–101] peritoneal dialysis,[24,102,103] and hemodynamic pressure monitoring.[84–87]

Gastrointestinal Endoscopy and Bronchoscopy Procedures

Despite the fact that numerous outbreaks related to gastrointestinal endoscopy and bronchoscopy procedures have been reported in both the inpatient and outpatient settings,[9,70, 104,105] many personnel in endoscopy suites do not follow appropriate protocols for reprocessing scopes.[106,107] Because endoscopes are complex instruments that are difficult to clean and disinfect, staff responsible for processing them must be instructed to follow meticulously the recommended guidelines, such as those developed by the American Society for Gastrointestinal Endoscopy (ASGE)[108,109] and the Association for Professionals in Infection Control and Epidemiology (APIC).[110] (Both of these organizations have World Wide Web sites: http://www.asge.org and http://www.apic.org, respectively.) Since outbreaks involving endoscopy and bronchoscopy procedures are generally traced to contaminated devices or solutions, several examples of these epidemics are noted in Table 3–6.

Hemodialysis and Peritoneal Dialysis

Nosocomial infections are well-recognized complications of hemodialysis.[97] Outbreaks in hemodialysis centers have occurred as a result of improper handling or inadequate cleaning and disinfection of reusable dialysers[98–100]; cross-contamination of blood tubing by

Table 3–6 Selected Device-Related Outbreaks and Associated Infection Control or Technical Errors

Outbreak	Year(s) Reported (Reference No.)	Device	Infection Control or Technical Error
Hepatitis B	1986[88]	Jet gun injector	Nozzle tip contaminated with blood; was not properly disinfected
Mycobacterium tuberculosis	1989[78]	Bronchoscope	Suction valve of bronchoscope not disinfected despite rigorous cleaning and disinfection
Pseudomonas aeruginosa infection and colonization after UGI* endoscopy	1991[72]	Upper GI endoscope	Flawed automatic disinfector
Bloody diarrhea associated with endoscopy	1992[95]	Endoscope	Residual gluteraldehyde in improperly rinsed endoscope
Proctitis following endorectal ultrasound examination	1993[96]	Endoscope	Residual gluteraldehyde in improperly rinsed endoscope
Pseudomonas aeruginosa and Enterobacteriaceae bacteremia after ERCP*	1993[71]	Endoscope	Flawed automatic disinfector
Pseudomonas cepacia respiratory tract colonization/infection and bacteremia	1993[82]	Reusable electronic ventilator probes	Improper disinfection solution used
Gram-negative bacteremia	1996[84]	Hemodynamic pressure-monitoring equipment	Pressure-monitoring equipment left uncovered overnight in the operating room
Hepatitis C	1997[75]	Colonoscope	Improper cleaning and disinfection of colonoscope
Multidrug-resistant *Mycobacterium tuberculosis*	1997[81]	Bronchoscope	Inadequate cleaning and disinfection of bronchoscope
Multidrug-resistant *Pseudomonas aeruginosa* urinary tract infection and urosepsis	1997[92]	Urodynamic transducer	Improperly processed transducer used for urodynamic testing
Hepatitis B in a hospital and a nursing home	1997[90]	Fingerstick blood-sampling devices	Disposable component of device became contaminated with blood and was not routinely changed between patients
Bloodstream infections caused by multiple pathogens	1998[94]	Hemodialysis equipment	Attachment used to drain spent priming saline became contaminated

*UGI = upper gastrointestinal; ERCP = endoscopic retrograde cholangiopancreatography.

ultrafiltrate waste[94]; sharing of staff, equipment, supplies, and medications between patients[101]; failure to isolate patients with chronic hepatitis B[101]; and failure to vaccinate susceptible hemodialysis patients against hepatitis B virus.[101] Guidelines to prevent transmission of infectious agents in the hemodialysis setting have been published by the CDC[111] and the Association for the Advancement of Medical Instrumentation.[112] Infection control recommendations for hemodialysis units can be found in Appendix G and can be downloaded from the CDC Web site at http://www.cdc.gov/ncidod/hip/dialysis/dialysis.htm.

Care must be taken to ensure that hemodialysis personnel are familiar with the proper use and disinfection of the equipment they are using. One outbreak of bloodstream infections occurred in two outpatient hemodialysis centers affiliated with a hospital; it was associated with a change in the setup of the hemodialysis system. The reservoir was a newly installed, commercially marketed attachment used to drain spent saline. The attachment became heavily contaminated with multiple gram-positive, gram-negative, and fungal pathogens and served as a portal of entry into the blood tubing.[94]

Outbreaks related to peritoneal dialysis have been associated with contaminated peritoneal dialysis machines[102,103] and the use of intrinsically contaminated povidone-iodine solution.[20] Personnel responsible for cleaning, disinfecting, and handling equipment used for peritoneal dialysis must practice strict aseptic technique and carefully follow manufacturers' directions for the specific equipment they are using.

Outbreaks Associated with Surgery

Most surgical site infections are caused by endogenous or exogenous organisms that are introduced into the wound at the time of surgery. However, outbreaks associated with surgical procedures may be caused either by contaminated antiseptics,[113] dressings,[114–116] equipment,[84] medications, or solutions,[32,117] or by organisms disseminated by a personnel carrier. These outbreaks are generally recognized when a cluster of surgical site infections caused by the same organism is detected. The type of organism causing the infections will often provide a clue to a source or reservoir. Outbreaks of postoperative infections caused by S aureus or group A streptococci are invariably associated with a human carrier. Outbreaks caused by gram-negative organisms and fungi are frequently associated with an environmental source.[84]

In addition to surgery-related outbreaks caused by infectious agents, clusters of adverse events associated with exposure to chemicals have also been reported in surgical patients. In one report, six patients who had cardiac surgery developed postoperative bleeding, which was caused by residual detergent in reprocessed laparotomy sponges.[118] In another, an outbreak of corneal edema following cataract surgery was thought to be caused by inadequate rinsing of small-lumen surgical instruments that had been disinfected by soaking in gluteraldehyde.[119]

OUTBREAKS ASSOCIATED WITH HUMAN CARRIERS OR DISSEMINATORS

Human disseminators have been responsible for hospital outbreaks of S aureus, Streptococcus pyogenes (group A beta-hemolytic streptococci), Candida species, hepatitis A, hepatitis B, hepatitis C, and Salmonella. Many organisms have more than one mode of transmission. Al-

though hospital outbreaks caused by S aureus, group A streptococcus, and hepatitis A are often associated with a human carrier, each of these organisms can be spread either by direct person-to-person contact or by food that is contaminated by a carrier. Hepatitis B may be transmitted from person to person directly by a carrier or indirectly via contaminated medications or equipment. Salmonella may be transmitted directly from person to person or via contaminated food.

Staphylococcus aureus

Although cross-infection on the hands of personnel is thought to be the primary mode of transmission of S aureus in health care facilities, some outbreaks have been associated with colonized or infected health care workers. Health care workers commonly carry S aureus in their nares and on their hands.[120] Outbreaks of surgical site infections caused by S aureus have been associated with personnel carrying the organism on their skin and hair[121] and in their nares.[122] Staphylococcal outbreaks in nurseries[123] and intensive care units (ICU)[124] have also been associated with personnel carriers.

Outbreaks caused by methicillin-resistant S aureus are discussed in Chapter 7. Since the control measures for preventing the transmission of MRSA are essentially the same as those for methicillin-sensitive S aureus, the reader is referred to Chapter 7 for a review of control measures used to interrupt staphylococcal outbreaks.

S aureus was the second most frequently identified bacterial agent causing foodborne outbreaks in the United States, as reported to the CDC between 1975 and 1992.[125] Dietary personnel who have a staphylococcal infection may contaminate food and be the source of a foodborne outbreak. Hospital personnel who have boils or skin lesions known or suspected to be infected with S aureus—especially on the hands—should be restricted from patient care activities and from food handling until they have been treated and their infection has resolved. If investigators suspect a common source outbreak (i.e., a personnel carrier), they should examine personnel for evidence of skin breakdown or infection.

Group A Beta-Hemolytic Streptococcus

Group A beta-hemolytic streptococcus (GAS) can spread rapidly from person to person and can cause serious disease in the health care setting.[126] Numerous outbreaks of nosocomial group A streptococci have been reported.[126–138] More than 50 nosocomial outbreaks of GAS were reported between 1966 and 1995.[126] Historically, nosocomial outbreaks of group A beta-hemolytic streptococci have involved newborns,[134] postpartum women,[126–131] patients in burn units[126,133] and in geriatric units, postoperative surgical patients, and residents of long-term care facilities.[126,137] Outbreaks have also been reported in medical units[135] and in critical care units.[136] In addition to person-to-person spread, GAS may be transmitted by contaminated food. An outbreak of streptococcal pharyngitis in a hospital pediatric clinic was traced to food that had been contaminated by a health care worker who was a GAS carrier.[138]

Nosocomial outbreaks are frequently associated with colonized or infected health care personnel. The CDC[17] and Weber et al[126] have published guidelines to assist in managing personnel with pharyngitis or suspected GAS infection. Although nasopharyngeal carriers are thought to be particularly likely to transmit GAS, personnel implicated in group A streptococcal surgical wound infection outbreaks, as reported in the past two decades, have usually been found to carry the organism in their scalp,[127] vagina,[128,129] or anus.[130,131] In one report, an outbreak of group A streptococcal surgical site infections was associated with an asymptomatic anesthesiologist who was a pharyngeal carrier.[132] The outbreak resulted from the exposure of the anesthesiologist to his infected daughter. In several reported outbreaks, the source of infection or colonization in hospital personnel was a household contact.[126,127,129,132] It should be noted that health care workers either may serve as the index case or may become infected through contact with infected patients or other health care workers during the course of an outbreak. An important measure for preventing and interrupting GAS outbreaks is the recognition by personnel of signs and symptoms, such as pharyngitis, that are consistent with GAS infection.

Because nosocomial infections caused by group A beta-hemolytic streptococcus are relatively rare, the occurrence of one nosocomial GAS infection at any site should prompt a search for other cases to detect a potential outbreak. This search can be done by reviewing laboratory reports and by asking hospital surgeons if they are aware of any GAS postoperative surgical site infections.

Candida and *Nocardia* Species

Several outbreaks of postoperative surgical site infections caused by *Candida* species have been associated with personnel carriers. One outbreak of *Candida albicans* sternal wound infections following cardiac surgery was associated with a scrub nurse who had recurrent vaginal infections,[139] and an outbreak of *Candida tropicalis* sternal wound infections was also associated with a scrub nurse.[140]

Several clusters of surgical site infections caused by *Nocardia farcinica* have been reported.[141,142] In one, the source was not determined,[142] and in the other the source was determined to be a colonized anesthesiologist.[141]

Hepatitis B Virus

Clusters of hepatitis B infection have been traced to transmission from infected obstetricians, gynecologists, and surgeons to their patients during surgery.[143–146] Of the three most commonly recognized bloodborne pathogens—hepatitis B virus (HBV), hepatitis C virus (HCV), and human immunodeficiency virus (HIV)—HBV is the most easily transmitted from person to person because an infected person can carry more than a billion HBV particles per milliliter of blood.[101] Risk factors associated with transmission of HBV from health care worker to patient include the presence of hepatitis B e antigen in the health care worker's blood, the type of surgical procedure (such as vaginal hysterectomy, cardiac surgery, and major pelvic surgery), and the potential for injury of the health care worker (such as needlestick during suturing) during the invasive procedure.[143] Recommendations for preventing transmission of hepatitis B have been published by the CDC[146] and in a position paper by the AIDS/TB (Acquired Immunodeficiency Syndrome/Tuberculosis) Committee of the Society for Healthcare Epidemiology of America (SHEA).[143] Because barriers such as gloves may not prevent transmission of HBV from health care provider to patient, the SHEA position paper recommends that HBV-infected health care workers who are e antigen-positive routinely wear double gloves when caring for patients and that they avoid performing those procedures, such as vaginal hysterectomy and cardiac surgery, that have been epidemiologically linked to transmission of HBV from health care worker to patient.[143] The CDC recommendations for preventing transmission of HBV and HIV to patients during exposure-prone procedures[146] can be obtained by accessing the *Morbidity and Mortality Weekly Report* (MMWR) Recommendations and Reports section of the CDC Web site (http://www.cdc.gov).

Not all cases of nosocomial hepatitis B are associated with personnel carriers. Transmission of hepatitis B virus associated with contaminated equipment and medications in hemodialysis units has long been recognized and is generally due to poor infection control techniques.[111] Because HBV in human plasma can survive for at least 1 week in the environment,[147] inanimate objects contaminated with blood can serve as vehicles for the transmission of the virus. When a cluster of nosocomial HBV infections unrelated to surgery is detected, the mode of transmission is most likely via contact with a contaminated inanimate object rather than through contact with an infected health care worker. HBV has also been transmitted by the reuse of contaminated needles and syringes.[148] When investigating an outbreak of HBV, investigators must review and observe infection control practices involving the use of needles, syringes, and multidose vials because the improper use of these items can result in the transmission of bloodborne pathogens from patient to patient.[149] Personnel who administer parenteral medications and vaccines should be instructed in the proper infection control technique, as recommended by the CDC:[149(p.970)]

- A needle or syringe that previously has been used to inoculate a patient is considered contaminated and should not be used to aspirate medication or vaccine from a multidose vial if any of the contents of the vial will subsequently be administered to another patient.
- All hypodermic needles, as well as the lumens of syringes used to administer parenteral substances, should be sterile. Needles and syringes manufactured for single use only should be discarded and should not be reprocessed or reused on a different patient because the reprocessing method may not sterilize the internal surfaces and/or may alter the integrity of the device.
- Reusable needles and syringes should be cleaned and then sterilized by standard heat-based sterilization methods (e.g., steam autoclave or dry-air oven) between

uses. Reprocessing of reusable needles and syringes by use of liquid chemical germicides cannot guarantee sterility and is not recommended.

Hepatitis C Virus

The epidemiology of nosocomial HCV is poorly understood; however, the risk for health care worker-to-patient transmission appears to be low.[143,150] There is one report of nosocomial transmission that occurred in five patients who had surgery performed by an HCV-infected cardiothoracic surgeon in Spain.[151]

The CDC[150] and SHEA[143] do not currently support restricting the professional activities of health care workers with HCV infection. Both organizations stress the need for all health care workers to follow routine infection control measures, such as the use of standard precautions, to prevent the transmission of bloodborne pathogens such as HBV, HCV, and HIV. The CDC recommendations for prevention and control of HCV infection[150] can be obtained from the MMWR Recommendations and Reports section of the CDC Web site (http://www.cdc.gov).

Human Immunodeficiency Virus

In 1990 there was a highly publicized transmission of HIV from an infected dentist to his patients.[152,153] To date, transmission of HIV from an infected surgeon has been reported only once—from a French orthopaedic surgeon to a patient.[154]

Guidelines for preventing transmission of HIV during surgical procedures have been published by the CDC,[146] the American Academy of Orthopedic Surgeons,[155] and the American College of Obstetricians and Gynecologists.[156] Guidelines for managing HIV-infected personnel have been published by SHEA.[143] All of these guidelines support the use of standard precautions to minimize the exposure of patients and personnel to blood and bloodborne pathogens.

Salmonella Species

Most reported hospital *Salmonella* outbreaks have been caused by improper handling of contaminated foods[125,157]; however, several epidemics have been traced to symptomatic dietary[158] and nursing personnel[159] and to infected patients.[160] In one outbreak, *Salmonella poona* was most likely introduced into a neonatal intensive care unit by an asymptomatic infant whose mother was infected with *S poona*. The organism was then transmitted to two other infants via cross-infection by personnel.[160] To prevent transmission of *Salmonella* in the health care setting, dietary and patient care personnel with acute gastrointestinal illness should be restricted from caring for patients and handling patient care items or food until symptoms subside.[17] Some health departments have regulations governing the restriction and culturing of health care workers and food handlers who have *Salmonella* infection.

Hepatitis A Virus

Hepatitis A virus (HAV) is most commonly transmitted in the hospital setting via the fecal-oral route by contact with feces or fecally contaminated items.[17] Transmission by ingestion of contaminated food or beverages is known to occur in hospitals but is rarely reported in the literature.[161,162] Transmission has also occurred by blood transfusion.[17,163–165] There is no chronic carrier state for hepatitis A virus as there is for hepatitis B and C virus. HAV is excreted in the stool, and transient viremia can occur.[166] Persons with HAV infection are most infectious during the prodromal stage, before the onset of jaundice.

Several outbreaks in nurseries were traced to neonates who received blood transfusions from a donor with HAV infection.[163–165] Once introduced into the unit, HAV was transmitted by cross-infection to other infants and personnel and to parents and relatives of the infected infants.[163–165] Activities that have been associated with nosocomial spread of HAV include eating and drinking in patient care areas[163,164,167,168] and failure to wash hands after caring for an infected infant.[167,168] In another outbreak, the source for nosocomial HAV was an adult patient with symptomatic HAV infection who was hospitalized for an unrelated reason, and HAV was transmitted to six health care workers and one patient.[169] Recommendations for preventing nosocomial transmission of HAV include hand washing and use of standard precautions.[17] The CDC Advisory Committee on Immunization Practices (ACIP) recommends that immune globulin be administered to close contacts of index patients only if an investigation indicates that nosocomial spread between patients or between patients and staff in a hospital has occurred.[166,170] The role of HAV vaccination in interrupting outbreaks in the hospital setting has not yet been determined.[166,170]

OUTBREAKS SPREAD FROM PERSON TO PERSON BY AIRBORNE AND DROPLET TRANSMISSION

Diseases Spread by Airborne Transmission

Outbreaks of airborne nosocomial infections have long been recognized in health care facilities,[17,171,172] although they are relatively uncommon compared to outbreaks spread by contact. Only a few diseases have been documented to be spread from person to person via a true airborne route (i.e., by airborne droplet nuclei, which are small particle residues of evaporated respiratory secretions that can remain suspended in the air and can be dispersed widely by air currents).[18,171] Three diseases caused by pathogens that can be truly airborne and have caused numerous epidemics in the health care setting are tuberculosis, measles, and varicella (chickenpox). Since tuberculosis outbreaks have been reported in a variety of health care settings, this disease is discussed in detail in Chapter 7.

Measles

Measles is one of the most contagious diseases in humans. Transmission of measles has occurred in hospitals, physicians' offices, and emergency rooms.[172–176] Measles may be introduced into a facility by infected patients or by health care workers and is easily transmitted either via contact with respiratory secretions of infected persons or via the airborne route.[17] Infected health care workers can transmit the disease to patients, to other health care workers, and to family members. Measles is readily spread because the virus may remain airborne for prolonged periods and because infected persons with measles may shed the virus in respiratory secretions during the prodromal period before the disease is recognized.[17] Transmission from patient to patient has occurred in physicians' offices even when direct contact did not occur. Fifteen of the 75 measles outbreaks reported in the United States during 1993–1996 involved transmission in a health care facility.[176] During 1989–1991, a major resurgence of measles occurred in the United States; however, in 1996 only 508 cases were reported, of which 65 were classified as international importations.[176]

Measures used to prevent transmission of measles in health care facilities have been published by the CDC[17,18,170,176] and include

- prompt recognition of persons with measles (Measles should be suspected in persons with a fever and rash.)
- prompt isolation of persons with suspected or known measles (Airborne precautions should be taken in a private room with negative airflow and nonrecirculating air.)[18]
- protocols to ensure measles immunity in all health care workers (Measles vaccine should be provided to all health care workers who cannot show proof of immunity, as follows:[17,170,176]
  1. health care workers born before 1957 are generally considered to be immune to measles
  2. health care workers born during or after 1957 are considered immune if they have one of the following:
     - documentation of physician-diagnosed measles
     - documentation of two doses of live measles vaccine on or after their first birthday
     - serologic evidence of measles immunity)

The ACIP recommendations regarding immunization of health care workers[170] and immunization for measles, mumps, and rubella[176] should be used when developing health care facility policies. The ACIP recommendations can be obtained by accessing the MMWR Recommendations and Reports section of the CDC Web site (http://www.cdc.gov). In addition, some state and local health departments require measles immunity for health care workers, and these requirements must be incorporated into a facility's policies.

The CDC Hospital Infection Control Practices Advisory Committee (HICPAC) recommendations for isolation precautions in hospitals[18] can also be obtained through the Internet at http://www.cdc.gov/ncidod/hip/isolat. Additional information on prevention and control of measles in the pediatric population can be found in the American Academy of Pediatrics *Red Book*.[177]

Because measles is highly communicable, one case in a facility (even a community-acquired case) should be considered a potential outbreak and should be accorded immediate action to prevent further transmission. Actions to be taken to interrupt measles transmission include the following:

- identification and prompt isolation of persons with measles

Note: The diagnosis of measles should be verified before exposure follow-up is conducted. Serologic testing is recommended to confirm the diagnosis; however, if measles is clinically diagnosed, exposure follow-up should begin before laboratory confirmation is received. Information on the clinical and laboratory diagnosis of measles is provided in Appendix D.

- compilation of a list of all potentially exposed personnel, patients, and visitors as soon as possible, especially if the suspected case is seen in the emergency room
- identification of all exposed personnel, patients, and visitors

Note: It is important to define "exposed person" before conducting contact tracing. Exposure may be defined as being in the same room (or area supplied by the same air-handling system) at the same time as a patient with measles or for up to 1 hour after the patient with measles left the room/area.

- evaluation of immunity in all exposed personnel and patients (Guidelines for evaluating immunity can be found in Appendix D.)
- restriction of susceptible exposed personnel from duty, from 5 days after the first exposure to 21 days after the last exposure to measles[17,176]
- isolation of exposed susceptible patients (airborne precautions in a private room with negative airflow and nonrecirculating air)[18] if they are still hospitalized, from 5 days after the first exposure to 21 days after the last exposure to measles
- prompt provision of measles vaccine to susceptible persons to halt disease transmission

Note: During an outbreak, serologic testing to identify susceptible persons is not necessary.[17,176] The vaccine should be provided to those born during or after 1957 who have no documentation of complete measles vaccination or physician-documented diagnosis of measles. Guidelines for providing the measles vaccine and immune globulin can be found in Appendix D and in the ACIP recommendations for measles, mumps, and rubella immunization.[176]

Community outbreaks can result in transmission into a health care facility,[178,179] and nosocomial transmission can spread into the community. One of the most important measures to prevent measles transmission is to ensure that all persons who work in a health care facility have acceptable evidence of measles immunity.[176,179]

Outbreaks of measles in health care facilities can be associated with significant morbidity. They are disruptive and costly to control due to (1) the time needed to conduct a contact investigation, (2) the lost workdays for restricted personnel who either acquire measles or who are exposed and are not immune, and (3) the cost of the measles vaccine for exposed personnel, patients, and visitors.

Varicella-Zoster Virus

Varicella-zoster virus (VZV) causes varicella (chickenpox) and zoster (shingles). Varicella is one of the most communicable diseases of humans and is readily spread from person to person via direct contact with infected lesions, droplet spread, or airborne transmission.[17,180,181] Nosocomial outbreaks of varicella in hospitals and physicians' offices have been well documented in the literature.[180–184] True airborne transmission has been documented in the hospital setting when susceptible patients have developed varicella even though they did not have face-to-face contact with the infected source patient.[182,184] Community outbreaks can result in nosocomial exposures and transmission.[183] VZV can easily be introduced into the health care setting by infected patients, personnel, and visitors (including the children of personnel) since infected persons may be contagious up to 2 days prior to the development of symptoms.[17]

Guidelines for prevention and control of VZV infections in health care facilities have been published by the CDC,[17,18,185] the American Academy of Pediatrics,[177] and others.[180,186,187] These guidelines should be reviewed when developing hospital policies.

Measures that should be implemented in health care facilities to prevent varicella transmission include

- implementation of protocols to ensure varicella immunity in personnel[185]
- prompt recognition of infected patients, personnel, and visitors

    Note: The diagnosis of chickenpox should be verified by infection control and/or employee health personnel before exposure follow-up and contact tracing is conducted.

- prompt and appropriate isolation of infected patients (airborne precautions in a private room with negative airflow and nonrecirculating air)[18]
- compilation of a list of all potentially exposed personnel, patients, and visitors as soon as possible, especially if the suspected case is seen in the emergency room
- prompt identification of exposed persons

    Note: It is important to define "exposed person" before conducting contact tracing. Weber et al define exposure as "being in an enclosed airspace with the source case (i.e., same room) or in intimate contact with the source in an open area during a potentially contagious stage of illness. Varicella is considered contagious beginning 48 hours prior to the onset of rash and until all lesions are dried and crusted."[180(p.699)]

- evaluation of immunity in all exposed personnel, patients, and visitors
- restriction of susceptible exposed personnel from duty beginning on the 8th day after the first exposure through the 21st day after the last exposure to chickenpox, or until all lesions are dried and crusted if varicella occurs[17]
- isolation of exposed susceptible patients if they are still hospitalized during the period of potential infectiousness (airborne precautions in a private room with negative airflow from 8 days after the first exposure through 21 days after the last exposure)[18]
- provision of the varicella vaccine to exposed personnel who are not immune (However, the vaccine's efficacy in preventing postexposure development of the disease is unknown, and the vaccinated personnel should be managed as if they were not immunized.)[17]

Varicella exposure management, follow-up, and contact tracing can result in considerable time expenditure by infection control and employee health staff, and the exclusion of exposed susceptible personnel from duty can lead to significant cost and disruption of services for a health care facility.[183] Much of this disruption can be prevented if persons with varicella are promptly identified and appropriately isolated and if health care facilities ensure that all of their personnel are immune to varicella.

Diseases Spread by Droplet Transmission

Diseases that are spread from person to person via droplet transmission are caused by pathogens that are expelled in large particle droplets of respiratory secretions by a person who is coughing, talking, or sneezing or by droplets that are produced during a procedure such as tracheal suctioning or bronchoscopy.[18] These droplets are not widely dispersed into the air and are generally said to travel about 3 feet before settling to the ground. Diseases that have caused outbreaks in health care facilities and that can be spread via droplet transmission include adenovirus infections,[172,188–190] mumps,[191,192] influenza, parvovirus B19 infection,[193–195] rubella,[196–198] *Mycoplasma pneumoniae* infection,[199] respiratory syncytial virus (RSV) infections,[200–210] and pertussis.[211–222] Although the influenza virus has been transmitted in the acute care setting, the majority of nosocomial outbreaks are reported in long-term care facilities. Influenza is therefore discussed in Chapter 4.

Respiratory Syncytial Virus

Respiratory syncytial virus infection is most common in infants and children and, although it can cause a severe pneumonia or bronchiolitis, it usually causes a mild disease. Community outbreaks of RSV disease are seasonal, generally occurring between December and March. RSV can be introduced into the hospital by infected patients, personnel, or visitors and can be easily transmitted directly from person to person via large particle aerosols during close contact with an infected person or indirectly via RSV-contaminated hands or articles.[19,200,201] The portal of entry for RSV is the conjunctiva or nasal mucosa, and transmission frequently occurs when contaminated hands touch the eyes or nose.[19] Hand washing is the most important measure for preventing the transmission of RSV. Outbreaks of RSV infection have most commonly been reported in pediatric units,[202] nurseries,[203,204] long-term care facilities,[205–206] and immunocompromised adults in bone marrow transplant units[207] and intensive care units.[208] RSV infection may occur concurrently with other respiratory tract infections, making outbreaks difficult to recognize.[209–210]

Measures used to control RSV epidemics have been published by the CDC[18,19] and include

- hand washing
- adherence to contact isolation precautions (gloves and gowns)

- use of private rooms for infected patients (When a private room is not available, patient may be placed in a room with a patient who has active infection with RSV but with no other infection [cohorting].)
- work restrictions for personnel who have symptoms of acute upper respiratory tract infection
- restriction on visitors with symptoms of upper respiratory tract infection from visiting pediatric, cardiac, and immunosuppressed patients

Pertussis

Pertussis (whooping cough) is generally considered to be a childhood disease; however, approximately 25 percent of cases reported in 1996 occurred in persons 15 years of age or older.[211] Disease in adults may be subclinical,[212] mild, or atypical,[213] and although it has been shown to be a common cause of prolonged cough in adults, it is probably frequently not recognized.[214,215] Pertussis is easily spread from person to person by direct contact with the respiratory droplets of infected persons. Multiple outbreaks of pertussis have been reported in acute care facilities[214,216–218] and have involved both patients and staff.[216,217] Outbreaks in the community may also involve hospital personnel.[219]

Guidelines for preventing the transmission of *Bordetella pertussis* and for managing pertussis exposures have been published by the CDC[17,18] and others[220–222] and include

- droplet precautions for infected patients (private room and use of masks for those coming within 3 feet of the patient) until 5 days after patient is started on effective therapy
- droplet precautions for suspected cases until pertussis is ruled out
- evaluation and appropriate therapy for exposed personnel who are symptomatic
- work restrictions for symptomatic personnel until 5 days of therapy are completed
- postexposure prophylaxis for exposed employees who are asymptomatic

The article by Haiduven et al contains a pertussis work-up checklist and pertussis exposure forms that can be used for managing exposures in patients and personnel.[222]

Exhibit 3–1 provides examples of diseases that have been responsible for outbreaks in hospitals and are

Exhibit 3–1 Airborne and Droplet-Spread Diseases Responsible for Outbreaks in Health Care Facilities

Airborne	*Droplet*
Measles	Adenovirus
Tuberculosis	Influenza
Varicella	Mumps
	Mycoplasma pneumoniae infection
	Parvovirus B19
	Pertussis
	Rubella
	Respiratory syncytial virus (RSV) infection

caused by organisms transmitted via the airborne and droplet routes. Since a detailed description of each of these diseases is beyond the scope of this chapter, for information on signs and symptoms, diagnosis, epidemiology, and infection prevention and control measures the reader is referred to the 1998 CDC Guideline for Infection Control in Health Care Personnel[17] and to the textbooks noted in the Suggested Reading section at the end of this chapter.

OUTBREAKS OF DISEASES THAT HAVE ENVIRONMENTAL RESERVOIRS

Legionnaires' disease and aspergillosis are two major nosocomial diseases that have airborne and droplet modes of transmission but have environmental, rather than human, reservoirs.

Legionnaires' Disease

Epidemiology

Legionella species are gram-negative bacilli that are ubiquitous in nature and live in aqueous habitats. They can be isolated from hot and cold tap water, ponds, streams, and the surrounding soil. Nosocomial cases of Legionnaires' disease (LD) were reported shortly after the etiologic agent of LD was identified in 1977,[223,224] and multiple nosocomial outbreaks and clusters have since been reported.[225–231] Nosocomial LD has generally been associated with contamination of the water in cooling systems[230,231] or the potable hot water systems in hospitals,[225–229] and these systems may remain colonized for prolonged periods.[229] In one hospital, persistent colonization of the water supply was associated with contaminated shock absorbers installed within the pipes to decrease noise.[227]

A 1994 community outbreak of *Legionella pneumophila* pneumonia in Wilmington, Delaware, was associated with the cooling towers of a hospital.[232] Although no hospitalized patients were affected, hospital staff and persons living in the area surrounding the hospital developed Legionnaires' disease.

Hospitals play an important role in the detection of outbreaks. Recognition of a cluster of community-acquired cases of Legionnaires' disease by the staff of a community hospital in the summer of 1994 led to the detection of an outbreak of LD among passengers of a cruise ship.[233] Since tests for *Legionella* species are not routinely performed, it is likely that many cases, both community acquired and nosocomial, are not recognized.

In one report, the CDC defined nosocomial Legionnaires' disease as follows:[229(p.416)]

> Definite nosocomial LD: was defined as a respiratory illness with a new infiltrate on chest roentgenogram occurring after greater than or equal to 10 days of continuous hospitalization for a nonpneumonia illness and laboratory confirmation of legionellae infection by at least one of the following: 1) isolation of legionellae from tissue or respiratory secretions, 2) detection of Legionella pneumophila serogroup 1 (Lp-1) antigens in urine by radioimmunoassay or enzyme immunoassay, or 3) a fourfold rise in Legionella serogroup-specific antibody titer to greater than or equal to 128 between acute- and convalescent-phase serum specimens.

> Possible nosocomial LD: was defined as onset of respiratory symptoms of LD after 2–9 days of continuous hospitalization (the incubation period for LD is usually 2–10 days).

Identification of one case of definite nosocomial LD or two cases of possible nosocomial LD in a 6-month period should prompt an epidemiologic investigation.[229] The investigation should include prospective surveillance for new cases, a retrospective review of laboratory reports (serologic and microbiologic) and postmortem results to identify any previously unrecognized cases, and a line-listing of cases by time, place, and person.[19,229]

Mode of Transmission

The mode of transmission for *Legionella pneumophila* is believed to be via inhalation of the organism in aerosolized water droplets that can be produced by cooling towers, showers, room air humidifiers, and respiratory therapy nebulization devices.[19,231]

Control Measures

To avoid transmission of *Legionella* in the hospital, sterile water (not tap or distilled water) should be used to rinse and fill respiratory therapy equipment. Measures that can be used to prevent nosocomial LD were published by the CDC in the 1994 Guideline for Prevention of Nosocomial Pneumonia.[19] This guideline includes information on procedures for decontaminating potable water and cooling systems and is available electronically on the CDC Web site: http://www.cdc.gov/ncidod/diseases/hip/pneumonia/pneu_mmw.htm. Control measures used to interrupt outbreaks in hospitals have included hyperchlorination and superheating of the hot water system, use of sterile water in nebulizers, and use of biocides in cooling towers.[227–229,231]

Aspergillosis

Epidemiology and Mode of Transmission

Aspergillus species are ubiquitous in nature and can easily be cultured from the hospital environment.[234] This fungus produces spores that are approximately 3 µm in size and that can remain suspended in air for prolonged periods.[235] The usual portal of entry is via inhalation of aerosolized spores.[19] However, primary cutaneous aspergillosis resulting from inoculation of spores onto nonintact skin has been reported.[29,47] Immunocompromised patients are at greatest risk of developing invasive pulmonary infection, which can result in significant morbidity and mortality.[236]

Multiple outbreaks of nosocomial aspergillosis have been reported in hospitals.[29,47,234,237–242] Most outbreaks have been associated with construction or renovation in, or adjacent to, the hospital.[29,234,238–240,242] In one outbreak, exposure to a radiology suite that was undergoing extensive renovation was the only common environmental factor found among six patients who developed nosocomial aspergillosis during a 1-month period.[242] Although most outbreaks involve pulmonary aspergillosis in immunosuppressed patients,[29,237–240] there are several reports of outbreaks of primary cuta-

neous aspergillosis due to contact with contaminated medical supplies, such as dressings[29,47] and intravenous arm boards.[241] In one report, an outbreak of cutaneous aspergillosis was recognized when three cases of extensive wound aspergillosis occurred in surgical and burn patients in a 3-week period. The source was traced to the outer packaging of dressing supplies (dressing trays, gauze, bandages, and tapes) that had become contaminated during renovation in the central inventory control area of the hospital.[29] In addition to outbreaks of infection, pseudo-outbreaks involving aspergillosis have been reported as a result of contamination of microbiology cultures in the laboratory.[243]

Control Measures

Measures used to prevent transmission of fungal spores to patients include implementation of protocols for protection against construction-related bioaerosols,[234,244] placement of high-risk patients (e.g., those with severe and prolonged granulocytopenia) in a protected environment,[19] routine inspection and maintenance of air-handling systems in high-risk patient care areas (such as operating rooms, nurseries, intensive care units, bone marrow or solid organ transplant units, and oncology units), and protection of sterile supplies from contamination.

Guidelines for controlling the airborne transmission of *Aspergillus* in the hospital have been published by the CDC,[19] Walsh and Dixon,[234] and Carter and Barr.[244] Measures used to control transmission of *Aspergillus* spores during construction and renovation projects include

- construction of impermeable barriers of plastic or drywall that extend from the floor to the ceiling to control the dissemination of dust and dirt and to separate the construction site from the patient care areas, the pharmacy, and areas where sterile supplies are stored
- frequent cleaning and vacuuming of the work site and the areas adjacent to the work site
- restriction of pedestrian traffic through the work area to prevent the tracking of dust and dirt through the facility
- careful attention to traffic patterns of the construction crew, personnel, patients, and visitors to avoid the spread of dirt and dust through the hospital and to reduce the risk of patient exposure to infectious agents
- evaluation of air patterns and air-handling systems in the work site and the surrounding areas to en-

sure that dust and spores are not disseminated through the facility via air currents

- ventilation of construction areas so they are at negative pressure to surrounding critical areas such as patient care units and clean and sterile supply rooms

Outbreaks and Pseudo-Outbreaks Associated with a Water Reservoir

Many outbreaks and pseudo-outbreaks in inpatient and outpatient health care facilities have been traced to a water reservoir,[245-251] including potable or drinking water, ice and ice machines, toilet water, and warm-water and sonicator baths. Table 3–7 lists several examples. Whenever outbreaks or pseudo-outbreaks are caused by nontuberculous mycobacteria or *Legionella, Pseudomonas, Flavobacterium,* or *Acinetobacter* species, an aqueous reservoir should be suspected.

Potable Water

Nontuberculous mycobacteria are commonly found in municipal water supplies and are frequent causes of pseudo-outbreaks. Sniadeck et al described an outbreak

of *Mycobacterium xenopi* pseudoinfections that occurred in 13 patients over a 1-year period.[252] Acid-fast bacilli (AFB) smears were negative and only a few colonies of the organism were isolated from each of the specimens (six sputa, two bronchial washings, four urines, and one stool). None of the patients had disease that was compatible with *M xenopi* infection. The source of the organism was believed to be the hospital's potable water system, which contaminated the specimens at the time of collection. A review of specimen collection and instrument disinfection procedures revealed the following:

1. Tap water was used to rinse a patient's mouth just prior to collecting a sputum specimen.
2. Tap water was used as a final rinse after cold sterilization of bronchoscopes.
3. Urine for mycobacterial culture was occasionally collected in previously used bedpans that had been rinsed with tap water.
4. Tap water was used for colonic irrigation.

This report highlights the need to instruct personnel to collect specimens for culture carefully in order to

Table 3–7 Outbreaks and Pseudo-Outbreaks Associated with a Water Reservoir

Outbreak	Reservoir	Source	Year(s) Reported (Reference No.)
Flavobacterium septicemia	Hospital potable water	Syringes cooled in ice from ice machine in intensive care unit	1975[246]
Pseudomonas septicemia	Hospital potable water	Contaminated water bath in the operating room used to thaw fresh-frozen plasma	1981[247]
Pseudomonas aeruginosa wound infections	Water in physical therapy department	Contaminated Hubbard tank; associated with discontinuation of using bleach to disinfect tank	1981[248]
Mycobacterium chelonae infections	Water supply in outpatient hemodialysis center	Hemodialyzers that were manually reprocessed using Renalin germicide	1990[249]
Pseudomonas pickettii bacteremia	Distilled water	Distilled water used by employee to replace Fentanyl during narcotic theft	1991[40]
Gram-negative bacteremia	Hospital potable water	Pressure-monitoring equipment left open and uncovered overnight in the operating room; contaminated by housekeeping personnel who sprayed a water-disinfectant mixture when cleaning	1996[84]
Legionellosis (one case prompted an investigation)	Hospital potable water	Contaminated ice machine	1997[250]
Pseudo-outbreak of *Pseudomonas aeruginosa*	Water in hospital toilet	Fecal specimens for surveillance cultures that were collected from the toilet	1997[251]

minimize microbial contamination, and to avoid using tap water as a final rinse when cleaning and disinfecting bronchoscopes.

Copepods and nonpathogenic freshwater microorganisms present in hospital drinking water have caused pseudo-outbreaks.[253,254] Copepods are small animals, such as *Cyclops*, that are the intermediate hosts of animal parasites of humans (e.g., the guinea worm, *Dracunculus medinensis*, and the fish tapeworm, *Diphyllobothrium latum*).

Ice

Contaminated ice machines and ice baths used to cool medical devices such as syringes have been responsible for nosocomial outbreaks.[245] An outbreak of bacteremia caused by *Flavobacterium* species was traced to syringes that were cooled in ice from the ice machine in an intensive care unit before being used to collect arterial specimens for blood gas determination.[246] Guidelines for minimizing the risk of transmission of infectious agents by ice and ice machines have been published by the CDC[255] and by Burnett et al.[256]

Water Baths

Warm-water baths have frequently served as the source of outbreaks.[245] Organisms present in water baths used to thaw blood components and peritoneal dialysis solutions can easily contaminate the outer surfaces of these items and can enter the container when it is opened or punctured. Items being thawed in water baths should be placed in an impermeable plastic wrapper to avoid contamination. Alternatively, peritoneal dialysis fluid can be warmed by using a dry-heat source or a microwave oven.

OUTBREAKS OF NOSOCOMIAL PNEUMONIA IN INTENSIVE CARE UNITS

Although most nosocomial pneumonias (NPs) arise from aspiration of endogenous oropharyngeal or gastric flora, outbreaks of NP in intensive care units have been caused by exogenously acquired organisms.[257] Epidemics of nosocomial pneumonia can be caused by a variety of bacteria, viruses, and fungi. Organisms causing NP can be transmitted by person-to-person contact or by health care workers or other patients through contact with contaminated respiratory therapy devices and equipment.[19,258–265] Examples of nosocomial pneumonia outbreaks in intensive care units that

were spread by contact are shown in Table 3–8. Control measures used to interrupt transmission of the pathogens are also shown.

Most outbreaks of nosocomial pneumonia that are spread by cross-infection can be controlled by implementation of routine infection control practices, such as contact isolation precautions, appropriate use of gloves and hand washing, and intensive surveillance.[257] It is often difficult to recognize clusters and outbreaks that are caused by common pathogens, such as *S aureus*, as these organisms may be causing endemic infections. Outbreaks caused by unusual gram-negative organisms, such as *Burkholderia* (formerly *Pseudomonas*) *cepacia* and *Stenotrophomonas* (formerly *Xanthomonas*) *maltophilia*, are more likely to be detected because these isolates are more likely to be noticed.

Outbreaks associated with bronchoscopy and respiratory therapy solutions and equipment, such as albuterol, mechanical ventilator circuits, and nebulizers, have been discussed previously in this chapter. Most of these outbreaks can be prevented by use of aseptic technique when handling fluids and by adherence to proper cleaning, disinfection, and sterilization protocols for devices and equipment.

Epidemics of *Legionella* and *Aspergillus* pneumonia associated with environmental reservoirs have occurred in ICU patients.[239,257,263–270] Control measures for these outbreaks depend on the specific reservoir and source of the organism, as outlined in Table 3–9. Information on outbreaks caused by these two pathogens was given in a previous section of this chapter.

For a comprehensive review of epidemics of nosocomial pneumonia reported in ICU patients, including a discussion of the steps used to investigate an outbreak of NP, the reader is referred to the article by Maloney and Jarvis.[257] The CDC Guideline for Prevention of Nosocomial Pneumonia provides information on the etiology, epidemiology, pathogenesis, diagnosis, risk factors, and control measures for preventing NP.[19] Guidelines for conducting outbreak investigations for specific pathogens are also included. Control measures recommended by the CDC include staff education on basic infection control practices, infection surveillance, sterilization or disinfection and proper handling of medical equipment and devices, installation and maintenance of special ventilation systems for patients at high risk for aspergillosis, and isolation precautions for patients with known or suspected infection.[19]

Table 3–8 Reported Epidemics of Nosocomial Pneumonia (NP) in Intensive Care Unit Patients Spread by Contact Transmission, 1982–1993

Pathogen	Author (Reference No.)	Year	Study Population	Number of Patients with NP/ Colonization	Risk Factors	Implicated Source		Control Measures*
						Patients/ Personnel	Respiratory Equipment	
Branhamella catarrhalis	Patterson et al[258]	1988	Intermediate care unit	8/2	Respiratory therapy Steroid use Ward location	X		1, 2, 5, 7
Influenza A virus	Centers for Disease Control[259]	1988	Med/Surg ICU**	3/NA*	NA			5
Methicillin-resistant *Staphylococcus aureus*	Locksley et al[260]	1982	Hospitalwide	15/1	Mechanical ventilation ICU/burn ward	X		1, 3, 5, 7, 8
Parainfluenza virus	Singh-Naz et al[261]	1990	Intermediate ICN**	6/1	NA	X		1, 2, 3, 5
Pseudomonas cepacia	Weems[82]	1993	General ICU	NA/120	Mechanical ventilation Respiratory therapy		X	6
	Conly et al[83]	1986	Medical ICU Surgical ICU	4/21	Mechanical ventilation Antimicrobial therapy	X	X	3, 4, 6
Respiratory syncytial virus and rhinovirus	Valenti et al[209]	1982	NICU/SCN**	7/1	Endotracheal or nasogastric intubation Mechanical ventilation	X		1, 3
Xanthomonas maltophilia	Villarino et al[262]	1992	CCU** Trauma ICU Med/Surg ICU	42/0	Trauma ICU Mechanical ventilation Antimicrobial therapy	X	X	1, 3, 4, 5, 6

*Control measures: 1 = isolation precautions; 2 = cohorting of infected patients; 3 = appropriate hand washing and glove use; 4 = staff education; 5 = prospective surveillance; 6 = high-level disinfection and sterile water for respiratory equipment; 7 = appropriate antimicrobial therapy; 8 = treatment of carrier state.

**Med/Surg = medical and surgical; ICU = intensive care unit; NA = not available; ICN = intensive care nursery; NICU/SCN = neonatal intensive care and special care nursery; CCU = critical care unit.

Source: Reprinted from the Investigation and Prevention Branch, Hospital Infections Program, National Center for Infectious Diseases, Centers for Disease Control and Prevention, Atlanta, Georgia.

Table 3–9 Outbreaks of NP Associated with Specific Environmental Reservoirs, 1978–1994

Pathogen	Author (Reference No.)	Year	Study Population	Number of Patients with NP	Risk Factors	Reservoir	Source	Control Measures*
Legionella species	Fisher-Hoch et al[263]	1981	General hospital	11	Immunosuppression; admission to new building	Water supply and cooling system	Tap water; cooling tower	1, 3
	Arnow et al[264]	1982	General hospital	5	Immunosuppressive therapy; jet nebulizer use	Water supply	Respiratory equipment	2, 3
	Brady[265]	1989	Pediatric hospital	7	Immunosuppressive therapy; chronic lung/kidney disease	Water supply	Showers; respiratory equipment	2, 4, and appropriate antimicrobial therapy
	Mastro et al[266]	1991	General hospital	13	Chronic lung disease; jet nebulizer use; >3 days in ICU**	Water supply	Respiratory equipment	1, 2
	Blatt et al[267]	1993	Military hospital	14	Immunosuppressive therapy; nasogastric tube use; antimicrobial therapy; bedbathing	Water supply	Tap water	2, 3
Aspergillus species	Arnow et al[239]	1978	Renal transplantation unit	2	Immunosuppressive therapy; proximity to construction	Construction	Surface dust	7, 8
	Weems et al[268]	1987	Pediatric hospital	5	Hematologic malignancy; construction activity	Construction	NA**	7, 8
	Arnow et al[269]	1991	General hospital	29	Malignancy; hematology/oncology ward	Ventilation system	Ventilator filters; surface dust	5, 6
	Buffington et al[270]	1994	Pediatric hospital	7	Hematologic malignancy; construction activity	Construction	NA	5, 7, 8

*Control measures: 1 = hyperchlorination and superheating of hospital water supply; 2 = sterile water for rinsing and use in respiratory equipment; 3 = prospective surveillance; 4 = staff education and shower prohibition; 5 = aggressive hospital cleaning and inspection; 6 = retrofitting of ventilation system; 7 = impermeable barriers around construction site; 8 = relocation of immunocompromised patients.

**ICU = intensive care unit; NA = not available.

Source: Reprinted from the Investigation and Prevention Branch, Hospital Infections Program, National Center for Infectious Diseases, Centers for Disease Control and Prevention, Atlanta, Georgia.

OUTBREAKS OF SICK BUILDING SYNDROME AND BUILDING-RELATED ILLNESS

Much has been published on "sick building syndrome" and indoor air pollution[271-274]; however, little has been published regarding noninfectious episodes of building-associated illnesses in health care facilities.[273,274] In one review of indoor air pollution, building-associated illnesses were linked to inadequate ventilation in approximately half of the cases studied and in many cases no causal factor was found.[272] Brandt-Rauf et al described an outbreak of eye and respiratory tract irritation in operating room personnel. The outbreak was attributed to emergency generator diesel exhaust emissions that entered the ventilation system for the operating room suite; however, personnel continued to complain of symptoms after this problem was rectified and a definitive etiology for the ongoing symptoms was not identified.[273]

Hospital personnel in infection control, employee health, and safety management are frequently called upon to investigate clusters of complaints of symptoms and illnesses by health care personnel, who often attribute the problems to exposure to some factor in the workplace. Infection control personnel who are asked to investigate such incidents should follow the epidemiologic principles used to investigate outbreaks of infection and other conditions as outlined in Chapter 8. In many cases of building-related complaints, it is difficult to determine if symptoms are truly a result of building-related exposures. A review article on indoor air pollution by Gold provides helpful information that can be used when evaluating building-related complaints, and Gold suggests that the following questions should be asked.[274]

1. Is the building tight?
2. Are there any significant levels of indoor air pollutants?
3. What is the overall prevalence of symptoms?
4. Are the symptoms clustered in any one work area?

When investigating building-related complaints, it is helpful to evaluate

1. the work exposure histories of the personnel involved (e.g., exposure to chemicals, paint fumes, exhaust fumes from nearby vehicles, photocopying machines, volatile organic substances from new carpets, or mold spores from wet carpets)
2. the time of day that the symptoms occur(red)
3. the time of day that exposure(s) to possible pollutants occur(red)
4. the temporal relationship between time of exposure and onset of symptoms
5. the relationship of symptoms at and away from work (do symptoms subside on weekends or when employees are away from the workplace?)
6. physical factors, such as poor lighting
7. psychological factors, such as job dissatisfaction, especially if no other causative factors can be found

It is important that employers listen to, and address, the concerns of personnel and demonstrate a genuine effort to identify the cause and implement corrective measures. Such support will encourage employee productivity and workplace satisfaction and will reduce the risk of legal or regulatory actions taken by personnel against the employer.

NEWLY RECOGNIZED AGENTS AND SOURCES FOR HEALTH CARE–ASSOCIATED OUTBREAKS

Candida Species

Epidemiology

The *Candida* species emerged in the 1980s as an important cause of nosocomial infection in severely ill and immunocompromised patients.[275-277] The most commonly reported *Candida* species causing infection in humans are *C albicans*, *C tropicalis*, *C (Torulopsis) glabrata*, *C parapsilosis*, *C krusei*, and *C lusitaniae*.[275,276] Risk factors for nosocomial candidiasis include intravenous therapy (especially total parenteral nutrition [TPN]), exposure to antibiotics, and neutropenia.[275] Although most *Candida* infections arise from a patient's endogenous flora, nosocomial transmission via contaminated intravenous fluids and medical devices and the hands of personnel has been documented.[275,277-280]

Although many reported clusters and outbreaks of *Candida* species have no identified source,[279,281] outbreaks have been associated with total parenteral nutrition,[281,282] intravenous blood pressure–monitoring devices,[283] and personnel carriers.[139,140] *Candida* species are important pathogens in neonatal intensive care units (NICU). Recent studies demonstrate that *Candida* can be acquired by the neonate either vertically from the mother or horizontally (nosocomially) in an NICU[278–281] and that a mother can carry different strains of *Candida albicans* at different body sites.[280] Studies show that TPN fluids can promote growth of *Candida* species and may serve as a reservoir for infection.[281] In one NICU, an outbreak of *Candida* bloodstream infections caused by *C albicans, C parapsilosis,* and *C tropicalis* was associated with a contaminated retrograde medication administration system used for TPN.[281]

Control Measures

Further epidemiologic studies are needed to identify and investigate common source outbreaks, nosocomial clusters, and instances of person-to-person transmission of *Candida* species so that the reservoirs and the modes of transmission for exogenously acquired candidiasis can be clarified.[280–284] Since little is known about the epidemiology of nosocomial *Candida* infections acquired from exogenous sources, it is difficult to identify control measures that can be used to interrupt transmission. Based on a review of the reports noted in this section, the following measures can be recommended to prevent the nosocomial spread of *Candida* species, to interrupt an outbreak, and to identify a possible cause in an outbreak:

- Since several investigators have associated outbreaks with transmission by personnel,[139,140] and since hand carriage of *Candida* species by health care workers has been documented,[285] careful hand washing should be practiced before and after patient care, especially when caring for neonates, severely ill patients, and immunocompromised patients, and before handling intravenous solutions and related equipment. If an outbreak is suspected, personnel should be reminded of the importance of proper hand washing.
- Since *Candida* outbreaks have been associated with total parenteral nutrition[281,282] and intravenous blood pressure-monitoring devices,[283] personnel preparing and infusing intravenous solutions, especially TPN, should be taught proper aseptic technique. If an outbreak is suspected, personnel practices should be observed to ensure that aseptic technique is being used.

- If a cluster or suspected increase in *Candida* infections occurs, an epidemiologic investigation should be conducted to verify the existence of an outbreak and to identify potential sources and modes of transmission (see Chapter 8). If an outbreak is suspected, the laboratory should be requested to save isolates from patients for possible future typing.
- If an epidemiologic investigation suggests an outbreak, control measures should be implemented based on the potential sources and possible modes of transmission identified.
- If initial control measures do not prevent transmission, culture surveys of patients, personnel, or an implicated source may be considered, based on the findings of the epidemiologic investigation; however, cultures should not be done unless the laboratory is involved in planning the specimen collection process and unless molecular typing will be done to determine the relatedness of any strains of *Candida* that are isolated.
- Because of the risk of contamination of retrograde medication administration systems, facilities using these systems need to evaluate carefully the practices used to maintain them.[281]
- Since clusters of *Candida* infections may be caused by more than one strain of *Candida*, laboratory typing methods must be chosen and interpreted carefully in conjunction with observational epidemiologic data.[286]

Identifying New Risk Factors and Sources for Infection

Emerging infectious diseases are considered to be those in which the incidence in humans increased in the 1970s through the 1990s or threatens to increase in the near future.[287] It is sobering to note that many of the diseases discussed in this text are considered emerging, or reemerging, infectious diseases: Legionnaires' disease, candidiasis, cryptosporidiosis, acquired immune deficiency syndrome, hepatitis B and C, and infections caused by methicillin-resistant *S aureus*, vancomycin-resistant *Enterococcus*, multidrug-resistant *Mycobacterium tuberculosis*, *Clostridium difficile*, human parvovirus B19, Norwalk and Norwalk-like agents, rotavirus, and *Pneumocystis carinii*.

In 1998 the CDC published *Preventing Emerging Infectious Diseases: A Strategy for the 21st Century*, a plan to combat infectious diseases.[288] One of the objectives of this plan is to "identify the behaviors, environments, and host factors that put people at increased risk for infectious diseases and their sequelae."[288(p.29)] One of the descriptive boxes listed in the plan shows a table of examples of new risk factors and sources for infections that were identified by CDC investigators from 1994 to 1998.[289–292] Four of the five examples given involved outbreaks of infections acquired as a result of health care activities in acute and home care settings (Table 3–10). An additional box indicated a new area for risk factor research—the relationship between health care practices and bloodstream infection rates in the acute and home care settings[290,293–296] (Exhibit 3–2). Infection surveillance, prevention, and control programs in health care facilities are an important compo-

nent in identifying the occurrence of infectious diseases, including their risk factors, sources, and prevention and control measures.

NOTE: Copies of the CDC plan can be obtained from the Office of Health Communication, National Center for Infectious Diseases, Centers for Disease Control and Prevention, Mailstop C-14, 1600 Clifton Road, Atlanta, GA 30333 or through the CDC Web site at http://www.cdc.gov/ncidod/emergplan.

Employee Health

Since health care workers (including personnel, physicians, volunteers, and students) play an important role in initiating and propagating outbreaks in health care facilities, each facility should have policies and

---

Table 3–10 Examples of New Risk Factors and Sources for Infection Identified by CDC Investigations, 1994–1998

Outbreak investigations provide some of the most important opportunities for identifying risk factors for disease. The investigations described below were conducted in collaboration with many partners in state and local health departments, other federal agencies, and other organizations.

Year	Location	Problem	Finding	Implications
1994	United States	Hepatitis C[289]	Strong association with particular lots of intravenous (IV) immuno-globulin from one company	Led to requirements for viral inactivation steps and new testing procedures to ensure safety of IV and intramuscular immunoglobulin products.
1994	Rhode Island	Bloodstream infections (BSIs)[290]	BSIs associated with use of inoculation devices. Findings led to CDC recommendations on the use and management of needleless devices.	First outbreak to link these devices with adverse outcomes in patients
1995	Democratic Republic of Congo	Ebola infection[291]	Transmission linked to direct contact with ill patients.	No evidence of airborne transmission. Led to updating of policies for managing patients with viral hemorrhagic fever in the United States.
1996	Indiana	Vancomycin-resistant Enterococci[292]	Illness linked to prior use of antibiotics. Implementation of control measures reduced transmission.	Highlighted rapid spread of this strain in the United States. Also showed feasibility and effectiveness of control measures to reduce the spread of antibiotic-resistant organisms in hospitals.
1997–1998	New York	human immunodeficiency virus (HIV)	Cluster of cases of HIV infection in women who had sex with one HIV-positive man	HIV detection and prevention programs need to be strengthened in rural communities.

Source: Reprinted from Centers for Disease Control and Prevention, *Preventing Emerging Infectious Diseases: A Strategy for the 21st Century,* p. 30, 1998, U.S. Department of Health and Human Services.

Exhibit 3–2 Bloodstream Infections in ICU and Home Health Care Patients

Since 1993, CDC has investigated three outbreaks of bloodstream infection (BSI)[293,294] among patients in intensive care units (ICUs) that were associated with decreases in nurse-to-patient ratios. In each of these outbreaks, rates of BSI increased when the number of health care workers per patient decreased or when the level of training of those workers decreased. The epidemiologic relationship between nursing staff numbers and training levels and the rates of BSIs remained significant even after controlling for other factors.

Since that time, CDC has also investigated three outbreaks of BSIs among patients receiving home infusion therapy.[290,295,296] Risk factors for these outbreaks include practices related to care of the intravenous line, the use of particular types of intravenous devices, and socioeconomic factors. Interventions that involve teaching and training home health care providers and families of home care patients are being evaluated.

Source: Reprinted from Centers for Disease Control and Prevention, *Preventing Emerging Infectious Diseases: A Strategy for the 21st Century,* p. 31, 1998, U.S. Department of Health and Human Services.

procedures that address personnel health and include hand washing and personal hygiene, standard precautions, immunization, and work restrictions for certain infectious diseases. Since many outbreaks involve vaccine-preventable diseases, such as hepatitis B, measles, and chickenpox, Appendix E contains a summary of the ACIP and HICPAC recommendations for the immunization of health care workers.[170] For guidance on developing policies relating to employee health, the reader is also referred to the ACIP recommendations on preventing varicella[185] and measles, mumps and rubella,[176] and the 1998 HICPAC guideline for infection control in health care personnel.[17] The HICPAC summary of recommended work restrictions for personnel can be found in Appendix F.

ADDITIONAL SOURCES OF INFORMATION ON OUTBREAKS IN HOSPITALS

Additional examples of reported outbreaks can be found by accessing the Centers for Disease Control and Prevention Web site at http://www.cdc.gov, as well as in the infection control textbooks edited by Wenzel,[297] Bennett and Brachman,[298] Olmsted,[299] and Mayhall.[300] Information on infection control guidelines and recommendations published by national agencies and organizations can be found in the text edited by Abrutyn, Goldmann, and Scheckler.[301]

REFERENCES

1. LaForce FM. The control of infections in hospitals: 1750 to 1950. In: Wenzel RP, ed. *Prevention and Control of Nosocomial Infections.* Baltimore: Williams & Wilkins; 1987:1–12.

2. Stamm WE, Weinstein RA, Dixon RE. Comparison of endemic and epidemic nosocomial infections. *Am J Med.* 1981;70:393–397.

3. Haley RW, Tenney JH, Lindsey JO, Garner JS, Bennett J. How frequent are outbreaks of nosocomial infection in community hospitals? *Infect Control.* 1985;6:233–236.

4. Jarvis WR, and the Epidemiology Branch, Hospital Infections Program, Centers for Disease Control. Nosocomial outbreaks: the Centers for Disease Control's Hospital Infections Program experience, 1980–1990. *Am J Med.* 1991;91:3B-101S–3B-106S.

5. Beck-Sague C, Jarvis W, Martone WJ. Outbreak investigations. *Infect Control Hosp Epidemiol.* 1997;18:138–145.

6. Jackson M, Fierer J. Infections and infection risk in residents of long-term care facilities: a review of the literature, 1970–1984. *Am J Infect Control.* 1985;13:63–77.

7. Nicolle LE, Garibaldi RA. Infection control in long-term-care facilities. *Infect Control Hosp Epidemiol.* 1995;16:348–353.

8. Smith P, Rusnak PG. Infection prevention and control in the long-term-care facility. *Am J Infect Control.* 1997;25:488–512.

9. Herwaldt LA, Smith SD, Carter CD. Infection control in the outpatient setting. *Infect Control Hosp Epidemiol.* 1998;19:41–74.

10. Bennett JV, Brachman P, eds. *Hospital Infections.* Boston: Little, Brown and Co; 1992:6.

11. Wenzel RP, Thompson RL, Landry SM, et al. Hospital-acquired infections in intensive care unit patients: an overview with emphasis on epidemics. *Infect Control.* 1983;4:371–375.

12. Lederberg J, Shope RE, Oaks SC, eds. *Emerging Infections: Microbial Threats to Health in the United States.* Washington, DC: National Academy Press; 1992.

13. Centers for Disease Control and Prevention. *Addressing Emerging Infectious Disease Threats: A Prevention Strategy for the United States.* US Dept of Health and Human Services; 1994.

14. Ostroff SM. Emerging infectious diseases in the institutional setting: another hot zone. *Infect Control Hosp Epidemiol.* 1996;17:484–489.

15. Wenger P, Tokars J, Brennan P, et al. An outbreak of *Enterobacter hormaechi* infection and colonization in an intensive care nursery. *Clin Infect Dis.* 1997;24:1243–1244.

16. American Public Health Association. *Control of Communicable Diseases Manual.* Benenson AS, ed. 16th ed. Washington, DC: American Public Health Association; 1995.

17. Centers for Disease Control and Prevention. Guideline for infection control in health care personnel, 1998. *Am J Infect Control.* 1998;26:289–354.

18. Centers for Disease Control and Prevention. Guideline for isolation precautions in hospitals. *Am J Infect Control.* 1996;24:24–52.

19. Centers for Disease Control and Prevention. Guideline for prevention of nosocomial pneumonia. *Am J Infect Control.* 1994;22:247–292.

20. Maki DG, Rhame FS, Mackel DC, Bennett JV. Nationwide epidemic of septicemia caused by contaminated intravenous products, I: epidemiologic and clinical features. *Am J Med.* 1976;60:471–485.

21. Centers for Disease Control and Prevention. Epidemiologic notes and reports: nosocomial bacteremias associated with intravenous fluid therapy—USA. *MMWR Morb Mortal Wkly Rep.* 1996;46:1227–1233.

22. Goldmann DA, Dixon RE, Fulkerson CC, et al. The role of nationwide infection surveillance in detecting epidemic bacteremia due to contaminated intravenous fluids. *Am J Epidemiol.* 1978;108:207–213.

23. Kaslow RA, Mackel DC, Mallison GF. Nosocomial pseudobacteremia: positive blood cultures due to contaminated benzalkonium chloride antiseptic. *JAMA.* 1976;236:2407–2409.

24. Wysowski DK, Flynt JW Jr, Goldfield M, Altman R, Davis AT. Epidemic neonatal hyperbilirubinemia and use of a phenolic disinfectant detergent. *Pediatrics.* 1978;61:165–167.

25. Berkelman RL, Lewin S, Allen JR, et al. Pseudobacteremia attributed to contamination of povidone-iodine with *Pseudomonas cepacia. Ann Intern Med.* 1981;95:32–36.

26. Panlilio AL, Beck-Sague CM, Siegel JD, et al. Infections and pseudoinfections due to povidone-iodine solution contaminated with *Pseudomonas cepacia. Clin Infect Dis.* 1992;14:1078–1083.

27. Sharbaugh RJ. Suspected outbreak of endotoxemia associated with computerized axial tomography. *Am J Infect Control.* 1980;8:26–28.

28. Cleary TJ, MacIntyre DS, Castro M. *Serratia marcescens* bacteremias in an intensive care unit. *Am J Infect Control.* 1998;9:107–111.

29. Bryce EA, Walker M, Scharf S, et al. An outbreak of cutaneous aspergillosis in a tertiary-care hospital. *Infect Control Hosp Epidemiol.* 1996;17:170–172.

30. Parrott PL, Terry PM, Whitworth EN, et al. *Pseudomonas aeruginosa* peritonitis associated with contaminated poloxamer-iodine solution. *Lancet.* 1982;2:683–685.

31. Martone WJ, Williams WW, Mortensen ML, et al. Illness with fatalities in premature infants: association with intravenous vitamin E preparation, E-Ferol. *Pediatrics.* 1986;78:591–600.

32. Safranek TJ, Jarvis WR, Carson LA, et al. *Mycobacterium chelonae* wound infections after plastic surgery employing contaminated gentian violet skin-marking solution. *N Engl J Med.* 1987;317:197–201.

33. Nakashima AK, McCarthy MA, Martone WJ, Anderson RL. Epidemic septic arthritis caused by *Serratia marcescens* and associated with a benzalkonium chloride antiseptic. *J Clin Microbiol.* 1987;25:1014–1018.

34. Centers for Disease Control. *Yersinia enterocolitica* bacteremia and endotoxin shock associated with red blood cell transfusion—United States, 1987–1988. *MMWR Morb Mortal Wkly Rep.* 1988;37:577–578.

35. Centers for Disease Control and Prevention. Red blood cell transfusions contaminated with *Yersinia enterocolitica*—United States, 1991–1996, and initiation of a national study to detect bacteria-associated transfusion reactions. *MMWR Morb Mortal Wkly Rep.* 1997;46:553–556.

36. Vargo LR, Le CT, Lee KK. Transfusion-acquired hepatitis A outbreak from fresh frozen plasma in a neonatal intensive care unit. Presented at: Third Decennial International Conference on Nosocomial Infections; July 31–August 3, 1990; Atlanta, GA. Abstract 61.

37. Centers for Disease Control. Postsurgical infections associated with an extrinsically contaminated intravenous anesthetic agent—Califor-

nia, Illinois, Maine, and Michigan, 1990. *MMWR Morb Mortal Wkly Rep.* 1990;39:426–427, 433.

38. Bennett SN, McNeil MM, Bland LA, et al. Postoperative infections traced to contamination of an intravenous anesthetic, propofol. *N Engl J Med.* 1995;333:147–154.

39. Kuehnert MJ, Webb RM, Jochimsen EM, et al. *Staphylococcus aureus* bloodstream infections among patients undergoing electroconvulsive therapy traced to breaks in infection control and possible extrinsic contamination by propofol. *Anesth Analg.* 1997;85:420–425.

40. Maki DG, Klein BS, McCormick R, et al. Nosocomial *Pseudomonas pickettii* bacteremias traced to narcotic tampering. *JAMA.* 1991;265:981–986.

41. Centers for Disease Control and Prevention. Outbreak of hepatitis C associated with intravenous immunoglobulin administration—United States, October 1993–June 1994. *MMWR Morb Mortal Wkly Rep.* 1994;43:505–509.

42. Hamill RJ, Houston ED, Georghiou PR, et al. An outbreak of *Burkholderia cepacia* respiratory tract colonization and infection associated with nebulized albuterol therapy. *Ann Intern Med.* 1995;122:762–766.

43. Reboli AC, Koshinski R, Arias K, et al. An outbreak of *Burkholderia cepacia* lower respiratory tract infection associated with contaminated albuterol nebulization solution. *Infect Control Hosp Epidemiol.* 1996;17:741–743.

44. Trilla A, Codina C, Salles M, et al. A cluster of fever and hypotension on a surgical intensive care unit related to the contamination of plasma expanders by cell wall products of *Bacillus stearothermophilus. Infect Control Hosp Epidemiol.* 1995;16:335–339.

45. File TM, Tan JS, Thomson RB, et al. An outbreak of *Pseudomonas aeruginosa* ventilator-associated respiratory infections due to contaminated food coloring dye—further evidence of the significance of gastric colonization proceeding nosocomial pneumonia. *Infect Control Hosp Epidemiol.* 1995;16:417–418.

46. Anglim AM, Collmer JE, Loving J, et al. An outbreak of needlestick injuries in hospital employees due to needles piercing infectious waste containers. *Infect Control Hosp Epidemiol.* 1995;16:570–576.

47. Larkin JA, Greene JN, Sandin RL, Houston SH. Primary cutaneous aspergillosis: case report and review of the literature. *Infect Control Hosp Epidemiol.* 1996;17:365–366.

48. Orth B, Frei R, Itin PH, et al. Outbreak of invasive mycoses caused by *Paecilomyces lilacinus* from a contaminated skin lotion. *Ann Intern Med.* 1996;125:799–806.

49. Axelrod P, St. John K, Palumbo A, et al. An outbreak of gram negative colonization and infection in a newborn ICU linked to contamination during formula preparation. Presented at: Seventh Annual Meeting of the Society for Healthcare Epidemiology of America; April 27–29, 1997; St. Louis, MO. Abstract 64.

50. Wang SA, Tokars JI, Carson LA, et al. Bacteremia associated with intrinsically contaminated human albumin. Presented at: Seventh Annual Meeting of the Society for Healthcare Epidemiology of America; April 27–29, 1997; St. Louis, MO. Abstract 65.

51. Shay DK, Fann LM, Jarvis WR. Respiratory distress and sudden death associated with receipt of a peripheral parenteral nutrition admixture. *Infect Control Hosp Epidemiol.* 1997;18:814–817.

52. Archibald LK, Shah B, Schulte M, et al. *Serratia marcescens* outbreak associated with extrinsic contamination of 1% chloroxylenol soap. *Infect Control Hosp Epidemiol.* 1997;18:704–709.

53. Chetoui H, Melin P, Struelens MJ, et al. Comparison of biotyping, ribotyping, and pulsed-field gel electrophoresis for investigation of a

common-source outbreak of *Burkholderia pickettii* bacteremia. *J Clin Microbiol.* 1997;35:1398–1403.

54. Mangam AJ, Archibald LK, Hupert M, et al. Nationwide outbreak of sterile peritonitis among continuous cycling peritoneal dialysis patients associated with intrinsically contaminated dialysis fluid. Presented at: Seventh Annual Meeting of the Society for Healthcare Epidemiology of America; April 27–29, 1997; St. Louis, MO. Abstract 48.

55. Van Laer F, Raes D, Vandamme P, et al. An outbreak of *Burkholderia cepacia* with septicemia on a cardiology ward. *Infect Control Hosp Epidemiol.* 1998;19:112–113.

56. Centers for Disease Control and Prevention. Nosocomial *Ralstonia pickettii* colonization associated with intrinsically contaminated saline solution—Los Angeles, California, 1998. *MMWR Morb Mortal Wkly Rep.* 1998;47:285–286.

57. Centers for Disease Control and Prevention. Endotoxin-like reactions associated with intravenous gentamicin—California, 1998. *MMWR Morb Mortal Wkly Rep.* 1998;47:877–880.

58. Centers for Disease Control and Prevention. *Enterobacter cloacae* bloodstream infections associated with contaminated prefilled saline syringes—California, November 1998. *MMWR Morb Mortal Wkly Rep.* 1998;47:959–960.

59. Centers for Disease Control and Prevention. Nosocomial *Burkholderia cepacia* infection and colonization associated with intrinsically contaminated mouthwash—Arizona, 1996–1998. *MMWR Morb Mortal Wkly Rep.* 1998;47:926–928.

60. Sautter RL, Mattman LH, Legaspi, RC. *Serratia marcescens* meningitis associated with a contaminated benzalkonium chloride solution. *Infect Control.* 1984;5:223–225.

61. Simmons BP. CDC guidelines for the prevention and control of nosocomial infections: guideline for hospital environmental control. *Am J Infect Control.* 1983;11:97–115.

62. Dixon RE, Kaslow RA, Mackel DC, et al. Aqueous quarternary ammonium antiseptics and disinfectants: use and misuse. *JAMA.* 1976;236:2415–2417.

63. Rutala WA. APIC guideline for selection and use of disinfectants. *Am J Infect Control.* 1996;24:313–342.

64. Donowitz LG. Benzalkonium chloride is still in use. *Infect Control Hosp Epidemiol.* 1991;12:186–187.

65. Larson EL, and the APIC Guidelines Committee. APIC guideline for handwashing and hand antisepsis in health care settings. *Am J Infect Control.* 1995;23:251–269.

66. France DR. Survival of *Candida albicans* in hand creams. *N Z J Med.* 1968;67:552–554.

67. Morse LJ, Williams HL, Grann FP, et al. Septicemia due to *Klebsiella pneumoniae* originating from a hand cream dispenser. *N Engl J Med.* 1967;277:472–473.

68. Morse LJ, Schonbeck LE. Hand lotions—a potential nosocomial hazard. *N Engl J Med.* 1968;278:376–378.

69. Anderson K. The contamination of hexachlorophene soap with *Pseudomonas pyocyanea. Med J Aust.* 1962;2:463.

70. Sprach DH, Silverstein FE, Stamm WE. Transmission of infection by gastrointestinal endoscopy and bronchoscopy. *Ann Intern Med.* 1993;118:117–128.

71. Struelens MJ, Rost F, Deplano A, et al. *Pseudomonas aeruginosa* and *Enterobacteriaceae* bacteremia after biliary endoscopy: an outbreak investigation using DNA macrorestriction analysis. *Am J Med.* 1993;95:489–498.

72. Alvarado CJ, Stolz SM, Maki DG. Nosocomial infections from contaminated endoscopes: a flawed automated endoscope washer: an investigation using molecular epidemiology. *Am J Med.* 1991;91: 272S–280S.

73. Schliessler KH, Rozendaal B, Taal C, Meawissen SGM. Outbreak of *Salmonella agona* after upper intestinal fiberoptic endoscopy. *Lancet.* 1980;2:1246.

74. Birnie GG, Quigley EM, Clements GB, Follet EAC, Watkinson G. Endoscopic transmission of hepatitis B virus. *Gut.* 1983;24:171–174.

75. Bronowicki JP, Venard V, Botte C, et al. Patient-to-patient transmission of hepatitis C virus during colonoscopy. *N Engl J Med.* 1997;337:237–240.

76. Allen JI, O'Connor AM, Olson MM, et al. *Pseudomonas* infection of the biliary system resulting from use of a contaminated endoscope. *Gastroenterology.* 1987;92:759–763.

77. Nelson KE, Larson PA, Schraufnagel DE, Jackson J. Transmission of tuberculosis by flexible fiberbronchoscopes. *Am Rev Respir Dis.* 1983;127:97–100.

78. Wheeler PW, Lancaster D, Kaiser AB. Bronchopulmonary cross-contamination and infection related to mycobacterial contamination of suction valves of bronchoscopes. *J Infect Dis.*1989;159:954–958.

79. Blanc DS, Parret T, Janin B, et al. Nosocomial infections and pseudoinfections from contaminated bronchoscopes: two-year follow-up using molecular markers. *Infect Control Hosp Epidemiol.* 1997;18:134–136.

80. Gubler JG, Salfinger M, von Graevenitz A. Pseudoepidemic of nontuberculous mycobacteria due to a contaminated bronchoscope cleaning machine: report of an outbreak and review of the literature. *Chest.* 1992;101:1245–1249.

81. Agerton T, Valway S, Gore B, et al. Transmission of a highly drug-resistant strain (Strain W1) of *Mycobacterium tuberculosis*: community outbreak and nosocomial transmission via a contaminated bronchoscope. *JAMA.* 1997;278:1073–1077.

82. Weems JJ. Nosocomial outbreak of *Pseudomonas cepacia* associated with contamination of reusable electronic ventilator temperature probes. *Infect Control Hosp Epidemiol.* 1993;14:583–586.

83. Conly JM, Klass L, Larson L, et al. *Pseudomonas cepacia* colonization and infection in intensive care units. *Can Med Assoc J.* 1986;134:363–366.

84. Rudnick JR, Beck-Sague CM, Anderson RL, Schable B, Miller JM, Jarvis WR. Gram-negative bacteremia in open-heart-surgery patients traced to probable tap-water contamination of pressure-monitoring equipment. *Infect Control Hosp Epidemiol.* 1996;17:281–285.

85. Weinstein RA, Emori TG, Anderson RL, Stamm WE. Pressure transducers as a source of bacteremia after open heart surgery: report of an outbreak and guidelines for prevention. *Chest.* 1976;69:338–344.

86. Beck-Sague CM, Jarvis WR. Epidemic bloodstream infections associated with pressure transducers: a persistent problem. *Infect Control Hosp Epidemiol.* 1989;10:54–59.

87. Centers for Disease Control and Prevention. Guideline for prevention of intravascular device-related infections. *Am J Infect Control.* 1996;24:262–293.

88. Centers for Disease Control. Hepatitis B associated with jet gun injection—California. *MMWR Morb Mortal Wkly Rep.* 1986; 35:373–376.

89. Centers for Disease Control. Nosocomial transmission of hepatitis B virus associated with a spring-loaded finger stick device—California. *MMWR Morb Mortal Wkly Rep.* 1990;39:610–613.

90. Centers for Disease Control and Prevention. Nosocomial hepatitis B virus infection associated with reusable fingerstick blood sampling devices—Ohio and New York City, 1996. *MMWR Morb Mortal Wkly Rep.* 1997;46:217–221.

91. Hamill RJ, Wright CE, Andres N, Koza MA. Urinary tract infection following instrumentation for urodynamic testing. *Infect Control Hosp Epidemiol.* 1989;10:26–32.

92. Climo MW, Pastor A, Wong ES. An outbreak of *Pseudomonas aeruginosa* related to contaminated urodynamic equipment. *Infect Control Hosp Epidemiol.* 1997;18:509–510.

93. Livornese L, Dias S, Samel C, et al. Hospital-acquired infection with vancomycin-resistant *Enterococcus faecium* transmitted by electronic thermometers. *Ann Intern Med.* 1992;117:112–116.

94. Arnow PM, Garcia-Houchins S, Neagle MB, Bova JL, Dillon JJ, Chou T. An outbreak of bloodstream infections arising from hemodialysis equipment. *J Infect Dis.* 1998;178:783–791.

95. Durante L, Zulty JC, Israel E, et al. Investigation of an outbreak of bloody diarrhea: association with endoscopic cleaning solution and demonstration of lesions in an animal model. *Am J Med.* 1992;92: 476–480.

96. Burtin P, Ruget O, Petit R, Boyer J. Gluteraldehyde-induced proctitis after anorectal ultrasound examination: a higher risk of incidence than expected? *Gastrointest Endosc.* 1993;39:859–860.

97. Favero MS, Alter MJ, Bland LE. Nosocomial infections associated with hemodialysis. In: Mayhall CG, ed. *Hospital Epidemiology and Infection Control.* Philadelphia: Williams & Wilkins; 1996:693–714.

98. Beck-Sague CM, Jarvis WR, Bland LA, Arduino MJ, Aguero SM, Verosic G. Outbreak of gram-negative bacteremia and pyrogenic reactions in a hemodialysis center. *Am J Nephrol.* 1990;10:397–403.

99. Welbel SF, Schoendorf K, Bland LA, et al. An outbreak of gram-negative bloodstream infections in chronic hemodialysis patients. *Am J Nephrol.* 1995;15:1–4.

100. Flaherty JP, Garcia-Houchins S, Chudy R, Arnow PM. An outbreak of gram-negative bacteremia traced to contaminated O-rings and reprocessed dialyzers. *Ann Intern Med.* 1993;119:1072–1078.

101. Centers for Disease Control and Prevention. Outbreaks of hepatitis B virus infection among hemodialysis patients—California, Nebraska, and Texas, 1994. *MMWR Morb Mortal Wkly Rep.* 1996;45:285–289.

102. Band JD, Ward JI, Fraser DW. Peritonitis due to a *mycobacterium chelonei*-like organism with intermittent chronic peritoneal dialysis. *J Infect Dis.* 1982;145:9–17.

103. Berkelman RL, Godley J, Weber JA, et al. *Pseudomonas cepacia* peritonitis associated with contamination of automatic peritoneal dialysis machines. *Ann Intern Med.* 1982;96:456–458.

104. Ayliffe GA. Nosocomial infection associated with endoscopy. In: Mayhall CG, ed. *Hospital Epidemiology and Infection Control.* Philadelphia: Williams & Wilkins; 1996:680–693.

105. Weber DJ, Rutala WA. Nosocomial infections associated with respiratory therapy. In: Mayhall CG, ed. *Hospital Epidemiology and Infection Control.* Philadelphia: Williams & Wilkins; 1996:748–758.

106. Kaczmarek RG, Moore RM, McCrohan J, et al. Multi-state investigation of the actual disinfection/sterilization of endoscopes in health care facilities. *Am J Med.* 1992;92:257–261.

107. Gorse GJ, Messner RL. Infection control practices in gastrointestinal endoscopy in the United States: a national survey. *Infect Control Hosp Epidemiol.* 1991;12:289–296.

108. American Society for Gastrointestinal Endoscopy. Infection control during gastrointestinal endoscopy: guidelines for clinical application. *Gastrointest Endosc.* 1988;34(suppl):37S–40S.

109. Members of the American Society for Gastrointestinal Endoscopy Ad Hoc Committee on Disinfection. Reprocessing of flexible gastrointestinal endoscopes: position statement. *Gastrointest Endosc.* 1996;43:540–546.

110. Martin MA, Reichelderfer M. APIC guideline for infection prevention and control in flexible endoscopy. *Am J Infect Control.* 1994;22:19–38.

111. Tokars JI, Miller ER, Alter MJ, Arduino MJ. National surveillance of dialysis-associated diseases in the United States, 1995. *Am Soc Artif Intern Organs J.* 1998;44:98–107.

112. Association for the Advancement of Medical Instrumentation. *Dialysis. AAMI Standards and Recommended Practices,* vol 3. Arlington, VA: AAMI; 1998.

113. Bassett DCJ, Stokes KJ, Thomas WRG. Wound infection with *Pseudomonas multivorans.* A waterborne contaminant of disinfectant solutions. *Lancet.* 1970;1:1188–1191.

114. Everett ED, Pearson S, Rogers W. *Rhizopus* surgical wound infection associated with elasticized adhesive tape dressing. *Arch Surg.* 1979;114:738–739.

115. Keys TF, Haldorson AM, Rhodes KH, Roberts GD, Fifer EZ. Nosocomial outbreak of *Rhizopus* infections associated with Elastoplast wound dressings—Minnesota. *MMWR Morb Mortal Wkly Rep.* 1978;27:33–34.

116. Pearson RD, Valenti WM, Steigbigel RT. *Clostridium perfringens* wound infections associated with elastic bandages. *JAMA.* 1980;244:1128–1130.

117. Mitchell RG, Hayward AC. Postoperative urinary tract infections caused by contaminated irrigating fluid. *Lancet.* 1966;1:793–795.

118. Geiss HK, Schmitt J, Frank SC. Bleeding after cardiovascular surgery caused by detergent residues in laparotomy sponges. *Infect Control Hosp Epidemiol.* 1997;18:579–581.

119. Courtright P, Lewallen S, Holland SP, Wendt TM. Corneal decompensation after cataract surgery: an outbreak investigation in Asia. *Ophthalmology.* 1995;102:1461–1465.

120. Wenzel RP. Healthcare workers and the incidence of nosocomial infection: can treatment of one influence the other?—a brief review. *J Chemother.* 1994;4:33–40.

121. Dineen P, Drudin L. Epidemics of postoperative wound infection associated with hair carriers. *Lancet.* 1973;2:1157–1159.

122. Kreiswirth BN, Kravitz GR, Schlievert PM, Novick RP. Nosocomial transmission of a strain of *Staphylococcus aureus* causing toxic shock syndrome. *Ann Intern Med.* 1986;105:704–707.

123. Belani A, Sheretz RJ, Sullivan ML, Russell BA, Reumen PD. Outbreak of staphylococcal infection in two nurseries traced to a single carrier. *Infect Control.* 1986;7:487–490.

124. Sheretz RJ, Reagan DR, Hampton KD, et al. A cloud adult: the *Staphylococcus aureus*-virus interaction revisited. *Ann Intern Med.* 1996;124:539–547.

125. Slutsker L. Villarino ME, Jarvis WR, Goulding J. Foodborne disease prevention in healthcare facilities. In: Bennett JV, Brachman PS, eds. *Hospital Infections.* 4th ed. Philadelphia: Lippincott-Raven Publishers; 1998:22–341.

126. Weber DJ, Rutala WA, Denny FW. Management of healthcare workers with pharyngitis or suspected streptococcal infections. *Infect Control Hosp Epidemiol.* 1996;17:753–761.

127. Mastro TD, Farley TA, Elliot JA, et al. An outbreak of surgical wound infections due to group A streptococcus carried on the scalp. *N Engl J Med.* 1990;32:968–972.

128. Stamm WE, Feeley JC, Facklam RR. Wound infections due to group A streptococcus traced to a vaginal carrier. *J Infect Dis.* 1978;138: 287–292.

129. Berkelman RL, Martin D, Graham DR, et al. Streptococcal wound infections caused by a vaginal carrier. *JAMA.* 1982;247:2680–2682.

130. Schaffner W, Lefkowitz LB Jr, Goodman JS, Koenig MG. Hospital outbreak of infections with group A streptococci traced to an asymptomatic anal carrier. *N Engl J Med.* 1969;280:1224–1225.

131. Viglionese A, Nottebart VF, Bodman HA, Platt R. Recurrent group A streptococcal carriage in a health care worker associated with widely separated nosocomial outbreaks. *Am J Med.* 1991;91(suppl 3B):329S–333S.

132. Paul SM, Genese C, Spitalny K. Postoperative group A beta-hemolytic streptococcus outbreak with the pathogen traced to a member of a healthcare worker's household. *Infect Control Hosp Epidemiol.* 1990;11:643–646.

133. Ridgway EJ, Allen KD. Clustering of group A streptococcal infections on a burns unit: important lessons in outbreak management. *J Hosp Infect.* 1993;25:173–182.

134. Isenberg HD, Tucci V, Lipsitz P, Facklam RR. Clinical laboratory and epidemiological investigations of a *Streptococcus pyogenes* cluster epidemic in a newborn nursery. *J Clin Microbiol.* 1984;19:366–370.

135. Ramage L, Green K, Pyskir D, Simor AE. An outbreak of fatal infections due to group A streptococcus on a medical ward. *Infect Control Hosp Epidemiol.* 1996;17:429–431.

136. Lannigan R, Hussain Z, Austin TW. *Streptococcus pyogenes* as a cause of nosocomial infection in a critical care unit. *Diagn Microbiol Infect Dis.* 1985;3:337–341.

137. Schwartz B, Elliott JA, Butler JC, et al. Clusters of invasive group A streptococcal infections in family, hospital, and nursing home settings. *Clin Infect Dis.* 1992;15:277–284.

138. Decker MD, Lavely GB, Hutcheson RH, Schaffner W. Foodborne streptococcal pharyngitis in a hospital pediatrics clinic. *JAMA.* 1985;253:679–681.

139. Pertowski CA, Baron RC, Lasker BA, Werner SB, Jarvis WR. Nosocomial outbreak of *Candida albicans* sternal wound infections following cardiac surgery traced to a scrub nurse. *J Infect Dis.* 1995;172:817–822.

140. Isenberg HD, Tucci V, Cintron F, et al. Single source outbreak of *Candida tropicalis* complicating coronary bypass surgery. *J Clin Microbiol.* 1989;27:2426–2428.

141. Wegener PN, Brown JM, McNeil MM, Jarvis WR. *Nocardia farcinica* sternotomy site infections in patients following open heart surgery. *J Infect Dis.* 1998;178:1539–1543.

142. Exmelin L, Malbruny B, Vergnaud M, Provost F, Boiron P, Morel C. Molecular study of nosocomial nocardiosis outbreak involving heart transplant recipients. *J Clin Microbiol.* 1996;34:1014–1016.

143. AIDS/TB Committee of the Society for Healthcare Epidemiology of America. Management of healthcare workers infected with hepatitis B virus, hepatitis C virus, human immunodeficiency virus, or other bloodborne pathogens. *Infect Control Hosp Epidemiol.* 1997;18:349–363.

144. Bell D, Shapiro CN, Chamberland ME, Ciesielski CA. Preventing bloodborne pathogen transmission from healthcare workers to patients: the CDC perspective. *Surg Clin North Am.* 1995;75:1189–1203.

145. Prentice MB, Flower AJE, Morgan GM, et al. Infection with hepatitis B virus after open heart surgery. *BMJ.* 1992;304:761–764.

146. Centers for Disease Control. Recommendations for preventing transmission of human immunodeficiency virus and hepatitis B virus to patients during exposure-prone invasive procedures. *MMWR Morb Mortal Wkly Rep.* 1991;40(RR-8):1–9.

147. Bond WW, Favero MS, Petersen NJ, Gravelle CR, Ebert JW, Maynard JE. Survival of hepatitis B virus after drying and storage for one week. *Lancet.* 1981;27:550–551.

148. Oren I, Hershow RC, Ben-Porath E, et al. A common-source outbreak of fulminant hepatitis B in a hospital. *Ann Intern Med.* 1989;110:691–698.

149. Centers for Disease Control and Prevention. Improper infection-control practices during employee vaccination programs—District of Columbia and Pennsylvania, 1993. *MMWR Morb Mortal Wkly Rep.* 1993;42:969–971.

150. Centers for Disease Control and Prevention. Recommendations for prevention and control of hepatitis C virus (HCV) infection and HCV-related chronic disease. *MMWR Morb Mortal Wkly Rep.* 1998;47(RR-19):1–39.

151. Esteban JI, Gomez J, Martell M, et al. Transmission of hepatitis C virus by a cardiac surgeon. *N Engl J Med.* 1996;334:555–560.

152. Centers for Disease Control. Update: transmission of human immunodeficiency virus infection during an invasive dental procedure—Florida. *MMWR Morb Mortal Wkly Rep.*1991;40:21–33.

153. Ciesielski CA, Marianos DW, Schochetman G, Witte JJ, Jaffe J. The 1990 Florida dental investigations: the press and the science. *Ann Intern Med.* 1994;121:886–888.

154. Lot F, Seguier JC, Fegueux S, et al. Probable transmission of HIV from an orthopedic surgeon to a patient in France. *Ann Intern Med.* 1999;130:1–6.

155. American Academy of Orthopedic Surgeons, Task Force on AIDS and Orthopedic Surgery. *Recommendations for the Prevention of Human Immunodeficiency Virus (HIV) Transmission in the Practice of Orthopedic Surgery.* Park Ridge, IL: American Academy of Orthopedic Surgeons; 1989.

156. Committee on Ethics, American College of Obstetricians and Gynecologists. Human immunodeficiency virus infection: physicians' responsibilities. *Obstet Gynecol.* 1990;75:1043–1045.

157. Centers for Disease Control. Foodborne nosocomial outbreak of *Salmonella reading*—Connecticut. *MMWR Morb Mortal Wkly Rep.* 1991;40:804–806.

158. Opal SM, Mayer KH, Roland F, Brondum J, Heelan J, Lyhte L. Investigation of a food-borne outbreak of salmonellosis among hospital employees. *Am J Infect Control.* 1989;17:141–147.

159. Perlino CA, Parrish CM, Terry PM. *Salmonella infantis* outbreak in neonates in an intermediate intensive care nursery. Presented at: Third Decennial International Conference on Nosocomial Infections; July 31–August 3, 1990; Atlanta, GA. Abstract 62.

160. Stone A, Shaffner M, Sautter R. *Salmonella poona* infection and surveillance in a neonatal nursery. *Am J Infect Control.* 1993;21:270–273.

161. Meyers JD, Romm FJ, Tihen WS, Bryan JA. Food-borne hepatitis A in a general hospital: epidemiologic study of an outbreak attributed to sandwiches. *JAMA.* 1975;231:1049–1053.

162. Eisenstein AB, Aach RD, Jacobsohn W, Goldman A. An epidemic of infectious hepatitis in a general hospital: probable transmission by contaminated orange juice. *JAMA.* 1963;185:171–174.

163. Rosenblum LS, Villarino ME, Naina OV, et al. Hepatitis A outbreak in a neonatal intensive care unit: risk factors for transmission and evidence of prolonged viral excretion among preterm infants. *J Infect Dis.* 1991;164:476–482.

164. Azimi PH, Roberto RR, Guralnik J, et al. Transfusion-acquired hepatitis A in a premature infant with secondary nosocomial spread in an intensive care nursery. *Am J Dis Child.* 1986;140:23–27.

165. Noble RC, Kane MA, Reeves SA, Roeckel I. Posttransfusion hepatitis A in a neonatal intensive care unit. *JAMA.* 1984;252:2711–2715.

166. Centers for Disease Control and Prevention. Prevention of hepatitis A through active or passive immunization: recommendations of the Ad-

visory Committee on Immunization Practices (ACIP). *MMWR Morb Mortal Wkly Rep.* 1996;45(RR-15):1–30.

167. Doebbeling BN, Li N, Wenzel RP. An outbreak of hepatitis A among health care workers: risk factors for transmission. *Am J Public Health.* 1993;83:1679–1684.

168. Drusin LM, Sohmer M, Groshen SL, Spiritos MD, Senterfit LB, Christenson WN. Nosocomial hepatitis A infection in a pediatric intensive care unit. *Arch Dis Child.* 1987;62:690–695.

169. Goodman RA, Carder CC, Allen JR, Orenstein WA, Finton RJ. Nosocomial hepatitis A transmission by an adult patient with diarrhea. *Am J Med.* 1982;73:220–226..

170. Centers for Disease Control and Prevention. Immunization of healthcare workers: recommendations of the Advisory Committee on Immunization Practices (ACIP) and the Hospital Infection Control Practices Advisory Committee (HICPAC). *MMWR Morb Mortal Wkly Rep.* 1997;46(RR-18):1–42.

171. Eickhoff TC. Airborne nosocomial infection: a contemporary perspective. *Infect Control Hosp Epidemiol.* 1994;15:663–672.

172. Sepkowicz KA. Occupationally acquired infections in health care workers, pt I. *Ann Intern Med.* 1996;125:826–834.

173. Atkinson WL. Measles and healthcare workers. *Infect Control Hosp Epidemiol.* 1994;15:5–7.

174. Gurevich I, Barzarga RA, Cuhna BA. Measles: lessons from an outbreak. *Am J Infect Control.* 1992;20:319–325.

175. Rank EL, Brettman L, Katz-Pollack H, DeHertogh D, Neville D. Chronology of a hospital-wide measles outbreak: lessons learned and shared from an extraordinary week in late March 1989. *Am J Infect Control.* 1992;20:315–318.

176. Centers for Disease Control and Prevention. Measles, mumps, and rubella—vaccine use and strategies for elimination of measles, rubella, and congenital rubella syndrome and control of mumps: recommendations of the Advisory Committee on Immunization Practices (ACIP). *MMWR Morb Mortal Wkly Rep.* 1998;47(RR-8):1–57.

177. American Academy of Pediatrics. Measles. In: American Academy of Pediatrics. *1997 Red book: Report of the Committee on Infectious Diseases.* Peter G, ed. 24th ed. Elk Grove Village, IL: American Academy of Pediatrics; 1997:334–357.

178. Rivera ME, Mason WH, Ross LA, Wright HT Jr. Nosocomial measles infection in a pediatric hospital during a community-wide epidemic. *J Pediatr.* 1991;119:183–186.

179. Houck P, Scott-Johnson G, Krebs L. Measles immunity among community hospital employees. *Infect Control Hosp Epidemiol.* 1991;12:663–668.

180. Weber DJ, Rutala WA, Hamilton H. Prevention and control of varicella-zoster infections in healthcare facilities. *Infect Control Hosp Epidemiol.* 1996;17:694–705.

181. Sawyer MH, Chamberlain CJ, Wu YN, Aintablian N, Wallace MR. Detection of varicella-zoster virus DNA in air samples from hospital rooms. *J Infect Dis.* 1994;169:91–94.

182. Leclair JM, Zaia JA, Levin MJ, Congdon RG, Goldmann DA. Airborne transmission of chickenpox in a hospital. *N Engl J Med.* 1980;302:450–453.

183. Faoagali JL, Darcy D. Chickenpox outbreak among the staff of a large, urban adult hospital: costs of monitoring and control. *Am J Infect Control.* 1995;23:247–250.

184. Gustafson TL, Lavely GB, Brawner ER, Hutcheson RH, Wright PF, Schaffner W. An outbreak of airborne nosocomial varicella. *Pediatrics.* 1982;70:550–556.

185. Centers for Disease Control and Prevention. Prevention of varicella: recommendations of the Advisory Committee on Immunization Practices (ACIP). *MMWR Morb Mortal Wkly Rep.* 1996;45(RR-11):1–36.

186. Brawley RL, Wenzel RP. An algorithm for chickenpox exposure. *Pediatr Infect Dis J.* 1984;3:502–504.

187. Stover BH, Bratcher DF. Varicella-zoster virus: infection, control and prevention. *Am J Infect Control.* 1998;26:369–381.

188. Levandowski RA, Rubenis M. Nosocomial conjunctivitis caused by adenovirus Type 4. *J Infect Dis.* 1981;143:28–31.

189. Brummit CF, Cherrington JM, Katzenstein DA. Nosocomial adenovirus infections: molecular epidemiology of an outbreak due to adenovirus 3a. *J Infect Dis.* 1988;158:423–432.

190. Birenbaum E, Linder N, Varsano N, et al. Adenovirus type 8 conjunctivitis outbreak in a neonatal intensive care unit. *Arch Dis Child.* 1993;68:610–611.

191. Wharton M, Cochi SL, Hutcheson RH, Schaffner W. Mumps transmission in hospitals. *Arch Intern Med.* 1990;150:47–49.

192. Fischer PR, Brunetti C, Welch V, Christenson JC. Nosocomial mumps: report of an outbreak and its control. *Am J Infect Control.* 1996;24:13–18.

193. Shishiba T, Matsunaga Y. An outbreak of erythema infectiosum among hospital staff members including a patient with pleural fluid and pericardial effusion. *J Am Acad Dermatol.* 1993;29:265–267.

194. Seng C, Watkins P, Morse D, et al. Parvovirus B19 outbreak on an adult ward. *Epidemiol Infect.* 1994;113:345–353.

195. Pillay D, Patou G, Hurt S, Kibbler CC, Griffiths PD. Parvovirus B19 outbreak in a children's ward. *Lancet.* 1992;339:107–109.

196. Poland GA, Nichol KL. Medical students as sources of rubella and measles outbreaks. *Arch Intern Med.* 1990;150:44–46.

197. Fliegel PE, Weinstein WM. Rubella outbreak in a prenatal clinic: management and prevention. *Am J Infect Control.* 1982;10:29–33.

198. Polk FB, White JA, DeGirolami PC, Modlin JF. An outbreak of rubella among hospital personnel. *N Engl J Med.* 1980;303:541–545.

199. Klausner JD, Passaro D, Rosenberg J, et al. Enhanced control of *Mycoplasma pneumoniae* pneumonia with azithromycin prophylaxis. *J Infect Dis.* 1998;177:161–166.

200. Hall CB. Nosocomial viral respiratory infections: perennial weeds on pediatric wards. *Am J Med.* 1981;70:670–676.

201. Hall CB, Douglas RG Jr. Possible transmission by fomites of respiratory syncytial virus. *J Infect Dis.* 1980;141:98–102.

202. Hall CB. Respiratory syncytial virus: its transmission in the hospital environment. *Yale J Biol Med.* 1982;55:219–223.

203. Hall CB. The nosocomial spread of respiratory syncytial viral infections. *Annu Rev Med.* 1983;34:311–319.

204. Snydman DR, Greer C, Meissner HC, McIntosh K. Prevention of nosocomial transmission of respiratory syncytial virus in a newborn nursery. *Infect Control Hosp Epidemiol.* 1988;9:105–108.

205. Falsey AR. Noninfluenza respiratory virus infection in long-term care facilities. *Infect Control Hosp Epidemiol.* 1991;12:602–608.

206. Sorvillo FJ, Huie SF, Strassburg MA, Butsumyo A, Shandera WAX, Fannin SL. An outbreak of respiratory syncytial virus pneumonia in a nursing home for the elderly. *J Infect.* 1984;9:252–256.

207. Harrington RD, Hooton TM, Hackman RC, et al. An outbreak of respiratory syncytial virus in a bone marrow transplant center. *J Infect Dis.* 1992;165:987–993.

208. Guidry GG, Black-Payne CA, Payne DK, Jamison RM, George RB, Bocchini JA Jr. Respiratory syncytial virus infection among intubated adults in a university intensive care unit. *Chest.* 1991;100:1377–1384.

209. Valenti WM, Clarke TA, Hall CB, et al. Concurrent outbreaks of rhinovirus and respiratory syncytial virus in an intensive care nursery: epidemiology and associated risk factors. *J Pediatr.* 1982;100:722–726.

210. Reed KL, Minnich LL, Hernandez JE. Control of a simultaneous outbreak of influenza A and respiratory syncytial virus in an inpatient rehabilitation unit. *Infect Control Hosp Epidemiol.* 1996;17:474. Abstract LB-4.

211. Centers for Disease Control. Summary of notifiable diseases, United States, 1996. *MMWR Morb Mortal Wkly Rep.* 1991;45:10,46–47.

212. Long SS, Welkon CJ, Clark JL. Widespread silent transmission of pertussis in families: antibody correlates of infection and symptomatology. *J Infect Dis.* 1990;161:480–486.

213. Black S. Epidemiology of pertussis. *Pediatr Infect Dis J.* 1997;16:S85–S89.

214. Weber DJ, Rutala WA. Pertussis: an underappreciated risk for nosocomial outbreaks. *Infect Control Hosp Epidemiol.* 1998;19:825–828.

215. Cherry JD. Nosocomial pertussis in the nineties. *Infect Control Hosp Epidemiol.* 1995;16:553–555.

216. Kurt TL, Yeager AS, Guenette S, Dunlop S. Spread of pertussis by hospital staff. *JAMA.* 1972;221:264–267.

217. Linneman CC Jr, Ramundo N, Perlstein PH, Minton SD, Englender GS. Use of pertussis vaccine in an epidemic involving hospital staff. *Lancet.* 1975;2:540–543.

218. Valenti WM, Pincus PH, Messner MK. Nosocomial pertussis: possible spread by a hospital visitor. *Am J Dis Child.* 1980;134:520–521.

219. Christie CD, Glover AM, Wilke MJ, Marx ML, Reising SF, Hutchinson NM. Containment of pertussis in the regional pediatric hospital during the greater Cincinnati epidemic of 1993. *Infect Control Hosp Epidemiol.* 1995;16:556–563.

220. Rutala WA, Weber DJ. Management of healthcare workers exposed to pertussis. *Infect Control Hosp Epidemiol.* 1994;15:411–415.

221. Strebel P. Pertussis. In: *APIC Infection Control and Applied Epidemiology: Principles and Practice.* St. Louis, MO: Mosby; 1996:71.1–71.5.

222. Haiduven DJ, Hench CP, Simpkins SM, Stevens DA. Standardized management of patients and employees exposed to pertussis. *Infect Control Hosp Epidemiol.* 1998;19:861–864.

223. Haley CE, Cohen ML, Halter J, Meyer RD. Nosocomial Legionnaires' disease: a continuing common-source epidemic at Wadsworth Medical Center. *Ann Intern Med.* 1979;90:583–586.

224. Thacker SB, Bennett JV, Tsai TF, et al. An outbreak in 1965 of severe respiratory illness caused by the Legionnaires' disease bacterium. *J Infect Dis.* 1978;138:512–519.

225. Mermel LA, Josephson SL, Giorgio CH, Dempsey J, Parentau S. Association of Legionnaires' disease with construction: contamination of potable water? *Infect Control Hosp Epidemiol.* 1995;16:76–81.

226. Doebbeling BN, Ishak MA, Wade BH, et al. Nosocomial *Legionella micdadei* pneumonia: 10 years experience and a case-control study. *J Hosp Infect.* 1989;13:289–298.

227. Memish ZA, Oxley C, Contant J, Garber GE. Plumbing system shock absorbers as a source of *Legionella pneumophila. Am J Infect Control.* 1992;20:305–309.

228. Venezia RA, Agresta MD, Hanley EM, Urquhart K, Schoonmaker D. Nosocomial legionellosis associated with aspiration of nasogastric feedings diluted in tap water. *Infect Control Hosp Epidemiol.* 1994;15:529–533.

229. Centers for Disease Control and Prevention. Sustained transmission of nosocomial Legionnaires' disease—Arizona and Ohio. *MMWR Morb Mortal Wkly Rep.* 1997;46:416–421.

230. Dondero TJ, Rendtorff RC, Mallison GF, et al. An outbreak of Legionnaires' disease associated with a contaminated cooling tower. *N Engl J Med.* 1980;302:365.

231. Arnow PM, Chou T, Weil D, et al. Nosocomial Legionnaires' disease caused by aerosolized tap water from respiratory devices. *J Infect Dis.* 1982;146:460–467.

232. Brown CM, Nuorti P, Fields B, et al. Community outbreak of Legionnaires' disease. Presented at: 44th Annual Epidemic Intelligence Service Conference; March 27–31, 1995; Atlanta, GA.

233. Guerrero IC, Filippone C. A cluster of Legionnaires' disease in a community hospital—a clue to a larger epidemic. *Infect Control Hosp Epidemiol.* 1996;17:177–178.

234. Walsh TJ, Dixon DM. Nosocomial aspergillosis: environmental microbiology, hospital epidemiology, diagnosis, and treatment. *Eur J Epidemiol.* 1989;5:131–142.

235. Cole EC, Cook CE. Characterization of infectious aerosols in health care facilities: an aid to effective engineering controls and preventive strategies. *Am J Infect Control.* 1998;26:453–464.

236. Pannuti CS, Gingrich RD, Pfaller MA, Wenzel RP. Nosocomial pneumonia in adult patients undergoing bone marrow transplantation: a 9-year study. *J Clin Oncol.* 1991;9:77–84.

237. Rotstein C, Cummings KM, Tidings J, et al. An outbreak of invasive aspergillosis among allogeneic bone marrow transplants: a case-control study. *Infect Control.* 1985;6:347–355.

238. Opal SM, Asp AA, Cannady PB Jr, Morse PL, Burton LJ, Hammer PG II. Efficacy of infection control measures during a nosocomial outbreak of disseminated aspergillosis associated with hospital construction. *J Infect Dis.* 1986;153:634–637.

239. Arnow PM, Anderson RL, Mainous D, et al. Pulmonary aspergillosis during hospital renovation. *Am Rev Respir Dis.* 1978;118:49–53.

240. Flynn PM, Williams BG, Hetherington SV, Williams BF, Giannini MA, Pearson TA. *Aspergillus terreus* during hospital renovation. *Infect Control Hosp Epidemiol.* 1993;14:363–365.

241. McCarty JM, Flam MJ, Pulen G, et al. Outbreak of primary cutaneous aspergillosis related to intravenous arm boards. *J Pediatr.* 1986;108:721–724.

242. Hopkins CC, Weber DJ, Rubin RH. Invasive *Aspergillus* infection: possible non-ward common source within the hospital environment. *J Hosp Infect.* 1989;13:19–25.

243. Hruszkewycz V, Ruben B, Hypes CM, Bostic GD, Staszkiewicz J, Band JD. A cluster of pseudofungemia associated with hospital renovation adjacent to the microbiology laboratory. *Infect Control Hosp Epidemiol.* 1992;13:147–150.

244. Carter CD, Barr BA. Infection control issues in construction and renovation. *Infect Control Hosp Epidemiol.* 1997;18:587–596.

245. Rutala WA, Weber DJ. Water as a reservoir of nosocomial pathogens. *Infect Control Hosp Epidemiol.* 1997;18:609–616.

246. Stamm WE, Colella JJ, Anderson RL, Dixon RE. Indwelling arterial catheters as a source of nosocomial bacteremia: an outbreak caused by *Flavobacterium* species. *N Engl J Med.* 1975;292:1099–1102.

247. Casewell MW, Slater NGP, Cooper JE. Operating theatre water baths as a cause of *Pseudomonas septicaemia. J Hosp Infect.* 1981;2:237–240.

248. McGuckin MB, Thorpe RJ, Abrutyn E. Hydrotherapy: an outbreak of *Pseudomonas aeruginosa* wound infections related to Hubbard tank treatments. *Arch Phys Med Rehabil.* 1981;62:283–285.

249. Lowry PW, Beck-Sague CM, Bland LA, et al. *Mycobacterium chelonae* infection among patients receiving high-flux dialysis in a hemodialysis clinic in California. *J Infect Dis.* 1990;161:85–90.

250. Graman PS, Quinlan GA, Rank JA. Nosocomial legionellosis traced to a contaminated ice machine. *Infect Control Hosp Epidemiol.* 1997;18:637–640.

251. Verweij PE, Bilj D, Melchers W, et al. Pseudo-outbreak of multiresistant *Pseudomonas aeruginosa* in a hematology unit. *Infect Control Hosp Epidemiol.* 1997;18:128–131.

252. Sniadack DH, Ostroff SM, Karlix MA, et al. A nosocomial pseudo-outbreak of *Mycobacterium xenopi* due to a contaminated potable water supply: lessons in prevention. *Infect Control Hosp Epidemiol.* 1993;14:636–641.

253. Van Horn KG, Tatz JS, Li KI, Newman L, Wormser GP. Copepods associated with a perirectal abscess and copepod pseudo-outbreak in stools for ova and parasite examinations. *Diagn Microbiol Infect Dis.* 1992;15:561–565.

254. Klotz SA, Normand RE, Kalinsky RG. "Through a drinking glass and what was found there": pseudocontamination of a hospital's drinking water. *Infect Control Hosp Epidemiol.* 1992;13:477–481.

255. Center for Disease Control. *Sanitary Care and Maintenance of Ice Chests and Ice Machines.* Atlanta, GA: Center for Disease Control; 1979. Publication. No. 00–2384.

256. Burnett IA, Weeks GR, Harris DM. A hospital study of ice-making machines: their bacteriology, design, usage, and upkeep. *J Hosp Infect.* 1994;28:305–313.

257. Maloney SA, Jarvis WR. Epidemic nosocomial pneumonia in the intensive care unit. *Chest.* 1995;16:209–223.

258. Patterson TF, Patterson JE, Masecar BL, et al. A nosocomial outbreak of *Branhamella catarrhalis* confirmed by restriction endonuclease analysis. *J Infect Dis.* 1988;157:996–1001.

259. Centers for Disease Control. Suspected nosocomial influenza cases in an intensive care unit. *MMWR Morb Mortal Wkly Rep.* 1988;37:3–4.

260. Locksley RM, Cohen ML, Quinn TC, et al. Multiply antibiotic-resistant *Staphylococcus aureus*: introduction, transmission, and evolution of nosocomial infection. *Ann Intern Med.* 1982;97:317–324.

261. Singh-Naz N, Willy M, Riggs N. Outbreak of para-influenza virus type 3 in a neonatal nursery. *Pediatr Infect Dis J.* 1990;9:31–33.

262. Villarino ME, Stevens, LE, Schable BS, et al. Risk factors for epidemic *Xanthomonas* infection/colonization in intensive care unit patients. *Infect Control Hosp Epidemiol.* 1992;13:201–206.

263. Fisher-Hoch SP, Tobin JO, Nelson AM, et al. Investigation and control of Legionnaires' disease in a district general hospital. *Lancet.* 1981;1:933–936.

264. Arnow PM, Chou T, Weil D, et al. Nosocomial Legionnaires' disease caused by aerosolized tap water from respiratory devices. *J Infect Dis.* 1982;146:460–467.

265. Brady MT. Nosocomial Legionnaires' disease in a children's hospital. *J Pediatr.* 1988;115:46–58.

266. Mastro TD, Fields BS, Breiman RF, et al. Legionnaires' disease and use of medication nebulizers. *J Infect Dis.* 1991;163:667–671.

267. Blatt SP, Parkinson MD, Pace E, et al. Nosocomial Legionnaires' disease: aspiration as a primary mode of disease acquisition. *Am J Med.* 1991;95:16–22.

268. Weems JJ, Davis BJ, Tablan OC, et al. Construction activity: an independent risk factor for invasive aspergillosis and zygomycosis in patients with hematologic malignancy. *Infect Control.* 1987;8:71–75.

269. Arnow PM, Sadigh M, Costas C, et al. Endemic and epidemic aspergillosis associated with in-hospital replication of *Aspergillus* organisms. *J Infect Dis.* 1991;164:998–1002.

270. Buffington J, Reporter R, Lasker B, et al. Investigation of an epidemic of invasive aspergillosis: utility of molecular typing with the use of random amplified polymorphic DNS probes. *Pediatr Infect Dis J.* 1994;13:386–393.

271. Samet JM, Marbury MC, Spengler JD. Health effects and sources of indoor air pollution, pt 1. *Am Rev Respir Dis.* 1987;136:1486–1508.

272. Samet JM, Marbury MC, Spengler JD. Health effects and sources of indoor air pollution, pt 2. *Am Rev Respir Dis.* 1988;137:221–242.

273. Brandt-Rauf PW, Andrews LR, Schwarz-Miller J. Sick-hospital syndrome. *J Occup Med.* 1991;33:737–739.

274. Gold DR. Indoor air pollution. *Clin Chest Med.* 1992;13:215–229.

275. Pfaller MA. Nosocomial candidiasis: emerging species, reservoirs, and modes of transmission. *Clin Infect Dis.* 1996;22(suppl 2):S89–S94.

276. Jarvis WR. Epidemiology of nosocomial fungal infections with emphasis on *Candida* species. *Clin Infect Dis.* 1995;20:1526–1530.

277. Pfaller MA. Epidemiology of candidiasis. *J Hosp Infect.* 1995;30(suppl):329–338.

278. Waggoner-Fountain LA, Whit Walker M, Hollis RJ, et al. Vertical and horizontal transmission of unique *Candida* species to premature newborns. *Clin Infect Dis.* 1996;22:803–808.

279. Fowler SL, Rhoten B, Springer SC, Messer SA, Hollis RJ, Pfaller MA. Evidence for person-to-person transmission of *Candida lusitaniae* in a neonatal intensive care unit. *Infect Control Hosp Epidemiol.* 1998;19:343–345.

280. Reef SE, Lasker BA, Butcher DS. Nonperinatal nosocomial transmission of *Candida albicans* in a neonatal intensive care unit: prospective study. *J Clin Microbiol.* 1998;36:1255–1259.

281. Sheretz RJ, Gledhill KS, Hampton KD, et al. Outbreaks of *Candida* bloodstream infections associated with retrograde medication administration in a neonatal intensive care unit. *J Pediatr.* 1992;120:455–461.

282. Solomon SL, Khabbaz R, Parker RH, et al. An outbreak of *Candida parapsilosis* bloodstream infections in patients receiving parenteral nutrition. *J Infect Dis.* 1984;149:96–102.

283. Solomon SL, Alexander H, Eley JW, et al. Nosocomial fungemia in neonates associated with intravascular pressure monitoring devices. *Pediatr Infect Dis J.* 1986;5:680–685.

284. Faix RG, Finkel DJ, Andersen RD, Hostetter MK. Genotypic analysis of a cluster of systemic *Candida albicans* infections in a neonatal intensive care unit. *Pediatr Infect Dis J.* 1995;14:1063–1068.

285. Strausbaugh LJ, Sewell DL, Ward TT, Pfaller MA, Heitzman T, Tjoelker R. High frequency of yeast carriage on hands of hospital personnel. *J Clin Microbiol.* 1994;32:2299–2300.

286. Khatib R, Thirumoorthi MC, Riederer KM, Sturm L, Oney LA, Baran J. Clustering of *Candida* infections in the neonatal intensive care unit: concurrent emergence of multiple strains simulating intermittent outbreaks. *Pediatr Infect Dis J.* 1998;17:130–134.

287. Institute of Medicine. *Emerging Infections: Microbial Threats to Health in the United States.* Washington, DC: National Academy Press; 1994.

288. Centers for Disease Control and Prevention. *Preventing Emerging Infectious Diseases: A Strategy for the 21st Century.* Atlanta, GA: US Dept of Health and Human Services; 1998.

289. Bresee JS, Mast EE, Coleman PJ, et al. Hepatitis C virus infection associated with administration of intravenous immune globulin: a cohort study. *JAMA.* 1996;276:1563–1567.

290. Danzig LE, Short LJ, Collins K, et al. Bloodstream infections associated with a needleless intravenous infusion system in patients receiving home infusion therapy. *JAMA.* 1995;273:1862–1864.

291. Dowell SF, Mukunu R, Ksiazek TG, Khan AS, Rollin PE, Peters CJ, and the Ebola Hemorrhagic Fever Study Group. Transmission of Ebola hemorrhagic fever: a study of risk factors in family members—Kikwit, Zaire. *J Infect Dis.* 1999;179:S87–S91.

292. Jochimsen EM, Fish L, Manning K, et al. Evaluation and control of vancomycin-resistant enterococci at an Indianapolis hospital. Presented at: Seventh Annual Meeting of the Society for Healthcare Epidemiology of America; April 27–29, 1997; St. Louis, MO. Abstract 54.

293. Fridkin SK, Pear SM, Williamson TH, Galgiani JN, Jarvis WR. The role of understaffing in central venous catheter-associated bloodstream infections. *Infect Control Hosp Epidemiol.* 1996;17:150–158.

294. Archibald LK, Manning ML, Bell LM, Banerjee S, Jarvis WR. Patient density, nurse-to-patient ratio and nosocomial infection risk in a pediatric cardiac intensive care unit. *Pediatr Infect Dis J.* 1997;16:1045–1048.

295. Kellerman S, Shay DK, Howard J, et al. Bloodstream infections in home infusion patients: the influence of race and needleless intravascular access devices. *J Pediatr.* 1996;129:711–717.

296. Do A, Ray B, Barnett B, et al. Evaluation of the role of needleless devices (ND) in bloodstream infections. Presented at: 1996 Annual Meeting of the American Society of Microbiology, 36th Interscience Conference on Antimicrobial Agents and Chemotherapy; September 1996; New Orleans, LA. Abstract J61.

297. Wenzel RP, ed. *Prevention and Control of Nosocomial Infections.* 3rd ed. Baltimore: Williams & Wilkins; 1997.

298. Bennett JV, Brachman PS, eds. *Hospital Infections.* 4th ed. Boston: Little, Brown and Co; 1997.

299. Olmsted RN, ed. *APIC Infection Control and Applied Epidemiology: Principles and Practice.* St. Louis, MO: Mosby–Year Book; 1996.

300. Mayhall CG. *Hospital Epidemiology and Infection Control.* Baltimore: Williams & Wilkins; 1996.

301. Abrutyn E, Goldmann DA, Scheckler WE, eds. *Saunders Infection Control Reference Service.* Philadelphia: WB Saunders; 1997.

SUGGESTED READING

American Academy of Pediatrics. *1997 Red Book: Report of the Committee on Infectious Diseases.* Peter G, ed. 24th ed. Elk Grove Village, IL: American Academy of Pediatrics; 1997.

American Public Health Association. *Control of Communicable Diseases Manual.* Benenson AS, ed. 16th ed. Washington, DC: American Public Health Association; 1995.

Block SS, ed. *Disinfection, Sterilization, and Preservation.* 4th ed. Philadelphia: Lea & Febiger; 1991.

Centers for Disease Control. Protection against viral hepatitis: recommendations of the Advisory Committee on Immunization Practices (ACIP). *MMWR Morb Mortal Wkly Rep.* 1990;39(RR-21):1–27.

Centers for Disease Control. Update: universal precautions for prevention of transmission of human immunodeficiency virus, hepatitis B virus, and other bloodborne pathogens in health-care settings. *MMWR Morb Mortal Wkly Rep.* 1988;37:377–382, 387–388.

Centers for Disease Control. Update on adult immunization: recommendations of the Immunization Practices Advisory Committee (ACIP). *MMWR Morb Mortal Wkly Rep.* 1991;40(RR-12):1–94.

Centers for Disease Control and Prevention. Guideline for infection control in health care personnel, 1998. *Am J Infect Control.* 1998;26:289–354.

Centers for Disease Control and Prevention. Guideline for prevention of intravascular device-related infections. *Am J Infect Control.* 1996;24:262–293.

Centers for Disease Control and Prevention. Guidelines for preventing the transmission of *Mycobacterium tuberculosis* in health-care facilities, 1994. *MMWR Morb Mortal Wkly Rep.* 1994;43(RR-13):1–132.

Centers for Disease Control and Prevention. Immunization of health-care workers: recommendations of the Advisory Committee on Immunization Practices (ACIP) and the Hospital Infection Control Practices Advisory Committee (HICPAC). *MMWR Morb Mortal Wkly Rep.* 1997;46(RR-18):1–42.

Centers for Disease Control and Prevention. *Preventing Emerging Infectious Diseases: A Strategy for the 21st Century.* Atlanta, GA: US Dept of Health and Human Services; 1998.

Centers for Disease Control and Prevention. Public Health Service (PHS) guidelines for the management of health-care worker exposures to HIV and recommendations for post-exposure prophylaxis. *MMWR Morb Mortal Wkly Rep.* 1998;47(RR-7):1–28.

Centers for Disease Control and Prevention, Hospital Infection Control Practices Advisory Committee. Guideline for prevention of nosocomial pneumonia. *Infect Control Hosp Epidemiol.* 1994;15:587–627.

Centers for Disease Control and Prevention, National Institutes of Health. *Biosafety in Microbiological and Bio-Medical Laboratories.* 3rd ed. Atlanta, GA: US Dept of Health and Human Services, Public Health Service; 1993.

Garner JS, and Hospital Infection Control Practices Advisory Committee. Guideline for isolation precautions in hospitals. *Infect Control Hosp Epidemiol.* 1996;17:53–80.

Garrett L. *The Coming Plague: Newly Emerging Diseases in a World Out of Balance.* New York: Farrar, Straus & Giroux; 1994.

Institute of Medicine. *Emerging Infections: Microbial Threats to Health in the United States.* Washington, DC: National Academy Press; 1994.

U.S. Department of Labor, Occupational Safety and Health Administration. Occupational Exposure to Bloodborne Pathogens (Final Rule). 1910 C.F.R. § 1030 (1991).

PROFESSIONAL ORGANIZATIONS

The following national agencies and organizations have guidelines, position papers, or standards that can be used for developing infection control programs in the acute care setting. Information on obtaining copies of these guidelines can be obtained by telephoning the organization or accessing the listed Web site.

American Society for Gastrointestinal Endoscopy (ASGE)
13 Elm St
Manchester, MA 01944-1314
Telephone: 978-526-8330
Internet: http://www.asge.org
(Note: the ASGE guidelines cited in the references section can be accessed through this Web site.)

Association for Professionals in Infection Control and Epidemiology (APIC)
1275 K St NW, Suite 1000
Washington, DC 20005-4006
Telephone: 202-789-1890
Internet: http://www.apic.org

Association for the Advancement of Medical Instrumentation (AAMI)
3330 Washington Blvd, Suite 400
Arlington, VA 22201-4598
Telephone: 800-332-2264, ext. 217
Internet: http://www.aami.org
(AAMI has standards and recommended practices for hemodialysis and for sterilization in health care facilities.)

Association of Operating Room Nurses (AORN)
2170 South Parker Rd, Suite 300
Denver, CO 80231-5711
Telephone: 800-755-2676
Internet: http://www.aorn.org

Centers for Disease Control and Prevention (CDC)
Hospital Infections Program
1600 Clifton Rd
Atlanta, GA 30033
Internet: http://www.cdc.gov
(Note: The *Morbidity and Mortality Weekly Report (MMWR)* and most of the CDC guidelines noted in this chapter can be downloaded from this web site.)

CHAPTER 4

Outbreaks Reported in the Long-Term Care Setting

Kathleen Meehan Arias

INTRODUCTION

The term "long-term care facility" (LTCF) encompasses a variety of institutions: nursing homes (NHs), psychiatric hospitals, rehabilitation centers, and facilities for the mentally retarded. Of the estimated 2.5 million Americans who reside in long-term care facilities, approximately 1.6 million elderly and disabled residents receive care in nearly 17,000 nursing homes in the United States.[1] These numbers are expected to increase as the baby boom generation ages. An estimated 25 to 43 percent of persons who reach the age of 65 will likely spend some time in a nursing home.[2,3] Persons admitted to a nursing home generally have a chronic disease or a disability or have reached an advanced age and require nursing and medical care, and 90 percent of those who reside in nursing homes are over 65.[4]

The purpose of this chapter is to review reports of outbreaks that have occurred in long-term care facilities. These reports were identified by conducting a MEDLINE search of English-language publications from 1985 through 1998, by reviewing the table of contents of selected journals, and by reading the references listed in relevant articles and infection control textbooks. Almost all of the identified outbreaks occurred in nursing homes. Perhaps this is because the frail, elderly population residing in nursing homes is more likely to develop a nosocomial (facility-acquired) infection than are the mostly younger, more mobile residents of other types of long-term care facilities. The reports of these outbreaks highlight the importance of having a routine surveillance program in an LTCF to recognize the occurrence of both nosoco-

mial and community-acquired infections. Personnel who are responsible for infection control and quality management programs in LTCFs should be familiar with the types of outbreaks that have been reported in long-term care facilities and should implement prevention and control measures to prevent similar occurrences in their facility.

Although this chapter describes outbreaks that occurred in long-term care facilities, many of the reported etiologic agents and disease syndromes, especially gastrointestinal and respiratory illnesses, are associated with endemic and epidemic infections in both long-term care and acute care settings. Therefore, practitioners in long-term care facilities should be familiar with outbreaks reported in a variety of health care settings, especially those reported in acute care settings.

The agents that commonly cause outbreaks in both long-term care facilities and hospitals (i.e., methicillin-resistant *Staphylococcus aureus* [MRSA], *Mycobacterium tuberculosis*, *Sarcoptes scabiei*, and *Clostridium difficile*) are discussed in Chapter 7. Vancomycin-resistant enterococcus (VRE), which has become endemic in many acute care and long-term care facilities, is also discussed in Chapter 7. There are many reports of outbreaks of VRE infection in hospitals—mostly among patients in intensive care units. Although VRE is responsible for causing sporadic infections in LTCF residents and is often found to colonize residents, as of May 1999 there were no published outbreaks of VRE infection in an LTCF.

The Suggested Reading list at the end of this chapter provides additional information on infectious diseases and infection control in long-term care facilities.

ENDEMIC INFECTIONS

Elderly patients in hospitals and LTCFs are particularly susceptible to infection, and nosocomial infections (NIs) have long been recognized in this population.[4-9] The overall NI rates reported in LTCFs vary widely because of differences in definitions used to classify infections, duration of study, data collection methods, format for data presentation (incidence versus prevalence), population characteristics, and level of nursing intensity (e.g., intermediate versus skilled nursing facilities). Reported overall prevalence rates range from 1.6 to 32.7 infections per 100 residents per month,[4,6,10] and incidence rates range from 10.7 to 20.7 percent or 2.6 to 7.1 infections per 1,000 resident days.[4] An estimated 1.6 million to 3.8 million NIs per year occur in NH patients in the United States.[11] It is important to remember that "classification of an infection as nosocomial does not imply that the LTCF caused the infection, that the infecting organism was acquired in the LTCF, or that it was preventable, but simply that it occurred in the LTCF."[4(p 490)]

The most common endemic infections in LTCFs are urinary tract infections (UTIs; cystitis and pyelonephritis); respiratory tract infections (pneumonia, bronchitis, and influenza); skin and soft tissue infections (cellulitis and infected pressure ulcers); gastroenteritis; and conjunctivitis.[4,8]

Risk Factors for Infection

Factors that place residents at risk for infection include indwelling urinary catheters (UTI); incontinence (infected pressure ulcers); decreased mental status (aspiration pneumonia and pressure ulcers); age-related decline in cell-mediated immunity (reactivation of latent infections such as tuberculosis or herpes zoster); decreased cough reflex (aspiration pneumonia); and underlying diseases such as congestive heart failure, chronic obstructive pulmonary disease, and diabetes mellitus.[4,5] Invasive devices such as intravascular catheters, tracheostomy tubes, feeding tubes, and mechanical ventilators, which are well-recognized risk factors for nosocomial infections, are commonly used in many LTCFs. Other factors that predispose LTCF residents to infection include poor nutritional status, functional impairment leading to decreased mobility, epidermal thinning, poor vascular circulation, and decreased gastric acidity. In addition, the LTCF is the

resident's home and socializing, which increases direct contact with other residents and health care workers, is encouraged.

EPIDEMIC INFECTIONS

The majority of reported infectious disease outbreaks in LTCFs involve respiratory and gastrointestinal infections.[5,6,9,10] Table 4–1 lists the types of infections and etiologic agents responsible for outbreaks in long-term care facilities.

Outbreaks in long-term care facilities are frequently reported to local and state health departments, although the proportion of NIs that occur in LTCFs as a result of an epidemic appears to be small when compared to endemic infections. In 1988 the Centers for Disease Control (CDC) and four state epidemiology offices con-

Table 4–1 Etiologic Agents of Outbreaks Reported in Long-Term Care Facilities

Body Sites	Etiologic Agents
Respiratory Infections	*Bordetella pertussis*
	Group A streptococcus
	Hemophilus influenzae
	Influenza A and B
	Mycobacterium tuberculosis
	Neisseria meningitidis
	Parainfluenza virus
	Respiratory syncytial virus (RSV)
	Rhinovirus (common cold virus)
	Streptococcus pneumoniae
Skin Infections	Group A streptococcus
	Methicillin-resistant *Staphylococcus aureus*
	Scabies
Conjunctivitis	Group A streptococcus
Gastrointestinal Infections	*Aeromonas hydrophilia*
	Bacillus cereus (food poisoning)
	Campylobacter jejuni
	Clostridium botulinum (food poisoning)
	Clostridium difficile
	Clostridium perfringens (food poisoning)
	Entamoeba histolytica
	Escherichia coli O157:H7
	Giardia lamblia
	Norwalk-like viruses
	Rotavirus
	Salmonella species
	Shigella species
	Staphylococcus aureus (food poisoning)

ducted a five-month study to assess a computerized surveillance system for epidemics.[12] In this study, long-term care facilities accounted for 15 percent of the 79 reported outbreaks. From 1975 through 1987, 2 percent of the 6,695 foodborne outbreaks reported to the CDC occurred in nursing homes in 26 states.[13]

RECOGNIZING AND CONFIRMING AN OUTBREAK IN THE LONG-TERM CARE SETTING

An outbreak is defined as the occurrence of more cases of a disease or event than expected during a specified period of time in a given area or among a specific group of people. A cluster is a group of cases of a disease or health-related event that occurs closely related in time and place, although the number of cases in a cluster may or may not exceed the expected number. An ongoing surveillance program, as discussed in Chapter 2, is essential to detect an outbreak or a cluster in an LTCF. Methods that can be used to detect an outbreak in an LTCF are discussed in Chapter 8. There are few criteria for defining the occurrence of an outbreak, and outbreaks or clusters of disease in health care facilities may go undetected unless they result in considerable morbidity or mortality or are caused by an unusual organism. For some diseases, such as tuberculosis, the occurrence of one nosocomial case should prompt an investigation; however, it may be difficult to recognize an outbreak that is caused by an organism such as MRSA if it has become endemic in a facility.

Many state health departments have guidelines for identifying, confirming, and controlling outbreaks in LTCFs. Appendices H, I, and J contain the Maryland Department of Health and Mental Hygiene guidelines for investigating and controlling outbreaks of scabies, gastroenteritis, and acute respiratory illnesses in LTCFs. These guidelines contain (1) case definitions and outbreak definitions that can be used to identify and confirm an outbreak, (2) line-listing forms that can be used to record cases among residents and personnel, (3) information on collecting appropriate specimens to confirm a clinical diagnosis, and (4) control measures that can be used to interrupt an outbreak.

Very few LTCFs have on-site laboratories and radiology services, and, due to the nature of the population, diagnostic testing is not frequently performed. Many suspected infections are treated empirically, and a de-

finitive diagnosis may not be made. The imprecision in clinical and laboratory diagnosis inherent in long-term care facilities makes recognition and confirmation of an outbreak more difficult than in the acute care setting. In addition, investigations of outbreaks in facilities with an elderly, debilitated population are complicated by the fact that many of the residents cannot give a clear history of the development of symptoms or exposures to risk factors such as food or beverages consumed or contact with other residents. These facts should be kept in mind when conducting routine surveillance and when investigating a cluster or potential outbreak in an LTCF.

OUTBREAKS OF RESPIRATORY DISEASE

Outbreaks of respiratory disease in the long-term care setting have involved a variety of bacterial and viral agents: influenza A and B viruses, *M tuberculosis*, *Streptococcus pneumoniae*, group A streptococcus, *Rhinovirus*, respiratory syncytial virus, *Bordetella pertussis*, parainfluenza virus, and *Neisseria meningitidis*.[14-33] Examples of respiratory infectious disease outbreaks in LTCFs are shown in Table 4–2. Many cases of respiratory disease in LTCFs are not definitively diagnosed because bacterial and viral cultures and serologic studies are not routinely performed. Serologic and culture surveys performed in LTCFs have demonstrated that viral agents are often responsible for sporadic cases and epidemics of acute respiratory illness such as cough, nasal congestion, pharyngitis, or wheezing.[33-36]

Influenza

Epidemiology and Mode of Transmission

Influenza is characterized by abrupt onset of fever, chills, headache, severe malaise and myalgia, and by respiratory symptoms such as nonproductive cough, sore throat, and rhinitis.[37] It is transmitted from person to person by droplet nuclei (small particle aerosols) and by contact with respiratory droplets from an infected person.[37] In the United States and other countries with temperate climates, epidemics of influenza usually occur during the winter months (usually December through April). Outbreaks in the community can result in introduction of the virus into a health care facility by personnel, visitors, or newly admitted or transferred patients or residents. Once introduced into a population, influenza can spread rapidly because it is highly

Table 4–2 Outbreaks of Respiratory Disease Reported in Long-Term Care Facilities

Agent	Major Symptoms or Disease Reported	Comments	Year Reported/ Reference
Influenza A	Cough, coryza, sore throat, fever	28% attack rate (11/39 NH residents) with 55% mortality rate; no staff members ill.	1995[14]
Influenza A	Cough, coryza, sore throat, fever	First cases occurred in 5 unvaccinated nurses; 11% attack rate (34/309) in personnel and 13% attack rate (25/192) in residents in one building; 2 residents died.	1999[15]
Influenza B	Cough, runny nose, sore throat	Outbreak occurred in a highly immunized (>85%) NH population during season when circulating and vaccine strains of influenza were well matched.	1997[17]
Streptococcus pneumoniae	Pneumonia, fever, bacteremia	Three outbreaks described: mortality rate ranged from 20% to 28%; <5% of residents aged ≥65 years had documentation of receipt of pneumococcal vaccine.	1997[18]
Streptococcus pneumoniae-antibiotic resistant	Pneumonia, bacteremia	Cluster of three cases of penicillin-resistant pneumococcus in an NH with no identified common exposures; organisms not characterized by serotyping or molecular analysis; only 2% of residents had received pneumococcal vaccine prior to the outbreak.	1998[19]
Myco-bacterium tuberculosis	Persistent cough	Source was highly infectious NH resident; 30% (49/161) of tuberculin-negative residents became infected and 8 developed tuberculosis; 15% (21/138) of tuberculin-negative employees became infected and one developed clinical tuberculosis.	1981[21]
Myco-bacterium tuberculosis		Skin testing program detected new infections in 8 patients (1 with unsuspected progressive primary tuberculosis) and 2 staff members in a chronic care Veterans Administration medical center; an additional three patients who were tuberculin skin test converters were thought to have been infected by transmission of mycobacteria via window air conditioning units.	1988[22]
Group A streptococ-cus	Invasive streptococcal disease: pneumonia, sepsis, toxic shock-like syndrome	Spatial clustering of cases occurred in one outbreak that affected 16/80 NH residents (20%) and 3/45 staff (7%); no evidence of common source infection.[23] In another outbreak spatial clustering of cases occurred in an ICF and major mode of transmission was thought to be direct contact between residents; contact with an infected staff member was also thought to play a role; attack rate was 2.4% (14/577).[24]	1992[23,24]
Group A streptococ-cus	Noninvasive streptococcal disease: cutaneous infection, upper respiratory infection	Separate outbreaks in an NH affected residents of a locked mental health unit and residents of a skilled nursing care area. A nurse with pharyngitis and a positive throat culture for group A streptococcus was implicated as the source of mental health unit outbreak that affected 24/46 (52%) residents.	1992[25]
Respiratory syncytial virus (RSV)	Rhinorrhea, cough, fever, pneumonia, malaise, anorexia	Outbreaks of RSV in NHs result in considerable morbidity and mortality.	1984[26] 1990[27]
Bordetella pertussis	Prolonged cough	NH outbreak occurred during a community outbreak; 38 residents were seropositive (9 ill, 29 asymptomatic) and 7 employees were seropositive (5 ill, 2 asymptomatic).	1991[28]

continues

Table 4–2 Continued

Agent	Major Symptoms or Disease Reported	Comments	Year Reported/ Reference
Rhinovirus	Upper respiratory: cough, nasal/ sinus congestion, sore throat, coryza; lower respiratory: productive cough, dyspnea, hoarseness; gastrointestinal: nausea, vomiting, diarrhea, anorexia; systemic: fatigue, myalgia	Epidemiologic study showed geographic clustering of rhinovirus-infected residents; rhinovirus produced severe illness in some residents; mode of transmission was not studied.	1995[29]
Parainfluenza virus	Cough, fever, pneumonia	Outbreaks affected residents and employees and resulted in considerable morbidity and mortality.	1997[30,31]
Neisseria meningitidis	Fever, bacteremia, meningitis	First published report of an LTCF as the setting for a meningococcal outbreak; index case was a nurse with respiratory illness and meningitis; 2 patients developed meningococcemia (1 died) and a nursing assistant developed meningitis.	1998[32]

NH, nursing home; ICF, intermediate care facility; LTCF, long-term care facility.

contagious and has a fairly short incubation period (usually 1 to 3 days). Persons over 65 years and those of any age with certain medical conditions (e.g., pulmonary and cardiovascular disorders) are at risk for complications and death from influenza.[37]

Although nosocomial transmission of influenza has been reported in both acute care[38] and long-term care facilities, outbreaks of influenza are more commonly reported in the long-term care setting.[14–17,39–43] In the LTCF, influenza can be spread from resident to resident,[14] from health care personnel to residents,[15,40] from residents to health care personnel, and among health care personnel.[33,42] Influenza outbreaks in LTCFs can result in considerable morbidity and mortality, with clinical attack rates as high as 70 percent and mortality rates averaging over 10 percent.[4] In one nursing home outbreak the attack rate among residents was 28 percent (11/39) with a 55 percent case-fatality rate.[14] Although most infected persons exhibit respiratory symptoms, asymptomatic infection can occur.

Control Measures

Control measures to prevent transmission of influenza in health care facilities have been published by the Centers for Disease Control and Prevention (CDC),[37,44–47] the Association for Professionals in Infection Control and Epidemiology (APIC) and the So-

ciety for Healthcare Epidemiology of America (SHEA),[4] Gravenstein et al.,[48] Gomolin et al.,[49] and many state health departments.[50] The most important measure used to control transmission of influenza in the health care setting is annual immunization of all patients for whom the vaccine is recommended, all residents of LTCFs, and health care workers.[37] It should be noted that, although studies have shown that immunization of residents in LTCFs reduces the risk of transmission of influenza,[37] outbreaks have been reported in nursing homes that had highly immunized populations.[15,17,40]

In addition to immunization, influenza-specific antiviral drugs (amantadine and rimantadine) are important components of an influenza prevention and control program. Amantadine and rimantadine have been shown to be 70 to 90 percent effective in preventing illness from influenza A when used as prophylaxis in healthy adults and children.[37] In addition, these drugs can reduce the duration and severity of illness when they are used to treat persons with influenza A.[37] Emergence of amantadine/rimantadine-resistant strains of influenza virus have been reported when these drugs are used for therapy, so it is important to periodically perform susceptibility tests on influenza isolates to detect resistance.[51]

The following measures have been recommended to reduce the risk of transmission in long-term care facilities:

- Develop and implement an influenza prevention and control program based on published recommendations.[37,38,44-50]
- Conduct routine surveillance for respiratory illness, especially during flu season, to identify residents and personnel with influenza-like symptoms so that control measures can be promptly taken.
- Promptly institute droplet precautions for residents suspected of having influenza. This includes restricting the resident to his or her room during the period of greatest communicability (at least three days after onset of symptoms) or cohorting ill residents, when possible, if private rooms are not available.[46,49]
- Annually vaccinate all residents and personnel, especially caregivers, prior to the influenza season. To avoid delay in vaccinating residents who may not be able to give consent, LTCFs should obtain consent from the resident or the health care decision maker at the time of admission to the facility. Ideally, all residents should be vaccinated annually at the same time, immediately preceding the influenza season. Residents who are admitted after completion of the annual vaccination program should be vaccinated at the time of their admission if they have not yet been immunized.
- Document the influenza vaccination status of all current residents and personnel. This allows rapid identification of unvaccinated individuals, who should be encouraged to receive the vaccine in the event of an outbreak. Whenever possible, develop a computer database to store this information so that it can be easily accessed.
- Educate personnel on the signs and symptoms of influenza, the safety and efficacy of the influenza vaccine, and the importance of not coming to work if they have an influenza-like illness.

In the event of an outbreak of influenza or influenza-like illness in an LTCF the following additional control measures have been recommended:

- Offer influenza vaccine to any unvaccinated residents or personnel.[37]
- Use rapid laboratory tests for influenza, such as the immunofluorescence assay (IFA) or the enzyme immunoassay (EIA) to confirm the diagnosis and establish the existence of an outbreak.[37,49] (Maryland Department of Health and Mental Hy-

giene guidelines for investigating influenza outbreaks in LTCFs define an outbreak as one laboratory-proven case of influenza or three or more clinically defined cases occurring in a facility within a seven-day period between October 1 and May 31).[50]
- Administer antiviral agents such as amantadine or rimantadine to all well and ill residents (regardless of vaccination status).[37] Dosing guidelines have been published by the CDC.[37] (Amantadine and rimantadine are not effective against influenza B.)
- Offer viral chemoprophylaxis (amantadine or rimantadine) to unvaccinated health care personnel for the duration of influenza activity or vaccinate unimmunized personnel and provide chemoprophylaxis for two weeks after vaccination (i.e., until immunity develops from the vaccination).[37,49]
- Report the outbreak to the local or state health department. (In some states, LTCFs are required to report outbreaks of acute lower respiratory illness, including influenza, to the health department.)
- Develop a line listing of residents and health care workers with suspected influenza (see Appendix H).[50]
- Collect viral cultures on a representative number of cases to identify the strain of virus responsible for the outbreak.[37,50]
- Consider closing the affected ward(s) to new admissions.
- Discourage visitors with influenza-like illness from visiting the facility by posting signs at the entrances of the facility.

Additional Information on Influenza

Appendix H contains the Maryland Department of Health and Mental Hygiene's Guidelines for the Prevention and Control of Upper and Lower Acute Respiratory Illnesses (including Influenza and Pneumonia) in Long Term Care Facilities. These guidelines provide information on preventing, detecting, investigating, and controlling an influenza outbreak and include a form for documenting influenza vaccine administration, information on laboratory tests that can be used to confirm a clinical diagnosis of influenza, and respiratory illness questionnaires for residents and employees.

The CDC guidelines on prevention and control of influenza,[37] surveillance summaries, and other information on influenza can be accessed at the Web site for the CDC's National Center for Infectious Diseases, Influenza Branch at http://www.cdc.gov/ncidod/diseases/flu/fluvirus.htm.

Streptococcus pneumoniae

Epidemiology and Mode of Transmission

S pneumoniae (the pneumococcus) is commonly found in the upper respiratory tract of children and adults worldwide. It can cause a variety of illnesses: invasive infections such as bacteremia and meningitis, lower respiratory tract infections such as pneumonia, and upper respiratory tract infections such as otitis media and sinusitis.[52] Children 2 years and younger and adults 65 years and older are at increased risk for pneumococcal infection. Persons who have chronic cardiovascular, pulmonary, or liver diseases are also at risk for developing pneumococcal infection and frequently develop severe disease and complications.[52] *S pneumoniae* is the most common bacterial cause of community-acquired and nursing home-acquired pneumonia.[18,52,53] The organism is transmitted from person to person by direct oral contact, by droplet spread, or by contact with articles that have been freshly soiled with respiratory secretions.[54]

Despite the fact that *S pneumoniae* is the most common cause of bacterial pneumonia in the long-term care setting, there are few published reports of outbreaks of pneumococcal disease in long-term care facilities. The attack rates among residents in these outbreaks ranged from 7.4 to 23 percent[18–20,55] and deaths resulting from pneumococcal infections were reported in five of the six facilities affected. In all of the reported outbreaks, less than 7 percent of the residents had previously received the pneumococcal vaccine.

Control Measures

The most important measure in preventing pneumococcal disease is immunization of those at greatest risk of infection, including all persons more than 65 years of age and residents of nursing homes and other chronic care facilities.[52] Although there are few published recommendations for controlling outbreaks of pneumococcal disease in LTCFs, several reports indicate that prompt immunization of unvaccinated residents resulted in decreased transmission and termination of the outbreak.[18,20,52] Using information published by the CDC on preventing pneumococcal disease and measures reported to be effective in controlling the re-

ported outbreaks, the following measures are recommended to prevent and control the transmission of *S pneumoniae* in LTCFs:[18,20,52,55]

- Develop and implement a protocol for assessing vaccination status and for immunizing residents, if needed, at the time of admission.
- Document administration of pneumococcal vaccine in the resident's medical record. This will aid in the rapid assessment of susceptible residents if an outbreak occurs.
- Conduct routine surveillance for acute upper and lower respiratory tract illness in residents and employees. Use surveillance criteria/definitions for disease.[50,55]
- Whenever possible, encourage ill residents to cover their mouth and nose when coughing or sneezing and to wash their hands after coughing or sneezing.
- When possible, restrict employees with acute respiratory illness from direct care of residents. At the very least, instruct these employees to wash their hands before caring for a resident and to use tissues to cover their mouth and nose when coughing or sneezing.
- If pneumonia is suspected, or a resident has a febrile respiratory illness, perform appropriate diagnostic tests, such as chest X-ray and throat or sputum cultures, to establish the diagnosis and to determine the etiologic agent.
- Keep an updated, ongoing surveillance log of residents and employees who meet the case definition for an acute respiratory disease.[50]
- If an outbreak is suspected, develop a line listing of residents with pneumococcal disease.[50]
- Use standard precautions when caring for a resident with pneumococcal disease.[46]

Additional information on investigating cases of pneumococcal pneumonia can be found in Appendix H.[50]

Neisseria meningitidis

Epidemiology and Mode of Transmission

Neisseria meningitidis (the meningococcus) causes sporadic and epidemic disease, principally meningitis and sepsis (meningococcemia), and it is the leading cause of bacterial meningitis in children and young adults in the United States.[56] *N meningitidis* is transmitted from person to person via direct contact with respiratory secretions and droplets.[54,56]

Outbreaks of meningococcal disease have long been recognized in communities and organizations such as schools, universities, military barracks, and correctional facilities[56]; however, a search of the literature uncovered only one published report of an outbreak of meningococcal disease in a health care facility, and that occurred in a skilled nursing facility in Florida in December 1997.[32] The index case in that outbreak was a nurse who was hospitalized with confusion and fever and suspected meningitis after a two-week illness. Shortly after his hospitalization, a 90-year-old patient in the wing where the nurse was assigned developed meningococcemia and died and a 56-year-old nursing assistant developed meningococcal meningitis. The nursing assistant had cared for the 90-year-old case patient. Ciprofloxacin prophylaxis was administered to all 114 of the facility's staff members and all but one of the 104 residents. Shortly thereafter, the one patient who refused prophylaxis was hospitalized with meningococcemia. At the recommendation of a community physician, the facility provided antibiotic prophylaxis to approximately 250 visitors and collected nasopharyngeal cultures from all available patients post prophylaxis—all cultures were negative for *N meningitidis*. The CDC investigators noted that mass prophylaxis was justified for the facility's staff and patients but was not needed for the 250 casual contacts and that culturing of patients or staff was an inappropriate response to the outbreak.[32]

Control Measures

Two measures that can be used to prevent meningococcal disease are chemoprophylaxis and vaccination. For information on the use of chemoprophylaxis and vaccination, the reader is referred to the CDC Advisory Committee on Immunization Practices (ACIP) recommendations on control and prevention of meningococcal disease.[56] The primary tool that is used to prevent the development of disease is the identification and chemoprophylaxis of close contacts of persons with meningococcal disease.

Based on the ACIP recommendations and the findings from the report of the nursing home outbreak, the following measures are recommended to identify and control an outbreak of meningococcal disease in a health care facility:

- Conduct routine surveillance to identify persons with meningococcal disease (case definitions are given in the ACIP recommendations[56] and in Appendix C).
- Identify close contacts of a patient with meningococcal disease. Close contacts are defined as persons "directly exposed to the patient's oral secretions (e.g., through kissing, mouth-to-mouth resuscitation, endotracheal intubation, or endotracheal tube management)."[56(p 4)]
- Provide chemoprophylaxis as soon as possible to close contacts—usually either rifampin twice daily for two days (600 mg every 12 hours for adults, 10 mg/kg of body weight every 12 hours for children 1 month old or older, or 5 mg/kg of body weight every 12 hours for infants less than 1 month old) or ciprofloxacin (a single 500-mg oral dose) is recommended.[56]
- Report cases of laboratory-confirmed meningococcal disease to the local or state health department. (In many states meningococcal disease should be reported immediately by telephone to the health department.)
- Use droplet precautions (private room and masks) for persons with known or suspected meningococcal meningitis, meningococcal pneumonia, or meningococcemia (meningococcal sepsis) until 24 hours after appropriate antimicrobial therapy is given.[46]
- Instruct the laboratory to type (serogroup) the organism and to save the isolate(s) of *N meningitidis* for confirmation of serogrouping and possible subtyping.[56]
- Do not collect oropharyngeal or nasopharyngeal cultures from residents, contacts, or personnel as cultures are not needed when investigating outbreaks or for determining who should receive antimicrobial prophylaxis.[56]

Other Organisms Causing Outbreaks of Respiratory Disease

Other organisms that have been reported to cause outbreaks of respiratory disease in long-term care facilities include respiratory syncytial virus (RSV),[26,27] *Rhinovirus* (common cold virus),[29] *B pertussis*,[28] and parainfluenza virus.[30,31] Each of these agents can affect both residents and personnel and can result in significant morbidity. Both endemic and epidemic infections caused by these organisms are likely to go unrecognized because specific diagnostic testing is rarely done.[35] Control measures to prevent transmission of these agents include recognition of illness in both residents and employees and consistent use of good hygienic practices such as hand washing and using tissues to cover the mouth and nose when coughing or sneezing.

Pertussis should be suspected in persons who have a prolonged cough (regardless of age), especially if pertussis is reported in the community.[28] Since oral erythromycin is used as prophylaxis to prevent development of disease in close contacts of persons with pertussis, early recognition of this disease is important.[57]

OUTBREAKS OF GASTROINTESTINAL DISEASE

Sporadic and epidemic cases of diarrhea occur frequently in LTCFs and can be associated with significant morbidity and mortality.[6,9,13] Outbreaks of infectious gastroenteritis in the long-term care setting have been caused by a variety of bacteria, viruses, and parasites: *Salmonella* species, *C difficile*, *Shigella* species, *Bacillus cereus*, *Aeromonas hydrophilia*, *S aureus*, *Campylobacter jejuni*, *Clostridium perfringens* and *botulinum*, *Escherichia coli* O157:H7, Norwalk-like viruses, *Rotavirus*, *Giardia lamblia*, and *Entamoeba histolytica*.

The organisms that cause epidemic diarrhea in LTCFs can be spread by contact with a contaminated item (such as soiled laundry), by contact with an infected or colonized person, or by consumption of contaminated food or beverages. Some organisms, such as *Salmonella* and *G lamblia*, can be transmitted by both the contact and foodborne routes.

Foodborne outbreaks in nursing homes and other LTCFs accounted for 2 percent of all foodborne outbreaks and 19 percent of outbreak-related deaths reported to the CDC from 1975 through 1987.[13] *Salmonella* is the most commonly reported pathogen responsible for foodborne outbreaks in LTCFs.[13] Outbreaks of gastrointestinal illness in LTCFs are difficult to investigate because diagnostic tests are infrequently performed to identify an infectious agent and those tests that are done are frequently negative. In addition, many residents in LTCFs are poor historians and are unable to remember risk factors for infection such as consumption of a particular food or contact with an infectious resident.

Each LTCF should have an ongoing education program to instruct personnel in how to properly handle, prepare, and store food and when, why, and how to wash their hands and use standard precautions.[4] The identification, investigation, and control of outbreaks of gastrointestinal disease are discussed in detail in Chapter 7. The Maryland Department of Health and Mental Hygiene's Guidelines for the Epidemiological Investigation of Gastroenteritis Outbreaks in Long-Term Care Facilities are reprinted in Appendix I.

OUTBREAKS OF CONJUNCTIVITIS

Although conjunctivitis is a common nosocomial ailment in long-term care facilities, outbreaks of conjunctivitis are rarely reported. Endemic episodes of conjunctivitis are seen in nursing home patients, and the reported incidence varies widely from 0.075 to 3.5 per 1,000 patient-days.[58] In several reports, conjunctivitis appeared to occur most often in debilitated patients.[7,58] Conjunctivitis may be due to microbial pathogens, allergies, or other irritative responses. The etiology of infective conjunctivitis in long-term care residents has not been well elucidated. Boustcha and Nicolle reported that *S aureus* and *Branhamella catarrhalis* were the most commonly isolated bacterial pathogens during a prospective study of episodes of conjunctivitis in residents of a long-term care facility.[58] They noted that no bacterial pathogen was isolated from the majority of cases and these may possibly have been caused by viruses or *Chlamydia* (laboratory tests for these agents were not performed).

There are only a few published reports of outbreaks of conjunctivitis associated with long-term care facilities and these were outbreaks of group A streptococcus in nursing homes in which residents developed conjunctivitis in concurrence with a widespread outbreak of group A streptococcal disease.[25,59] Brennen and Muder studied the clinical characteristics of 20 episodes of MRSA-associated conjunctivitis that occurred in 19 patients over a three-year period in a 432-bed long-term care facility.[60] These were infections that occurred in a facility in which MRSA had been endemic for at least six years, and nine of the patients who developed conjunctivitis from which MRSA was isolated had documented prior colonization of other body sites with MRSA.[60]

Control measures for outbreaks caused by group A streptococcus are discussed below and infections caused by MRSA are discussed in Chapter 7. In reports of outbreaks of conjunctivitis that occurred in ambulatory care settings (primarily in ophthalmology clinics), the most successful measures shown to interrupt an outbreak were appropriate hand washing by health care workers, recognition of an outbreak, and use of aseptic technique when providing eye care.[61]

OUTBREAKS CAUSED BY GROUP A STREPTOCOCCUS

Epidemiology and Mode of Transmission

Although group A beta-hemolytic streptococcus (*Streptococcus pyogenes*) most commonly causes pharyngitis, it can also cause invasive disease such as pneumonia, sepsis, cellulitis, wound infection, and toxic shock-like syndrome. Some serotypes of group A streptococci are primarily associated with pharyngeal and minor skin infections such as impetigo, while others readily cause invasive diseases such as sepsis and pneumonia.[62] The elderly are particularly prone to developing invasive disease, and mortality rates from group A streptococcal bacteremia have been reported to be as high as 60 percent in this population.[23] Person-to-person transmission generally occurs by direct contact with an infected or colonized person, although foodborne outbreaks of streptococcal pharyngitis have also occurred.[54] Little has been published on the risk factors for acquisition, mode of transmission, and effective control measures to prevent transmission of group A streptococci in long-term care facilities.

Outbreaks of invasive and noninvasive group A streptococcal infections in LTCFs have been reported.[23-25,59,62-67] The reports of these outbreaks identified several risk factors for nosocomial acquisition and disease: sharing a room with an infected resident, being bedridden, requiring extensive nursing care, having contact with a culture-positive nurse or with an infected resident, and having decubitus ulcers.[23, 62] Unlike reports of outbreaks of group A streptococcal postoperative infections in hospitals,[68] none of the reported LTCF outbreaks were associated with a personnel disseminator. In all of the LTCF outbreaks, the organism was thought to be spread by direct contact with an infected or colonized person or by cross-infection due to poor infection control practices, such as lack of hand washing or failure to change gloves between residents. In two outbreaks nursing personnel with symptomatic group A streptococcal pharyngitis had direct contact with residents who subsequently became infected, and these personnel may have been responsible for introducing the organism into their facilities.[24,62]

Control Measures

The following measures are recommended to recognize and control outbreaks of group A streptococcus in a long-term care facility:[23,24,59]

- Conduct routine ongoing surveillance for nosocomial group A streptococcal infections so that single cases, clusters, and outbreaks can be detected and control measures can be promptly implemented.
- Provide timely diagnosis and antimicrobial therapy for persons with pharyngitis or other streptococcal infections.
- Educate personnel about the importance of reporting pharyngitis.
- Restrict personnel with group A streptococcal infections from resident care activities until 24 hours after they have received appropriate therapy.[44]
- Use standard precautions for all wound care; however, if a resident has a group A streptococcal wound infection that cannot be covered or has drainage that cannot be contained, use contact precautions (private room or cohort with another resident with known or suspected group A streptococcal infection, gloves for direct care, proper hand washing, and a gown for substantial contact with the resident) in addition to standard precautions. Contact precautions are needed only until 24 hours after appropriate antimicrobial therapy has been given.[46]
- Use standard precautions for mild cutaneous and other streptococcal infections.[46]
- Enforce good infection control practices (hand washing and glove use for wound care), especially when caring for an infected resident.
- Initiate an outbreak investigation if two nosocomial group A streptococcal infections occur in a short time period among residents of an LTCF.
- Instruct the laboratory to save group A streptococcal isolates for serotyping if an outbreak or cluster occurs (i.e., more than two nosocomial cases).
- Obtain assistance in conducting an outbreak investigation from the local or state health department.
- Consider prophylactic antimicrobials if an outbreak is ongoing or involves severe infections.[23]

- Use a case definition[23] and construct a line listing of infected and colonized persons. Case definitions for streptococcal toxic-shock syndrome and invasive group A streptococcal disease can be found in Appendix C.

SUMMARY

Residents and patients in long-term care facilities are at risk for developing NIs; however, only a small proportion of these infections appear to be related to recognized outbreaks in LTCFs. Infection control and quality management personnel in LTCFs should implement a routine surveillance, prevention, and control program to reduce the risk of infection in residents and personnel.[4,6,9,37,47,52,69] An effective surveillance program should be able to detect and quantify the occurrence of NIs and other adverse health-related events so that clusters and outbreaks can be identified and control measures can be instituted to prevent new cases from occurring.

REFERENCES

1. Health Care Financing Administration (HCFA). Medicare Fact Sheet, May 16, 1999. HCFA Online Information Clearinghouse (http://www.HCFA.gov/facts).

2. American Medical Association. White paper on elderly heath. *Arch Intern Med.* 1990;150:2459–2472.

3. Kemper P, Murtaugh CM. Lifetime use of nursing home care. *N Engl J Med.* 1991;324:595–600.

4. Smith PW, Rusnak PG. Infection prevention and control in the long-term care facility. *Am J Infect Control.* 1997;25:488–512.

5. Jackson MM, Fierer J. Infections and infection risk in residents of long-term care facilities: a review of the literature, 1970–1984. *Am J Infect Control.* 1985;13:63–77.

6. Nicole LE, Garibaldi RA. Infection control in long-term care facilities. *Infect Control Hosp Epidemiol.* 1995;16:348–353.

7. Garbaldi RA, Brodine S, Matsumiya S. Infections among patients in nursing homes—policies, prevalence, and problems. *N Engl J Med.* 1981;305:731–735.

8. Yoshikawa TT, Norman DC. Approach to fever and infection in the nursing home. *J Am Geriatr Soc.* 1996;44:74–82.

9. Bennett RG. Diarrhea among residents of long-term care facilities. *Infect Control Hosp Epidemiol.* 1993;14:397–404.

10. Smith PW, Daly PB, Roccaforte JS. Current status of nosocomial infection control in extended care facilities. *Am J Med.* 1991;91:3B-281S–3B-285S.

11. Strausbaugh LJ. Infection control in long-term care: news from the front. *Am J Infect Control.* 1999;27:1–3.

12. Centers for Disease Control. Surveillance for epidemics—United States. *MMWR Morb Mortal Wkly Rep.* 1989;38:694–696.

13. Levine WC, Smart JF, Archer DL, Bean NH, Tauxe RV. Foodborne disease outbreaks in nursing homes, 1975 through 1987. *JAMA.* 1991;266:2105–2109.

14. Morens DM, Rash VM. Lessons from a nursing home outbreak of influenza A. *Infect Control Hosp Epidemiol.* 1995;16:275–280.

15. Centers for Disease Control and Prevention. Update: influenza activity—United States, 1998–99 season. *MMWR Morb Mortal Wkly Rep.* 1999;48:177–181.

16. Libow LS, Neufeld RR, Olson E, Breuer B, Starer P. Sequential outbreak of influenza A and B in a nursing home: efficacy of vaccine and amantadine. *J Am Geriatr Soc.* 1996;44:1153–1157.

17. Drinka PJ, Gravenstein S, Krause P, Schilling M, Miller BA, Shult P. Outbreak of influenza A and B in a highly immunized nursing home population. *J Fam Pract.* 1997;45:509–514.

18. Centers for Disease Control and Prevention. Outbreaks of pneumococcal pneumonia among unvaccinated residents in chronic-care facilities—Massachusetts, October 1995, Oklahoma, February 1996, and Maryland, May–June 1996. *MMWR Morb Mortal Wkly Rep.* 1997;46:60–62.

19. McNeeley DF, Lyons J, Conte S, Labowitz A, Layton M. A cluster of drug-resistant *Streptococcus pneumoniae* among nursing home patients. *Infect Control Hosp Epidemiol.* 1998;19:476–477.

20. Sheppard DC, Bartlett KA, Lampiris HW. *Streptococcus pneumoniae* transmission in chronic-care facilties: description of an outbreak and review of management strategies. *Infect Control Hosp Epidemiol.* 1998;19:851–853.

21. Stead WW. Tuberculosis among elderly persons: an outbreak in a nursing home. *Ann Intern Med.* 1981;94:606–610.

22. Brenner C, Muder RR, Muraca PW. Occult endemic tuberculosis in a chronic care facility. *Infect Control Hosp Epidemiol.* 1988;9:548–552.

23. Auerbach SB, Schwartz B, Williams D, et al. Outbreak of invasive group A streptococcal infections in a nursing home. *Arch Intern Med.* 1992;152:1017–1022.

24. Harkness GA, Bentley DW, Mottley M, Lee J. *Streptococcus pyogenes* outbreak in a long-term care facility. *Am J Infect Control.* 1992;20:142–148.

25. McNutt LA, Casiano-Colon AE, Coles FB, et al. Two outbreaks of primarily noninvasive group A streptococcal disease in the same nursing home, New York, 1991. *Infect Control Hosp Epidemiol.* 1992;13:748–751.

26. Sorvillo FJ, Huie SF, Strassburg M, Butsumyo A, Shandera WX, Fannin SL. An outbreak of respiratory syncytial virus pneumonia in a nursing home for the elderly. *J Infect.* 1984;9:252–259.

27. Osterweil D, Norman D. An outbreak of influenza-like illness in a nursing home. *J Am Geriatr Soc.* 1990;38:659–662.

28. Addiss DG, Davis JP, Meade BD. A pertussis outbreak in a Wisconsin nursing home. *J Infect Dis.* 1991;164:704–710.

29. Wald TG, Shult P, Krause P, Miller BA, Drinka P, Gravenstein S. A *Rhinovirus* outbreak among residents of a long-term care facility. *Ann Intern Med.* 1995;123:588–593.

30. Brady G, Kenny D, Ackman D, Duncan R. An outbreak of parainfluenza type 1 in a long-term care facility. *Infect Control Hosp Epidemiol.* 1997;18:P27. [Abstract 45]

31. Patel A, Hernandez JM, Przykucki JM, et al. Parainfluenza 1 virus outbreak at an extended care facility, June 1996. *Infect Control Hosp Epidemiol.* 1997;18:P27. [Abstract 46]

32. Centers for Disease Control and Prevention. Outbreaks of group B meningococcal disease—Florida, 1995 and 1997. *MMWR Morb Mortal Wkly Rep.* 1998;47:883–837.

33. Gross PA, Rodstein M, LaMontagne JR, et al. Epidemiology of acute respiratory illness during an influenza outbreak in a nursing home. *Arch Intern Med.* 1988;148:559–561.

34. Arroya JC, Jordan W, Milligan L. Upper respiratory tract infection in nursing home residents. *Am J Infect Control.* 1988;16:152–158.

35. Falsey AR, Treanor JJ, Betts RF, Walsh EE. Viral respiratory infections in the institutionalized elderly: clinical and epidemiologic findings *J Am Geriatr Soc.* 1992;40:115–119.

36. Falsey AR. Noninfluenza respiratory virus infection in long-term care facilities. *Infect Control Hosp Epidemiol.* 1991;12:602–608.

37. Centers for Disease Control and Prevention. Prevention and control of influenza: recommendations of the Advisory Committee on Immunization Practices (ACIP). *MMWR Morb Mortal Wkly Rep.* 1999;48(RR-04):1–28.

38. Evans ME, Hall KL, Berry SE. Influenza control in acute care hospitals. *Am J Infect Control.* 1997;25:357–362.

39. Taylor JN, Dwyer DM, Coffman T, Groves C, Patel J, Israel E. Nursing home outbreak of influenza A (H3N2): evaluation of vaccine efficacy and influenza case definitions. *Infect Control Hosp Epidemiol.* 1992;13:93–97.

40. Coles FB, Balzano GJ, Morse DL. An outbreak of influenza A (H3N2) in a well-immunized nursing home population. *J Am Geriatr Soc.* 1992;40:589–592.

41. Degelau J, Somani SK, Cooper SL, Guay DR, Crossley KB. Amantadine-resistant influenza A in a nursing facility. *Arch Intern Med.* 1992;152:390–392.

42. Patriarca PA, Weber JA, Parker RA, et al. Risk factors for outbreaks in nursing homes. A case-control study. *Am J Epidemiol.* 1986;124:114–119.

43. Staynor K, Foster G, McArthur M, McGeer A, Petric M, Simor AE. Influenza A outbreak in a nursing home: the value of early diagnosis and the use of amantadine hydrochloride. *Can J Infect Control.* 1994;9:109–111.

44. Centers for Disease Control and Prevention. Guideline for infection control in health care personnel, 1998. *Am J Infect Control.* 1998;26:289–354.

45. Centers for Disease Control and Prevention, Hospital Infection Control Practices Advisory Committee. Guideline for prevention of nosocomial pneumonia. *Infect Control Hosp Epidemiol.* 1994;15:587–627.

46. Garner JS, Hospital Infection Control Practices Advisory Committee. Guideline for isolation precautions in hospitals. *Infect Control Hosp Epidemiol.* 1996;17:53–80.

47. Centers for Disease Control and Prevention. Immunization of health-care workers: recommendations of the Advisory Committee on Immunization Practices (ACIP) and the Hospital Infection Control Practices Advisory Committee (HICPAC). *MMWR Morb Mortal Wkly Rep.* 1997;46(RR-18):1–42.

48. Gravenstein S, Miller BA, Drinka P. Prevention and control of influenza A outbreaks in long-term care facilities. *Infect Control Hosp Epidemiol.* 1992;13:49–54.

49. Gomolin IH, Leib HB, Arden NH, Sherman FT. Control of influenza outbreaks in the nursing home: guidelines for diagnosis and management. *J Am Geriatr Soc.* 1995;43:71–74.

50. Maryland Department of Health and Mental Hygiene. Guideline for the prevention and control of upper and lower acute respiratory illnesses (including influenza and pneumonia) in long term care facilities, December 1997.

51. Houck P, Hemphill M, LaCroix S, Hirsh D, Cox N. Amantadine-resistant influenza A in nursing homes. Identification of a resistant virus prior to drug use. *Arch Intern Med.* 1995;155:533–537.

52. Centers for Disease Control and Prevention. Prevention of pneumococcal disease: recommendations of the Advisory Committee on Immunization Practices (ACIP). *MMWR Morb Mortal Wkly Rep.* 1997;46(RR-8):1–24.

53. Marrie TJ, Slater KL. Nursing home-acquired pneumonia. Treatment options. *Drugs Aging.* 1996;8:338–348.

54. Benenson AS, ed. *Control of Communicable Diseases Manual.* Washington, DC: American Public Health Association; 1995.

55. Quick RE, Hoge CW, Hamilton DJ, Whitney CJ, Borges M, Kobayaski JM. Underutilization of pneumococcal vaccine in nursing homes in Washington state: report of a serotype-specific outbreak and a survey. *Am J Med.* 1993;94:149–152.

56. Centers for Disease Control and Prevention. Control and prevention of meningococcal disease: recommendations of the Advisory Committee on Immunization Practices (ACIP). *MMWR Morb Mortal Wkly Rep.* 1997;46(RR-5):1–51.

57. Weber DJ, Rutala WA. Management of healthcare workers exposed to pertussis. *Infect Control Hosp Epidemiol.* 1994;15:411–415.

58. Boustcha E, Nicolle LE. Conjunctivitis in a long-term care facility. *Infect Control Hosp Epidemiol.* 1995;16:210–216.

59. Ruben FL, Norden CW, Heisler B, Korica Y. An outbreak of *Streptococcus pyogenes* infections in a nursing home. *Ann Intern Med.* 1984;101:494–496.

60. Brennen C, Muder RR. Conjunctivitis associated with methicillin-resistant *Staphylococcus aureus* in a long-term-care facility. *Am J Med.* 1990;88:5-14N–5-17N.

61. Buehler JW, Finton RJ, Goodman RA, et al. Epidemic keratoconjunctivitis: report of an outbreak in an ophthalmology practice and recommendations for prevention. *Infect Control.* 1984;390–394.

62. Schwartz B, Ussery XT. Group A streptococcal outbreaks in nursing homes. *Infect Control Hosp Epidemiol.* 1992;13:742–747.

63. Rahman M. Outbreak of *Streptococcus pyogenes* in a geriatric hospital and control by mass treatment. *J Hosp Infect.* 1981;2:63–69.

64. Barnham M, Kerby J. *Streptococcus pyogenes* in residential homes: probable spread of infection from the staff. *J Hosp Infect.* 1981;2:255–257.

65. Reid RI, Briggs RS, Seal DV, Pearson AD. Virulent *Streptococcus pyogenes*: outbreak and spread within a geriatric unit. *J Infect.* 1983;6:219–225.

66. Ruben FL, Norden CW, Heisler B, Korica Y. An outbreak of *Streptococcus pyogenes. Ann Intern Med.* 1984;101:494–496.

67. Pritchard VG, Kerry CS. Streptococcal outbreak. *J Gerontol Nurs.* 1988;14:19–23.

68. Berkelman RL, Martin D, Graham DR, et al. Streptococcal wound infections caused by a vaginal carrier. *JAMA.* 1982;247:2680–2682.

69. Ahlbrecht H, Shearen C, Degelau J, Guay DRP. Team approach to infection prevention and control in the nursing home setting. *Am J Infect Control.* 1999;27:64–70.

SUGGESTED READING

Smith PW, ed. *Infection Control in Long-Term Care Facilities*. 2nd ed. Albany, NY: Delmar Publishers Inc; 1994.

Smith PW, Rusnak PG. Infection prevention and control in the long-term care facility. *Am J Infect Control*. 1997;25:488–512.

Strasbaugh LF, Joseph C. Epidemiology and prevention of infections in long-term care facilities. In: Mayhall G, ed. *Hospital Epidemiology*. Baltimore, MD: Williams & Wilkins; 1996.

CHAPTER 5

Outbreaks Reported in the Ambulatory Care Setting

Kathleen Meehan Arias

INTRODUCTION

Despite the general belief that the risk of transmission of infectious diseases and other illnesses in the ambulatory health care setting is low, numerous outbreaks caused by a variety of bacterial, fungal, viral, and chemical agents have been reported in outpatient areas.[1,2] Many therapeutic, diagnostic, and surgical procedures formerly performed in the inpatient hospital setting are now routinely done in free-standing or hospital-sponsored outpatient facilities such as ambulatory surgery centers. As more health care services move from inpatient to outpatient facilities, the potential for nosocomial infections and other adverse events in the ambulatory care setting increases.

This chapter reviews outbreaks that have been reported in ambulatory care settings. One can use the findings of these outbreak investigations to identify risk factors that may be contributing to a similar outbreak and to identify prevention and control measures. For the purposes of this chapter, the ambulatory care setting is defined as one in which a patient does not remain overnight for health care services. Examples include physicians' offices, ambulatory surgery centers, dental offices, hemodialysis and peritoneal dialysis centers, chemotherapy facilities, outpatient clinics, and procedure suites (e.g., gastrointestinal endoscopy and bronchoscopy).

Little is known about the incidence of nosocomial infections in the outpatient setting because surveillance is not generally conducted and the populations at risk (i.e., the denominator numbers needed to calculate rates) are often difficult to define. Unlike the routine surveillance methods used to detect nosocomial infections in hospitalized patients, no standardized surveillance methodology has yet been developed for the ambulatory care setting. Therefore, it is likely that many infectious diseases and other illnesses transmitted in these settings go undetected unless they affect large numbers of patients or cause significant morbidity. The risk of disease transmission in the outpatient setting varies according to the services provided and the populations served. For instance, the risk of transmission of infectious agents in an internal medicine practice that does not perform invasive procedures is lower than the risk of infection in a hemodialysis center, where the transmission of bloodborne pathogens has been well defined. Table 5–1 contains examples of outbreaks that have occurred in a variety of outpatient settings.[3–17]

PHYSICIANS' OFFICES AND OUTPATIENT CLINICS

A literature review published by Goodman and Solomon in 1991 characterized 23 reports of case clusters and outbreaks that occurred in general medical offices, clinics, and emergency departments from 1961 through 1990.[1]

- Thirteen episodes involved common source transmission in which the agent was transmitted by a contaminated medical device (e.g., *Salmonella* via an endoscope and hepatitis B via acupuncture needles) or by contaminated fluids (e.g., disinfectants, benzalkonium chloride antiseptic, multidose medication vials, and multidose vials of influenza or diphtheria-

Table 5–1 Selected Outbreaks Occurring in Ambulatory Care Settings

Outbreak	Setting	Source/Cause	Year(s) Reported (Reference No.)
Group A beta-hemolytic streptococcus abscesses	Pediatrician's office	Contamination of multidose vial of DTP* vaccine	1985[3]
Measles	Pediatrician's office	12-year-old boy with cough and rash was in office for 1 hour	1985[4]
Hepatitis B	Weight reduction clinic	Jet injector gun—nozzle tip contaminated with blood was difficult to disinfect	1986[5]
Hepatitis B	Dentist's office	Dentist was asymptomatic carrier of hepatitis B	1986[6]
Septic arthritis caused by *Serratia marcescens*	Physician's office	Injection site and multidose vials cleansed with cotton balls soaked in contaminated benzalkonium chloride antiseptic	1987[7]
MDR-TB* in health care workers and HIV-infected* patients	Outpatient HIV clinic and hospital	HIV-infected patients with MDR-TB	1990[8]
Mycobacterium tuberculosis infection	Public health clinic	Patients with pulmonary tuberculosis; associated with aerosolized pentamidine therapy	1989[9]
Legionella pneumophila pneumonia	Outpatient clinic	Contaminated air-conditioning unit	1990[10]
Pseudomonas (currently *Burkholderia*) *cepacia* bacteremia	Oncology clinic	Contaminated 500-ml bag of 5% dextrose solution used to prepare heparin flush solution over a 2-week period	1993[11]
Patient-to-patient transmission of HIV	Private surgeon's office	Unknown	1993[12]
Adenovirus type 8 EKC*	Outpatient eye clinic	Inadequate hand washing by personnel; inadequate disinfection of instruments	1993[13]
Acremonium kiliense endophthalmitis	Ambulatory surgery center	Air contaminated by *A kiliense* in ventilation system humidifier water	1996[14]
Pseudomonas putida pseudopneumonia	Pulmonary clinic	Bronchoscope contaminated by improper maintenance of automated bronchoscope washer	1996[15]
Pseudomonas aeruginosa urinary tract infections	Urodynamic suite	Improper reuse and disinfection of single-use urodynamic testing equipment	1996[16]
Epidemic keratoconjunctivitis (EKC)	Eye care clinic	Lack of hand washing by personnel; inadequate decontamination of diagnostic lenses	1998[17]

*DTP = diphtheria-tetanus-pertussis; HIV = human immunodeficiency virus; MDR-TB = multidrug-resistant tuberculosis; EKC = epidemic keratoconjunctivitis.

tetanus-pertussis vaccines); in 10 of these outbreaks the mode of transmission was via injection and the causative agents were *Mycobacterium chelonae,* group A beta-hemolytic streptococci, *Pseudomonas cepacia, Serratia marcescens, Mycobacterium abscessus,* or *Mycobacterium fortuitum.*[5,7,18–28]

- Nine episodes involved organisms transmitted via the airborne or droplet route (*Mycobacterium tuberculosis,* measles, Epstein-Barr virus, and rubella).[4,8,9,29–34]
- One report documented person-to-person (staff-to-patient) transmission of epidemic keratocon-

junctivitis caused by adenovirus type 8 in an emergency department.[35]

Outbreaks Associated with Products and Devices (Common Source Outbreaks)

Many common source outbreaks in outpatient clinics and private physicians' offices have been associated with the use of intrinsically or extrinsically contaminated fluids.[36–41] Intrinsic contamination (i.e., contamination of the product before it reaches the consumer) is rarely reported; however, extrinsic contamination (i.e., that which occurs during use or preparation of a product) is documented often. Many users are not aware that antiseptic and disinfectant solutions may be intrinsically contaminated or may become extrinsically contaminated during use.

Intrinsically Contaminated Products

Intrinsic contamination of povidone-iodine solutions has caused outbreaks and pseudo-outbreaks in health care facilities.[38–40] The first report of intrinsic contamination of povidone-iodine was in 1981, when *Pseudomonas cepacia* pseudobacteremias in four New York City hospitals were associated with use of a povidone-iodine solution from a single manufacturer.[38]

Other fluids that are sold as sterile have also been found to be intrinsically contaminated. In 1998, 10 children who received outpatient therapy at a hospital-based hematology/oncology service developed sepsis caused by *Enterobacter cloacae*.[36] The source of the outbreak was traced to intrinsically contaminated prefilled saline syringes, and the manufacturer initiated a recall of the product.

These incidents illustrate the importance of recognizing clusters and outbreaks of infection and other adverse events and the possibility that they are related to the use of a product. Infections or pseudoinfections believed to be due to intrinsic (not extrinsic) contamination should be reported immediately to the facility's pharmacy, the manufacturer, and the Food and Drug Administration's Medical Products Reporting Program at 800-332-1088 (or Web site at http://www.fda.gov/medwatch).

Extrinsically Contaminated Products

Extrinsically contaminated fluids that have been the cause of outbreaks in the ambulatory care setting include vaccines,[3] benzalkonium chloride antiseptic,[7] 5% dextrose intravenous fluid,[11] and gentian violet skin-marking solution.[37] Benzalkonium chloride antiseptic has been responsible for many outbreaks and is not recommended for use in the health care setting because of the ease with which it may become contaminated during use.[7,41–45] One outbreak related to use of benzalkonium chloride involved 10 patients who developed *Serratia marcescens* joint infections after being treated by two orthopaedic surgeons who shared an office.[7] All of the patients had received injections of methylpredniso-

lone and lidocaine in the office. The reservoir of the organism was determined to be a canister of cotton balls soaking in benzalkonium chloride. Two previously used vials of methylprednisolone were also culture-positive for *S marcescens*. The outbreak terminated when the physicians' office discontinued the use of the benzalkonium chloride solution. Facilities using this antiseptic should find an alternative product. Information on choosing antiseptic agents has been published by the Association for Professionals in Infection Control and Epidemiology,[46] and the Centers for Disease Control and Prevention (CDC—formerly Centers for Disease Control until October 27, 1992, Center for Disease Control between 1970 and 1980, and Communicable Disease Center from 1946 to 1970).[42]

An outbreak of *Mycobacterium chelonae* postoperative surgical site infections occurred in eight patients who had cosmetic plastic surgery in a dermatologist's office. The source of the organism was traced to a contaminated gentian violet solution used to demarcate the incision site.[37] The investigators concluded that only sterile skin-marking agents should be used in surgical procedures.

Contaminated Devices

Contaminated medical devices that have been associated with outbreaks in outpatient care facilities include jet gun injectors,[5,28] bronchoscopes,[15] and urodynamic testing equipment.[16] There are several reports of outbreaks associated with the use of jet gun injectors. An outbreak of hepatitis B (31 clinical cases) occurred from January 1984 to November 1985 in a weight reduction clinic where attendees received parenteral human chorionic gonadotrophin given by jet injection.[5] One factor that contributed to this outbreak was the design of the jet gun nozzle tip, which made it difficult to clean and disinfect once it became contaminated with blood. An outbreak of *Mycobacterium chelonae* foot infections occurred in eight patients of a podiatry office. The infections were associated with use of a jet injector used to administer lidocaine. The source of the organism was a distilled water/quaternary ammonium disinfectant solution in which the jet injector was soaked between procedures.[28] These two outbreaks emphasize the need to clean carefully these devices and to disinfect them with a high-level disinfectant. Guidelines for choosing an appropriate disinfectant have been published by the Association for Professionals in Infection Control and Epidemiology.[44]

Control Measures for Preventing Product- and Device-Related Outbreaks

The following measures should be used to prevent the transmission of infection by contaminated products and devices:

- Personnel handling fluids must be instructed in and adhere to proper aseptic technique to prevent extrinsic contamination of solutions.
- Reusable equipment must be cleaned thoroughly, according to the manufacturer's directions, to remove dirt and organic debris before disinfection or sterilization in order to prevent transmission of infectious agents by devices.
- Semicritical items—those that come in contact with mucous membranes or nonintact skin—must be free of microbial contamination. If reusable, these items must be either sterilized or disinfected with a high-level disinfectant.[44] Examples of semicritical devices are bronchoscopes, gastrointestinal endoscopes, vaginal specula, and cervical diaphragm fitting rings.
- An appropriate disinfectant (a germicide formulated to inactivate microorganisms on inanimate surfaces) should be chosen based on the composition and the use of the item being disinfected.[44]
- Devices that enter tissues or the vascular system, such as surgical instruments, cardiac and urinary catheters, and implants and needles, must be sterile. If these devices are reusable, they must be mechanically cleaned and then sterilized after each use and wrapped and stored properly so they are not contaminated by dirt or microorganisms.
- Directions on the labels of cleansers, antiseptics, and disinfectants should be followed carefully. Care must be taken to ensure that cleansers (solutions formulated to remove dirt and debris) or antiseptic solutions (solutions formulated to inactivate microorganisms on skin and tissues) are not used as disinfectants to decontaminate devices and equipment because they will not be effective at destroying microbial pathogens present on these surfaces.
- Single-use items, especially needles and syringes, should be used only once and discarded.
- Benzalkonium chloride solution should not be used as a skin antiseptic in the health care setting because it is easily contaminated and has been associated with numerous outbreaks.[45] An alternative product should be chosen.

Outbreaks associated with products and devices are also discussed in Chapter 3. Infection control and quality management personnel should be familiar with products and devices causing outbreaks in all types of health care settings, since many products and devices may be used in acute care, long-term care, and outpatient facilities.

Outbreaks Associated with Patient-to-Patient Transmission

In addition to common source transmission, pathogens may also be transmitted from patient to patient via direct contact or the airborne route.

Transmission via Direct Contact

Hlady et al reported a large outbreak of hepatitis B transmitted to approximately 300 patients in a dermatology practice in Florida from 1985 through 1991.[47] The outbreak was detected when personnel at a county health department recognized that eight patients with acute hepatitis B infection reported between 1985 and 1991 had visited the same dermatologist prior to onset of their symptoms. An investigation revealed that the dermatologist routinely operated without gloves, did not wash his hands between patients, used a common needle that remained in a multidose vial to access medications (although he did use a separate syringe for each patient), and reused electrocautery tips without cleaning them between patients. Because the dermatologist was not found to be a hepatitis B virus (HBV) carrier, the investigators concluded that transmission occurred from patient to patient due to the physician's failure to use universal (standard) precautions or sterile surgical technique.

Patient-to-patient transmission of human immunodeficiency virus (HIV) has been documented in a private surgical practice in Australia, although the mode of transmission was not identified.[12] Investigators concluded that a breach in infection control precautions was responsible for the transmission of HIV from an infected patient to four other patients who had minor surgery on the same day.

Transmission via the Airborne Route

Measles and tuberculosis are two diseases spread via the airborne route that have caused outbreaks in ambulatory and acute care settings.

Measles. Measles is highly communicable from person to person via the airborne route, and transmission in medical facilities has been well documented.[4,29,30,33,34] The virus that causes measles can remain airborne for prolonged periods. In an outbreak that occurred in a pediatrician's office, infection developed in three children who arrived at the office an hour or more after a child with measles had left.[34]

Strategies for preventing transmission of measles in physicians' offices include

- prompt recognition of patients with measles (measles should be considered in any patient, whether an adult or a child, who has fever and a rash)
- separation of patients with known or suspected measles from other patients (this may be difficult due to ease of airborne spread and lack of adequate ventilation in many physicians' offices)
- postexposure prophylaxis of potentially exposed contacts, such as patients, persons accompanying patients, and medical personnel
- postexposure immunization of patients and personnel according to the recommendations of the Advisory Committee on Immunization Practices[48,49]

Guidelines for preventing transmission of measles have been published by the CDC[50,51] and the American Academy of Pediatrics.[52] Measles outbreaks and prevention and control measures are discussed in detail in Chapter 3. Because the incidence of measles in the United States is low,[48] one case of measles should be considered an outbreak and should be promptly reported by telephone to the local health department so that measures to prevent further spread can be implemented as soon as possible. Appendix D contains a protocol for controlling an outbreak of measles in a health care facility, including a physician's office.

Tuberculosis. Transmission of tuberculosis (TB) in the ambulatory care setting is well recognized.[8,9,53–55] Multiple outbreaks of TB infection and disease, including multidrug-resistant tuberculosis (MDR-TB), occurred in the United States in the late 1980s and early 1990s, and several involved patients and personnel in outpatient treatment facilities.[8,9,54] There are also reports of TB outbreaks among emergency room personnel who were exposed to patients with pulmonary tuberculosis.[53,56] In 1996, the CDC investigated patients who were seen by a pediatrician diagnosed with infectious pulmonary tuberculosis; at least five children were found to be infected as a result of exposure to the physician, who continued to work despite the fact that he was symptomatic.[55]

Information on the epidemiology and mode of transmission of *Mycobacterium tuberculosis* and on control measures used to prevent the spread of TB in health care facilities can be found in Chapter 7. The CDC[57] has published guidelines for preventing the transmission of tuberculosis in health care facilities. In any health care setting, the most important control measures for preventing the transmission of *M tuberculosis* include

- prompt recognition of persons (patients and personnel) with pulmonary TB
- prompt isolation of patients with known or suspected pulmonary TB in a private room with negative airflow and air exhausted to the outside
- prompt and appropriate diagnostic work-up for persons with signs and symptoms of pulmonary tuberculosis (i.e., medical history and physical, chest radiograph, tuberculin skin testing, and smear and culture of sputum for acid-fast bacilli)
- use of respiratory protection by personnel caring for a patient with known or suspected TB
- prompt treatment of patients with antituberculosis medications

Patients who come to an ambulatory care facility with signs and symptoms suggestive of pulmonary tuberculosis should be instructed to wear a mask and should be separated from other patients until the diagnosis is confirmed or ruled out.

DENTAL OFFICES

Outbreaks in dental offices have long been recognized.[1,6,58] Hepatitis B virus is the most common agent involved in reported outbreaks. Goodman and Solomon reviewed 13 reports of infectious disease transmission that occurred in dental practices between 1961 and 1990.[1]

- Nine were reports of transmission of hepatitis B virus from an infected dentist or oral surgeon to patients.[6,58–65]
- One involved gingivostomatitis caused by herpes simplex transmitted by a dental hygienist with herpetic whitlow.[66]

- One investigated a presumed transmission of human immunodeficiency virus from an infected dentist to his patients.[67]
- One involved oral abscesses caused by *Pseudomonas aeruginosa* from a contaminated dental unit water system.[68]
- One involved intraoral and pulmonary tuberculosis transmitted by a dentist with infectious pulmonary TB.[69]

Most of the reports of the investigations of the hepatitis B virus outbreaks suggested that the virus was transmitted directly from an infected dentist or oral surgeon to the patient(s).[6,58–65] There was no evidence in these reports of transmission from patient to patient via contaminated instruments or equipment.

One of the most highly publicized events involving transmission of an infection from a health care provider to a patient was the 1990 report of HIV transmitted to a patient by a dentist with acquired immune deficiency syndrome (AIDS).[70] Further investigation linked the Florida dentist to HIV infection in six of his patients[67,71,72]; however, the mode of transmission of HIV was not determined.

Measures Used To Prevent Transmission of Infection in Dental Offices

Control measures for preventing transmission of infectious agents, including HIV, HBV, and other bloodborne pathogens, in the dental setting have been published by the CDC[73] and the American Dental Association[74–76] and include

- development and implementation of a comprehensive infection control program
- use of protective attire and standard (universal) precautions by personnel[73–76]
- use of aseptic technique by personnel
- immunization of susceptible dental personnel with HBV vaccine[49,75]
- appropriate cleaning, disinfection, and sterilization of instruments and equipment[75]
- decontamination of environmental surfaces[75,76]

HEMODIALYSIS AND PERITONEAL DIALYSIS CENTERS

Numerous outbreaks have been reported in hemodialysis and peritoneal dialysis centers.[77–91] Many of these have been caused by hepatitis B virus, although hepatitis C virus, HIV, fungi, bacteria, and bacterial endotoxins have also been responsible, as shown in Table 5–2. In addition, improperly processed hemodialyzers have caused anaphylactoid reactions,[82] and improperly installed filters in a water treatment system have caused hypotension.[86]

Several factors help to promote the transmission of HBV in the dialysis setting.

- HBV may be present in high titers ($\geq 10^9$ virus particles per milliliter) in the blood and body fluids of infected patients.[78]
- HBV survives well in the environment.[92]
- Equipment and surfaces in dialysis facilities can easily become contaminated with blood.

The majority of outbreaks of hepatitis B infection in hemodialysis facilities are associated with lack of adherence to recommended infection control practices for preventing the transmission of bloodborne pathogens. The following factors have contributed to hemodialysis outbreaks[78]:

- failure to use separate rooms for hemodialyzing patients with chronic HBV infection
- failure to use dedicated machines, medications, supplies, and staff for patients with chronic hepatitis B
- failure to abide by standard cleaning and disinfection procedures
- failure to restrict sharing of medications and supplies between patients

Measures Used To Prevent Transmission of Infection in Dialysis Centers

Recommendations to prevent the transmission of HBV in dialysis centers were originally published by the CDC in 1977,[93] and recommendations to use universal (standard) precautions[73] and to vaccinate all susceptible hemodialysis patients[94,95] have since been added. The CDC has a series of "Prevention Guidelines" that are accessible through the CDC's Web site (http://www.cdc.gov). These include the following recommendations for preventing the transmission of bloodborne pathogens in hemodialysis settings[78]:

- use of universal (standard) precautions by personnel
- requirement of monthly testing of serum specimens from all susceptible patients for hepatitis B

Table 5–2 Selected Outbreaks Reported in Dialysis Facilities

Outbreak	Source/Cause	Year(s) Reported (Reference No.)
Hepatitis B	Shared multidose vial used by patient with chronic HBV*	1983[80]
Hepatitis B	Failure to isolate patient with chronic HBV; shared equipment and staff	1989[79]
Hypotension	Ultrafilters preserved in sodium azide not rinsed prior to installation in dialysis center water treatment system; dialysis water became contaminated with sodium diazide	1990[86]
Anaphylactoid reactions	Reuse of hollow-fiber hemodialyzers reprocessed with automated reprocessing system	1992[82]
Bacteremia with gram-negative organisms and *Enterococcus casseliflavus*	Venous blood tubing cross-contaminated with ultrafiltrate waste from hemodialysis system	1992[87]
Hepatitis C virus	No common source or person-to-person mode of transmission documented; probable cause was lack of adequate infection control precautions	1992[81]
HIV*	Reusable needle used on patient with HIV then improperly processed with benzalkonium chloride by soaking in a common pan with needles used on other patients	1995[85]
Pyrogenic reactions	*Candida parapsilosis* colonization of the membranes in dialysis machine balance chamber; associated with use of contaminated white distilled vinegar used to descale the machines	1996[83]
Hepatitis B, Texas	Lack of separation of patients with chronic HBV infection from other patients; lack of review of monthly HBsAg* results; lack of use of standard precautions; poor compliance with HBV recommendations	1996[78]
Culture-negative peritonitis	Dialysate used for continuous cyclic peritoneal dialysis contaminated with endotoxin	1997[88]
Bloodstream infections caused by multiple pathogens	Contamination of newly installed attachment used to drain spent priming saline in hemodialysis system	1998[91]

*HBV = hepatitis B virus; HIV = human immunodeficiency virus; HBsAg = hepatitis B surface antigen.

---

surface antigen (HbsAg) and prompt review of the results of this testing

- isolation of HbsAg-positive patients by room, machines, instruments, medications, supplies, and staff
- avoidance of sharing instruments, medications, and supplies between patients
- preparation of multidose medication vials in a clean centralized area away from areas used for patient care, laboratory work, or waste disposal

- implementation of routine cleaning and disinfection protocols
- separation of areas used to store clean supplies and handle contaminated items
- storage of blood specimens in designated areas away from medication preparation or clean supply areas
- use of hepatitis B vaccine for susceptible hemodialysis patients[94,95]

For additional information on infection control practices in the hemodialysis setting, the reader is referred to the chapters by Garcia-Houchins,[96] Band,[97] and Favero et al.[98] and to Appendix G.

OPHTHALMOLOGY OFFICES AND CLINICS

Many reports of outbreaks of nosocomial epidemic keratoconjunctivitis (EKC) have been published.[1,2,17,99–108] Goodman and Solomon reviewed 11 reports of infectious disease outbreaks in ophthalmology offices and eye clinics[1]: 10 were outbreaks of EKC caused by adenovirus transmitted by inadequately disinfected equipment (frequently a tonometer) and/or by poor hand-washing practices by physicians and other health care personnel,[99–108] and one episode was a cluster of cases of *Mycobacterium chelonei* keratitis associated with invasive procedures in which a contaminated solution was the likely source of the organism.[109]

Person-to-person transmission of adenovirus occurs via direct contact with an infected person or with infective secretions, such as those on the hands of a health care worker or on contaminated fomites. In a report of an outbreak involving 63 patients at a large university medical center ophthalmology clinic, the CDC noted that exposure to a particular health care worker or exposure to pneumotonometry were risk factors for acquiring EKC.[110] Contaminated ocular devices, particularly tonometers, are frequently implicated in nosocomial outbreaks. Since tonometers vary in design, it is important that methods used for cleaning and disinfecting or sterilizing these instruments allow for adequate disinfection/sterilization of the instrument's tip and adjacent parts after each patient use.[110]

Measures Used To Prevent Spread of Epidemic Keratoconjunctivitis

Recommendations for preventing the spread of infection and for controlling EKC outbreaks in ophthalmology practices have been published by the American Academy of Ophthalmology,[111] the CDC,[110] Buehler et al,[99] and Montessori et al.[17] Prevention and control measures to limit the spread of adenovirus and other infectious agents include

- appropriate hand-washing practices both before and after examining patients
- proper cleaning and disinfection or sterilization protocols for the types of equipment used[110]

- cleaning and disinfection/sterilization of equipment after each patient
- triage of patients with signs and symptoms of conjunctivitis (e.g., eye discharge or redness)
- meticulous administration of eye drops to avoid contaminating the dropper and the medication
- careful cleaning and disinfection of environmental surfaces
- use of gloves for contact with infective eye secretions (e.g., when a patient has clinical signs and symptoms of conjunctivitis and during an EKC outbreak)
- restriction of personnel with conjunctivitis from direct contact with patients (for up to 14 days for personnel with viral conjunctivitis)[110]

The CDC recommends that tonometer tips "be cleaned with soap and water or with another cleansing agent suggested by the manufacturer and disinfected by soaking for at least 10 minutes in a solution containing 500–5,000 ppm chlorine (e.g., a 1:100–1:10 dilution of household bleach) or in any commercial germicidal solution that is registered with the Environmental Protection Agency as a 'sterilant' and is compatible with the tonometer. The soaking time in commercial germicides necessary to achieve high-level disinfection (which includes inactivation of adenovirus type 8 and bacteria that are pathogenic to the eye) varies by type and concentration of solution and should be indicated by the germicide manufacturer on the product label."[110(p.600)] When using any commercially available cleaner or disinfectant, it is important to read carefully the indications for use and to follow the directions on the label. The CDC recommendations for preventing EKC in ophthalmology services[110] can be downloaded from the CDC Web site at http://www.cdc.gov/epo/mmwr/preview/mmwrhtml/00001741.htm.

GASTROINTESTINAL ENDOSCOPY AND BRONCHOSCOPY PROCEDURE SUITES

Numerous outbreaks associated with endoscopic procedures have been reported in inpatient and outpatient settings. Most of these were caused by failure to clean adequately and to disinfect endoscopes or by contamination of automated endoscope processors. Outbreaks related to endoscopic procedures, including prevention and control measures, are discussed in Chapter 3.

AMBULATORY SURGERY CENTERS

A search of the MEDLINE database from 1985 through 1998 revealed only two outbreaks reported in ambulatory surgery centers.

1. An outbreak of *Proteus mirabilis* surgical site infections occurred in patients who underwent outpatient podiatric surgery.[112] An investigation traced the source to inadequately sterilized bone drills. The cluster of infections was recognized in part because it was caused by an uncommon strain of *P mirabilis*.
2. An outbreak of *Acremonium kiliense* endophthalmitis occurred following cataract surgery in four patients in an ambulatory surgical center.[14] An epidemiologic study discovered that the infected patients had surgery either on the first operative day of the week or soon after the operating room opened. Cultures of perioperative medications and environmental samples were negative for *A kiliense* except for water from a grossly contaminated humidifier reservoir in the heating, ventilation, and air-conditioning (HVAC) system. Further investigation revealed that the HVAC system was routinely turned off after the last case on Thursday and switched back on when surgery resumed the following Tuesday. The investigators concluded that the HVAC system was contaminated by the humidifier water, and agitation of the system probably dislodged fungal spores when the system was turned on. The spores were then carried on air currents into the operating room. No further cases occurred after the HVAC system was left running 7 days a week and the humidifier was removed.

Because the incidence of surgical site infections associated with the types of procedures performed in ambulatory care centers is low, most surgical centers do not routinely conduct surveillance for surgical site infections. Therefore, it is likely that clusters and outbreaks of infection in this setting may not be detected unless they are caused by an unusual organism or result in significant morbidity. As more procedures are moved from the inpatient to the outpatient setting, consideration should be given to implementing infection surveillance in ambulatory surgery settings.[113,114]

CONCLUSIONS

Risk Factors Associated with Infectious Disease Outbreaks in the Ambulatory Care Setting

Many outbreaks in the ambulatory care setting occur because (1) the responsibility for implementing an infection control program is often not assigned to a specific individual and (2) personnel working in these settings are frequently not familiar with basic infection control practices that are routinely used in acute care facilities. By reviewing the reports of the outbreaks discussed in this chapter, one can identify the following risk factors as causing or contributing to infectious disease outbreaks in the outpatient care setting:

- inadequate cleaning, disinfection, sterilization, and storage of instruments and equipment
- inappropriate use of barrier precautions, such as gloves, by health care personnel
- inadequate hand-washing practices by health care workers
- failure to use aseptic technique
- failure to use appropriate isolation precautions for infected patients
- lack of temporary work restriction on infected health care personnel
- lack of familiarity with established infection control practices on the part of ambulatory care personnel

Measures Used To Prevent Transmission of Infectious Agents in the Ambulatory Care Setting

The specific measures that should be implemented to prevent the transmission of infectious agents in each practice setting will depend on the types of patients, the procedures performed, and the equipment and devices that are used.

However, all ambulatory care settings should have an infection control program that addresses the following:

- assignment of responsibility for coordinating and implementing the program to specific individuals
- process for identifying the types of patients and procedures performed and the risk for infection and other adverse events
- infection control policies and procedures that are site specific

- protocols for implementing standard (universal) precautions[51,73,74]
- identification of the types of reusable devices and instruments used and determination of whether they must be disinfected or sterilized[42,44]
- protocols for cleaning and disinfection or sterilization of reusable devices and instruments in accordance with the manufacturer's instructions and the recommendations of relevant organizations (e.g., the Association for Professionals in Infection Control and Epidemiology,[44,115] the Association of Operating Room Nurses,[116] the American Academy of Ophthalmology,[111] and the American Society for Gastrointestinal Endoscopy[117,118])
- protocols for monitoring the effectiveness of the sterilization process, if a sterilizer is used[116]
- protocols for identifying and isolating infected patients[51,52,57]
- protocols for restricting infected personnel from direct patient contact[50]
- policies for the immunization of health care workers[49]

- protocols for handling multidose medication vials
- education of ambulatory care personnel on basic infection control practices, such as standard precautions, triage and isolation of infected patients, separation of clean and dirty items, and the use of aseptic technique

ADDITIONAL INFORMATION ON OUTBREAKS AND INFECTION CONTROL IN THE AMBULATORY CARE SETTING

For comprehensive reviews of outbreaks that have been reported in a variety of outpatient settings, including the infection control deficiencies that contributed to their occurrence and measures that can be used to prevent them, the reader is referred to the articles by Goodman and Solomon[1] and by Herwaldt, Smith, and Carter.[2] A review of infection control practices in the dental setting has been written by Molinari.[119] Additional information on outbreaks and infection control can also be found in relevant chapters in the infection control texts noted in the Suggested Reading section at the end of this chapter.

REFERENCES

1. Goodman RA, Solomon SL. Transmission of infectious diseases in outpatient health care settings. *JAMA.* 1991;265:2377–2381.
2. Herwaldt LA, Smith LA, Carter CD. Infection control in the outpatient setting. *Infect Control Hosp Epidemiol.* 1998;19:41–74.
3. Stetler HC, Garbe PL, Dwyer DM, et al. Outbreaks of group A streptococcal abscesses following diphtheria-tetanus toxoid-pertussis vaccination. *Pediatrics.* 1985;75:299–303.
4. Bloch AB, Orenstein WA, Ewing WM, et al. Measles outbreak in a pediatric practice: airborne transmission in an office setting. *Pediatrics.* 1985;75:676–683.
5. Centers for Disease Control. Hepatitis B associated with jet gun injection. *MMWR Morb Mortal Wkly Rep.* 1986;35:373–376.
6. Shaw F Jr, Barrett CL, Hamm R, et al. Lethal outbreak of hepatitis B in a dental practice. *JAMA.* 1986;255:3260–3264.
7. Nakashima AK, McCarthy MA, Martone WJ, Anderson RL. Epidemic septic arthritis caused by *Serratia marcescens* and associated with a benzalkonium chloride antiseptic. *J Clin Microbiol.* 1987;25:1014–1018.
8. Centers for Disease Control. Nosocomial transmission of multidrug-resistant tuberculosis to health care workers and HIV-infected patients in an urban hospital—Florida. *MMWR Morb Mortal Wkly Rep.* 1990;39:718–722.
9. Centers for Disease Control. *Mycobacterium* tuberculosis transmission in a health clinic—Florida, 1988. *MMWR Morb Mortal Wkly Rep.* 1989;38:256–258, 263–264.
10. O'Mahoney MC, Stanwell-Smith RE, Tillett HE, et al. The Stafford outbreak of Legionnaires' disease. *Epidemiol Infect.* 1990;104:361–380.
11. Pegues DA, Carson LA, Anderson RI, et al. Outbreak of *Pseudomonas cepacia* bacteremia in oncology patients. *Clin Infect Dis.* 1993;16:407–411.
12. Chant K, Lowe D, Rubin G, et al. Patient-to-patient transmission of HIV in private surgical consulting rooms [letter]. *Lancet.* 1993;342:1548–1549.
13. Jernigan JA, Lowry BS, Hayden FG, et al. Adenovirus type 8 epidemic keratoconjunctivitis in an eye clinic: risk factors and control. *J Infect Dis.* 1993;167:1307–1313.
14. Fridkin SK, Kremer FB, Bland LA, Padhye A, McNeil MM, Jarvis WR. *Acremonium kiliense* endophthalmitis that occurred after cataract extraction in an ambulatory surgical center and was traced to an environmental reservoir. *Clin Infect Dis.* 1996;22:222–227.
15. Umphrey J, Raad I, Tarrand J, Hill LA. Bronchoscopes as a contamination source of *Pseudomonas putida*. *Infect Control Hosp Epidemiol.* 1996;17(suppl):P42. Abstract M2.
16. Climo M, Pastor A, Wong E. Outbreak of *P. aeruginosa* infections related to contaminated urodynamic testing equipment. *Infect Control Hosp Epidemiol.* 1996;17(suppl):P48. Abstract M58.
17. Montessori V, Scharf S, Holland S, Werker DH, Roberts FJ, Bryce E. Epidemic keratoconjunctivitis outbreak at a tertiary referral eye care clinic. *Am J Infect Control.* 1998;26:399–405.
18. Beecham HJ, Cohen ML, Parkin WE. *Salmonella typhimurium* transmission by fiberoptic upper gastrointestinal endoscopy. *JAMA.* 1979;241:1013–1015.
19. Borghans JGA, Stanford JL. *Mycobacterium chelonei* in abscesses after injection of diphtheria-pertussis-tetanus-polio vaccine. *Am Rev Respir Dis.* 1973;107:1–8.

20. Edell TA. *Serratia marcescens* abscesses in soft tissue associated with intramuscular methylprednisolone injections. In: Program and abstracts of the 28th Annual Epidemic Intelligence Service Conference; April 2–6, 1979; Atlanta, GA.

21. Georgia Department of Human Resources. Abscesses in an allergy practice due to *Mycobacterium chelonae*. *Ga Epidemiol Rep.* April 1990.

22. Greaves WL, Hinman AR, Facklam RR, et al. Streptococcal abscesses following diphtheria-tetanus toxoid-pertussis vaccination. *Pediatr Infect Dis J.* 1982;1:388–390.

23. Inman PM, Beck A, Brown AE, Stanford JL. Outbreak of injection abscesses due to *Mycobacterium abscessus*. *Arch Dermatol.* 1969;100:141–147.

24. Kobler E, Schmuziger P, Hartmann G. Hepatitis nach Akupunktur. *Schweizerische Medizinische Woschenschrift.* 1979;109:1828–1829.

25. Kothari T, Reyes MP, Brooks N, Brown WJ, Lerner AM. *Pseudomonas cepacia* septic arthritis due to intra-articular injections of methylprednisolone. *Can Med Assoc J.* 1977;116:1230–1235.

26. Lowry PW, Jarvis WR, Oberle AD, et al. *Mycobacterium chelonae* causing otitis media in an ear, nose, and throat practice. *N Engl J. Med.* 1968;319:978–982.

27. Owen M, Smith A, Coultras J. Granulomatous lesions occurring at site of injections of vaccines and antibiotics. *South Med J.* 1963;56:949–952.

28. Wenger JD, Spika JS, Smithwick RW, et al. Outbreak of *Mycobacterium chelonae* infection associated with use of jet injectors. *JAMA.* 1990;264:373–376.

29. Centers for Disease Control. Measles—Washington, 1990. *MMWR Morb Mortal Wkly Rep.* 1990;39:473–476.

30. Davis RM, Orenstein WA, Frank JA Jr. Transmission of measles in medical settings, 1980 through 1984. *JAMA.* 1986;255:1295–1298.

31. Ginsburg CM, Henle G, Henle W. An outbreak of infectious mononucleosis among the personnel of an outpatient clinic. *Am J Epidemiol.* 1976;104:571–575.

32. Greaves WL, Orenstein WA, Stetler HC, et al. Prevention of rubella transmission in medical facilities. *JAMA.* 1982;248:861–864.

33. Istre GR, McKee PA, West GR, et al. Measles spread in medical settings: an important focus of disease transmission? *Pediatrics.* 1987;79:356–358.

34. Remington PL, Hall WN, Davis IH, Herald A, Gunn RA. Airborne transmission of measles in a physician's office. *JAMA.* 1985;253:1574–1577.

35. Richmond S, Burman R, Crosdale E, et al. A large outbreak of keratoconjunctivitis due to adenovirus type 8. *J Hygiene.* 1984;93:285–291.

36. Centers for Disease Control and Prevention. *Enterobacter cloacae* bloodstream infections associated with contaminated prefilled saline syringes—California, November 1998. *MMWR Morb Mortal Wkly Rep.* 1998;47:959–960.

37. Safranek TJ, Jarvis WR, Carson LA, et al. *Mycobacterium chelonae* wound infections after plastic surgery employing contaminated gentian violet skin-marking solution. *N Engl J Med.* 1987;317:197–201.

38. Berkelman RL, Lewin S, Allen JR, et al. Pseudobacteremia attributed to contamination of povidone-iodine with *Pseudomonas cepacia*. *Ann Intern Med.* 1981;95:32–36.

39. Panlilio AL, Beck-Sague CM, Siegel JD, et al. Infections and pseudoinfections due to povidone-iodine solution contaminated with *Pseudomonas cepacia*. *Clin Inf Dis.* 1992;14:1078–1083.

40. Parrott PL, Terry PM, Whitworth EN, et al. *Pseudomonas aeruginosa* peritonitis associated with contaminated poloxamer-iodine solution. *Lancet.* 1982;2:683–685.

41. Sautter RL, Mattman LH, Legaspi RC. *Serratia marcescens* meningitis associated with a contaminated benzalkonium chloride solution. *Infect Control.* 1984;5:223–225.

42. Simmons BP. CDC guidelines for the prevention and control of nosocomial infections: guideline for hospital environmental control. *Am J Infect Control.* 1983;11:97–115.

43. Dixon RE, Kaslow RA, Mackel DC, Fulkerson CC, Mallinson GF. Aqueous quaternary ammonium antiseptics and disinfectants: use and misuse. *JAMA.* 1976;236:2415–2417.

44. Rutala WA. APIC guideline for selection and use of disinfectants. *Am J Infect Control.* 1996;24:313–342.

45. Donowitz LG. Benzalkonium chloride is still in use. *Infect Control Hosp Epidemiol.* 1991;12:186–187.

46. Larson EL. APIC guideline for handwashing and hand antisepsis in health care settings. *Am J Infect Control.* 1995;23:251–269.

47. Hlady WG, Hopkins RS, Ogilby TE, Allen ST. Patient-to-patient transmission of hepatitis B in a dermatology practice. *Am J Public Health.* 1993;83:1689–1693.

48. Centers for Disease Control and Prevention. Measles, mumps, and rubella—vaccine use and strategies for elimination of measles, rubella, and congenital rubella syndrome and control of mumps: recommendations of the Advisory Committee on Immunization Practices (ACIP). *MMWR Morb Mortal Wkly Rep.* 1998;47(RR-08):1–57.

49. Centers for Disease Control and Prevention. Immunization of healthcare workers: recommendations of the Advisory Committee on Immunization Practices (ACIP) and the Hospital Infection Control Practices Advisory Committee (HICPAC). *MMWR Morb Mortal Wkly Rep.* 1997;46(RR-18):1–42.

50. Centers for Disease Control and Prevention. Guideline for infection control in health care personnel, 1998. *Am J Infect Control.* 1998;26:289–354.

51. Centers for Disease Control and Prevention. Guideline for isolation precautions in hospitals. *Am J Infect Control.* 1996;24:24–52.

52. American Academy of Pediatrics. *1997 Red Book: Report of the Committee on Infectious Diseases.* Peter G, ed. 24th ed. Elk Grove Village, IL: American Academy of Pediatrics; 1997.

53. Griffith DE, Hardeman JL, Zhang Y, Wallace RJ, Mazurek GH. Tuberculosis outbreak among healthcare workers in a community hospital. *Am J Respir Crit Care Med.* 1995;152:808–811.

54. Couldwell DL, Dore GJ. Harkness JL, et al. Nosocomial outbreak of tuberculosis in an outpatient HIV treatment room. *AIDS.* 1996;10:521–525.

55. Moore M, and the Investigative Team. Evaluation of transmission of tuberculosis in a pediatric setting—Pennsylvania. Presented at: 46th Annual Epidemic Intelligence Service Conference; April 14–18, 1997; Atlanta, GA; p. 53.

56. Sokolove PE, Mackey D, Wiles J, Lewis RJ. Exposure of emergency department personnel to tuberculosis: PPD testing during an epidemic in the community. *Ann Emerg Med.* 1994;24:418–421.

57. Centers for Disease Control and Prevention. Guidelines for preventing the transmission of *Mycobacterium tuberculosis* in health-care facilities, 1994. *MMWR Morb Mortal Wkly Rep.* 1994;43(RR-13):1–132.

58. Ahtone JL, Goodman RA. Hepatitis B and dental personnel: transmission to patients and prevention issues. *J Am Dent Assoc.* 1983;106:219–222.

59. Centers for Disease Control. Outbreak of hepatitis B associated with an oral surgeon—New Hampshire. *MMWR Morb Mortal Wkly Rep.* 1987;36:132–133.

60. Goodman RA, Ahtone JL, Flinton RJ. Hepatitis B transmission from dental personnel to patients: unfinished business. *Ann Intern Med.* 1982;96:119.

61. Goodwin D. An oral surgeon-related hepatitis B outbreak. *Calif Morbid.* April 16, 1976.

62. Hadler SC, Sorley DL, Acree KH, et al. An outbreak of hepatitis B in a dental practice. *Ann Intern Med.* 1981;95:133–138.

63. Levin ML, Maddrey WC, Wanda JR, Mendeloff AI. Hepatitis B transmission by dentists. *JAMA.* 1974;228:1139–1140.

64. Reingold AL, Kane MA, Murphy BL, et al. Transmission of hepatitis B by an oral surgeon. *J Infect Dis.* 1982;145:262–268.

65. Rimland D, Parkin WE, Miller GB Jr, Schrack WD. Hepatitis B outbreak traced to an oral surgeon. *N Engl J Med.* 1977;296:953–958.

66. Manzella JP, McConville JH, Valenti W, et al. An outbreak of herpes simplex virus type I gingivostomatitis in a dental hygiene practice. *JAMA.* 1984;252:2019–2022.

67. Centers for Disease Control. Update: transmission of HIV infection during an invasive dental procedure. *MMWR Morb Mortal Wkly Rep.* 1991;40:21–27, 33.

68. Martin MV. The significance of the bacterial contamination of dental unit water systems. *Br Dent J.* 1987;183:152–154.

69. Smith WHR, Mason KD, Davies D, Onions JP. Intraoral and pulmonary tuberculosis following dental treatment. *Lancet.* 1982;1:842–844.

70. Centers for Disease Control. Possible transmission of human immunodeficiency virus to a patient during an invasive dental procedure. *MMWR Morb Mortal Wkly Rep.* 1990;39:489–493.

71. Ciesielski CA, Marianos DW, Ou CY, et al. Transmission of human immunodeficiency virus to a patient during an invasive dental procedure. *MMWR Morb Mortal Wkly Rep.* 1990;39:489–493.

72. Ciesielski CA, Marianos DW, Schochetman G, Witte JJ, Jaffe J. The 1990 Florida dental investigations: the press and the science. *Ann Intern Med.* 1994;121:886–888.

73. Centers for Disease Control. Update: universal precautions for prevention of transmission of human immunodeficiency virus, and other bloodborne pathogens in health-care settings. *MMWR Morb Mortal Wkly Rep.* 1988;37:377–82,387–8.

74. Centers for Disease Control. Recommendations for preventing transmission of human immunodeficiency virus and hepatitis B virus to patients during exposure-prone invasive procedures. *MMWR Morb Mortal Wkly Rep.* 1991;40(RR-8):1–9.

75. Centers for Disease Control. Recommended infection-control practices for dentistry. *MMWR Morb Mortal Wkly Rep.* 1986;35:237–242.

76. American Dental Association, Council on Scientific Affairs and Council on Dental Practice. Infection control recommendations for the dental office and the dental laboratory. *J Am Dent Assoc.* 1996;127:672–680.

77. Tokars JI, Miller ER, Alter MJ, Arduino MJ. National surveillance of dialysis-associated diseases in the United States, 1995. *Am Soc Artif Intern Organs J.* 1998;44:98–107.

78. Centers for Disease Control and Prevention. Outbreaks of hepatitis B virus infection among hemodialysis patients—California, Nebraska, and Texas, 1994. *MMWR Morb Mortal Wkly Rep.* 1996;45:285–289.

79. Niu MT, Penberthy LT, Alter MJ, Armstrong CW, Miller GB, Hadler SC. Hemodialysis-associated hepatitis B: report of an outbreak. *Dial & Transplantation.* 1989;18:542–555.

80. Alter MJ, Ahtone J, Maynard JE. Hepatitis B virus transmission associated with a multiple-dose vial in a hemodialysis unit. *Ann Intern Med.* 1983;99:330–333.

81. Niu MT, Alter MJ, Kristensen C, Margolis HS. Outbreak of hemodialysis-associated non-A, non-B hepatitis and correlation with antibody to hepatitis C virus. *Am J Kidney Dis.* 1992;19:345–352.

82. Pegues DA, Beck-Sague CM, Woolleen SW, et al. Anaphylactoid reactions associated with reuse of hollow-fiber hemodialyzers and ACE inhibitors. *Kidney Int.* 1992;42:1232–1237.

83. Keroack MA, Rosen Kotilainen H. A cluster of pyrogenic reactions and yeast colonization of hemodialysis machines. *Infect Control Hosp Epidemiol.* 1996;17:474. Abstract LB-5.

84. Centers for Disease Control. Update: acute allergic reactions associated with reprocessed hemodialyzers—United States, 1989–1990. *MMWR Morb Mortal Wkly Rep.* 1991;40:147, 153–154.

85. Velandi M, Fridkin SK, Cardenas V, et al. Transmission of HIV in dialysis centre. *Lancet.* 1995;345:1417–1422.

86. Gordon SM, Drachman J, Bland LA, Reid MH, Favero M, Jarvis WR. Epidemic hypotension in a dialysis center caused by sodium azide. *Kidney Int.* 1990;37:110–115.

87. Longfeld RN, Wortham WG, Fletcher LL, Nauscheutz WF. Clustered bacteremias in a hemodialysis unit: cross-contamination of blood tubing from ultrafiltrate waste. *Infect Control Hosp Epidemiol.* 1992;13:160–164.

88. Hopkins DP, Cicirello H, Dievendorf G, Kondracki S, Morse D. An outbreak of culture-negative peritonitis in dialysis patients—New York. Presented at: 46th Annual Epidemic Intelligence Service Conference; April 14–18, 1997; Atlanta, GA; p. 40.

89. Flaherty JP, Garcia-Houchins S, Chudy R, Arnow PM. An outbreak of gram-negative bacteremia traced to contaminated O-rings and reprocessed dialysers. *Ann Intern Med.* 1993;119:1072–1078.

90. Beck-Sague CM, Jarvis WR, Bland LA, Arduino MJ, Aguero SM, Verosic G. Outbreak of gram-negative bacteremia and pyrogenic reactions in a hemodialysis center. *Am J Nephrol.* 1990;10:397–403.

91. Arnow PM, Garcia-Houchins S, Neagle MB, Bova JL, Dillon JJ, Chou T. An outbreak of bloodstream infections arising from hemodialysis equipment. *J Infect Dis.* 1998;178:783–791.

92. Favero MS, Maynard JE, Peterston NJ, et al. Hepatitis B antigen on environmental surfaces. *Lancet.* 1973;2:1455.

93. Center for Disease Control. Hepatitis: control measures for hepatitis B in dialysis centers. In: Hepatitis Surveillance Report no. 41. Atlanta, GA: US Dept of Health and Human Services, Public Health Service; 1977:12–17.

94. Centers for Disease Control. Hepatitis B virus: a comprehensive strategy for eliminating transmission in the United States through universal childhood vaccination—recommendations of the Immunization Practices Advisory Committee (ACIP). *MMWR Morb Mortal Wkly Rep.* 1991;40(RR-13):1–19.

95. Stevens CE, Alter MJ, Taylor PE, et al. Hepatitis B vaccine in patients receiving hemodialysis: immunogenicity and efficacy. *N Engl J Med.* 1984;311:496–501.

96. Garcia-Houchins S. Dialysis. In: Olmsted RN, ed. *APIC Infection Control and Applied Epidemiology: Principles and Practice, Part I, Section C: Practice Settings.* St. Louis, MO: Mosby–Year Book; 1996:89-1–89-15.

97. Band JD. Nosocomial infections associated with peritoneal dialysis. In: Mayhall CG, ed. *Hospital Epidemiology and Infection Control.* Philadelphia: Williams & Wilkins; 1996:714–725.

98. Favero MS, Alter MJ, Bland LE. Nosocomial infections associated with hemodialysis. In: Mayhall CG, ed. *Hospital Epidemiology and Infection Control.* Philadelphia: Williams & Wilkins; 1996:693–714.

99. Buehler JW, Finton RF, Goodman RA, et al. Epidemic keratoconjunctivitis: report of an outbreak in an ophthalmology practice and recommendations for prevention. *Infect Control Hosp Epidemiol.* 1984;5:390–394.

100. D'Angelo LJ, Hierholzer JC, Holman RC, Smith JD. Epidemic kerato-conjunctivitis caused by adenovirus type 8: epidemiologic and laboratory aspects of a large outbreak. *Am J Epidemiol.* 1981;113:44–49.

101. Keenlyside RA, Hierholzer JC, D'Angelo LJ. Keratoconjunctivitis associated with adenovirus type 37: an extended outbreak in an ophthalmologist's office. *J Infect Dis.* 1983;147:191–198.

102. Koo D, Bouvier B, Wesley M, et al. Epidemic keratoconjunctivitis in a university medical center ophthalmology clinic: need for re-evaluation of the design and disinfection of instruments. *Infect Control Hosp Epidemiol.* 1989;10:547–552.

103. Murrah WF. Epidemic keratoconjunctivitis. *Am J Ophthalmol.* 1988;20:36–38.

104. Nagington J, Sutehall GM, Whipp P. Tonometer disinfection and viruses. *Br J Ophthalmol.* 1983;67:674–676.

105. Warren D, Nelson KE, Farrar JA, et al. A large outbreak of epidemic keratoconjunctivitis: problems in controlling nosocomial spread. *J Infect Dis.* 1989;160:938–943.

106. Wegman DH, Guinee VF, Millian SJ. Epidemic keratoconjunctivitis. *Am J Public Health.* 1970;60:1230–1237.

107. Darougar S, Grey RHB, Thaker U, McSwiggan DA. Clinical and epidemiological features of adenovirus keratoconjunctivitis in London. *Br J Ophthalmol.* 1985;67:1–7.

108. Vastine DW, West CE, Yamashiroya H, et al. Simultaneous nosocomial and community outbreak of epidemic keratoconjunctivitis with types 8 and 19 adenovirus. *Trans Am Acad Ophthalmol Otolaryngol.* 1976;81:826–840.

109. Newman PE, Goodman RA, Waring GO, et al. A cluster of cases of *Mycobacterium chelonei* keratitis associated with outpatient office procedures. *Am J Ophthalmol.* 1984;97:344–348.

110. Centers for Disease Control. Epidemic keratoconjunctivitis in an ophthalmology clinic—California. *MMWR Morb Mortal Wkly Rep.* 1990;39:598–601.

111. American Academy of Ophthalmology. *Updated Recommendations for Ophthalmic Practice in Relation to Human Immunodeficiency Virus and Other Infectious Agents.* San Francisco: American Academy of Ophthalmology; 1992.

112. Rutala WA, Weber DJ, Thomann CA. Outbreak of wound infections following podiatric surgery due to contaminated bone drills. *Foot & Ankle.* 1987;7:350–354.

113. Manian FA. Surveillance of surgical site infections in alternative settings: exploring the current options. *Am J Infect Control.* 1997;25:102–105.

114. Manian FA, Meyer L. Comprehensive surveillance of surgical wound infections in outpatient and inpatient surgery. *Infect Control Hosp Epidemiol.* 1990;11:515–520.

115. Martin MA, Reichelderfer M. APIC guideline for infection prevention and control in flexible endoscopy. *Am J Infect Control.* 1994;22:19–38.

116. Association of Operating Room Nurses (AORN). *Standards, Recommended Practices, and Guidelines.* Denver, CO: AORN; 1998.

117. American Society of Gastrointestinal Endoscopy (ASGE) Ad Hoc Committee on Disinfection. Reprocessing of flexible gastrointestinal endoscopes. *Gastrointest Endosc.* 1996;43:540–546.

118. American Society of Gastrointestinal Endoscopy (ASGE). Infection control during gastrointestinal endoscopy. Manchester, MA; December 1998. Position statement.

119. Molinari JA. Dental office. In: Olmsted RN, ed. *APIC Infection Control and Applied Epidemiology: Principles and Practice, Part I, Section C: Practice Settings.* St. Louis, MO: Mosby–Year Book; 1996:88-1–88-20.

SUGGESTED READING

American Academy of Pediatrics. *1997 Red Book: Report of the Committee on Infectious Diseases.* Peter G, ed. 24th ed. Elk Grove Village, IL: American Academy of Pediatrics; 1997.

Bennett JV, Brachman PS, eds. *Hospital Infections.* 4th ed. Boston: Little, Brown and Co; 1997.

Block SS, ed. *Disinfection, Sterilization, and Preservation.* 4th ed. Philadelphia: Lea & Febiger; 1991.

Herwaldt LA, Smith SD, Carter CD. Infection control in the outpatient setting. *Infect Control Hosp Epidemiol.* 1998;19:41–74.

Mayhall CG. *Hospital Epidemiology and Infection Control.* Baltimore: Williams & Wilkins; 1996.

Olmsted RN, ed. *APIC Infection Control and Applied Epidemiology: Principles and Practice.* St. Louis, MO: Mosby–Year Book; 1996.

Wenzel RP, ed. *Prevention and Control of Nosocomial Infections.* 3rd ed. Baltimore: Williams & Wilkins; 1997.

PROFESSIONAL ORGANIZATIONS

The following national agencies and organizations have guidelines, position papers, or standards that can be used for developing infection control programs in the ambulatory care setting. Information on how to acquire copies of these guidelines can be obtained by accessing the organization's Web site.

American Academy of Ophthalmology
655 Beach St
PO Box 7424
San Francisco, CA 94120-7424
Telephone: 415-561-8500
Internet: http://www.eyenet.org

American Dental Association (ADA)
211 E Chicago Ave
Chicago, IL 60611
Telephone: 312-440-2500
Internet: http://www.ada.org
(The ADA recommendations for infection control for dental offices can be viewed at this Web site, which also contains many topics on infection control issues in the dental practice setting.)

American Society for Gastrointestinal Endoscopy (ASGE)
13 Elm St
Manchester, MA 01944-1314
Telephone: 978-526-8330

Internet: http://www.asge.org

(Note: the ASGE guidelines noted in the references section can be accessed through this Web site.)

Association for Professionals in Infection Control and Epidemiology (APIC)
1275 K St NW, Suite 1000
Washington, DC 20005-4006
Telephone: 202-789-1890
Internet: http://www.apic.org

Association for the Advancement of Medical Instrumentation (AAMI)
3330 Washington Blvd, Suite 400
Arlington, VA 22201-4598
Telephone: 800-332-2264, ext. 217
Internet: http://www.aami.org
(AAMI has standards and recommended practices for hemodialysis and for sterilization in health care facilities.)

Association of Operating Room Nurses (AORN)
2170 South Parker Rd, Suite 300
Denver, CO 80231-5711
Telephone: 800-755-2676
Internet: http://www.aorn.org

Centers for Disease Control and Prevention (CDC)
Hospital Infections Program
1600 Clifton Rd
Atlanta, GA 30033
Internet: http://www.cdc.gov
(Note: The *Morbidity and Mortality Weekly Report* (*MMWR*) and most of the CDC guidelines noted in this chapter can be downloaded from this Web site.)

CHAPTER 6

Pseudo-Outbreaks Reported in Health Care Facilities

Kathleen Meehan Arias

INTRODUCTION

Nosocomial pseudo-outbreaks, or pseudoepidemics, have long been recognized in the health care setting.[1-5] As used in this chapter, a pseudo-outbreak is defined as a real clustering of false infections or an artefactual clustering of real infections. Twenty-nine (11 percent) of the 265 nosocomial epidemics investigated by the Hospital Infections Program of the Center for Disease Control (CDC—currently Centers for Disease Control and Prevention) between 1956 and 1979 were actually pseudo-outbreaks.[3] A review of those pseudo-outbreaks found that the majority were traced to errors in collecting, handling, or processing specimens.[3] The processing errors that occurred in the laboratory were most frequently the result of a change in personnel, technique, or culture media.

Table 6–1 lists examples of pseudo-outbreaks that have been reported in health care facilities.[6-29]

In addition to errors in collecting and processing specimens, nosocomial pseudo-outbreaks have been traced to intrinsically contaminated iodine solutions[6,10] and organisms in hospital tap water.[12,14] Pseudo-outbreaks have also resulted from the improper categorization of an infection or other condition as being nosocomial rather than community aquired.[1,9,21]

Pseudoepidemics have been associated with a variety of microorganisms. They frequently involve blood cultures and respiratory tract specimens. False-positive cultures of blood or other normally sterile sites are more likely to be recognized because infections at these sites are closely monitored by clinicians and infection control personnel.

Many pseudoepidemics are the result of contamination of specimens or cultures. Specimens may be contaminated at the time of collection, during transport, or during processing in the laboratory. An example of a pseudo-outbreak that resulted from specimen contamination at the point of collection was reported by Verweij et al,[26] who investigated a cluster of multidrug-resistant *Pseudomonas aeruginosa* involving 10 neutropenic patients in a hematology unit. The epidemic strain was isolated from surveillance stool cultures. An epidemiologic investigation revealed that health care workers had collected the surveillance stool cultures by sampling feces that were in the toilet and were therefore contaminated by the toilet water. Isolates of *P aeruginosa* from the stool samples in the outbreak and from the toilet water were shown to be identical by genotyping. The "outbreak" subsided when personnel were instructed how properly to collect stool specimens for culture.

Common causes of pseudo-outbreaks are:

- errors in specimen collection or processing[16,18,24,26,29]
- cross-contamination in the laboratory[7,8,20,22,28]
- contaminated equipment, medical devices, or solutions[6,11,13,17,19,23,27]
- failure to recognize that patients' infections are community acquired rather than nosocomial[1,21]
- failure to use appropriate criteria to diagnose nosocomial infection[30]
- failure to recognize that an organism causing an outbreak or cluster may actually be several unrelated strains[31]

Table 6–1 Examples of Pseudo-Outbreaks Reported in Health Care Facilities

Pseudo-Outbreak	Year(s) Reported (Reference No.)	Source/Cause
Pseudomonas (currently *Burkholderia*) *cepacia* pseudobacteremia	1981[6]	Povidone-iodine intrinsically contaminated at manufacturing plant
Influenza A	1984[7]	Cross-contamination in the laboratory
Pseudobacteremia with *Enterococcus* and *Staphylococcus aureus*	1987[8]	Contaminated radiometric blood culture device
Senile hemangioma in a nursing home	1991[9]	Incorrect perception that lesions had recent and rapid onset
Pseudomonas (currently *Burkholderia*) *cepacia* pseudoinfections	1992[10]	Intrinsically contaminated povidone-iodine
Respiratory tract infections caused by nontuberculous mycobacteria	1992[11]	Contaminated bronchoscope cleaning machine and laboratory contamination of an antimicrobial solution
Copepod pseudo-outbreak in stool specimens	1992[12]	Copepods in hospital tap water
Bronchoscopy specimens positive for *Mycobacterium chelonae*	1992[13]	Flawed automatic endoscope disinfector
Pseudocontamination of hospital drinking water	1992[14]	Presence of nonpathogenic freshwater organisms
Enterobacter cloacae pseudobacteremia	1993[15]	Laboratory contamination during use of a new blood-culturing system
Mycobacterium xenopi	1993[16]	Specimen contamination by potable water containing *M xenopi*
Mycobacterium abscessus pseudoinfection	1994[17]	Inadequate disinfection by automated endoscope washer
Pseudomonas aeruginosa orthopaedic infections	1994[18]	Contaminated saline used in laboratory as diluent in processing specimens
Rhodotorula rubra	1995[19]	Improper disinfection and drying of bronchoscopes
Nontuberculous mycobacteria	1995[20]	Contaminated probe on automated lab instrument
Cluster of methicillin-resistant *Staphylococcus aureus*	1995[21]	Cluster suggesting nosocomial infection found to be coincidental
Pseudomonas (currently *Burkholderia*) *cepacia* pseudobacteremia	1996[22]	Contaminated blood gas analyzer
Mycobacterium chelonae respiratory tract pseudoinfections	1997[23]	Contaminated multidose lidocaine sprayers
Respiratory tract infections with *Acinetobacter* species	1997[24]	Laboratory errors in processing respiratory specimens
PPD* skin test conversions	1997[25]	Use of 250 TU* of PPD instead of 5 TU
Multiresistant *Pseudomonas aeruginosa*	1997[26]	Improper stool collection technique
Multidrug-resistant *Mycobacterium tuberculosis*	1997[27]	False-positive cultures due to inadequate cleaning and disinfection of bronchoscope
Mycobacterium tuberculosis	1998[28]	Specimen cross-contamination due to faulty ventilation in the laboratory
Cluster of *Alcaligenes xylosoxidans*	1998[29]	Contaminated saline used in laboratory as diluent in processing specimens

*PPD = purified protein derivative; TU = tuberculin unit.

PSEUDO-OUTBREAKS INVOLVING *MYCOBACTERIUM* SPECIES

There are multiple reports in the literature of clusters and pseudoepidemics involving *Mycobacterium tuberculosis* and nontuberculous mycobacteria. The majority of the reported pseudo-outbreaks were caused by laboratory errors,[20,28,32–34] false-positive tuberculin skin tests,[25] and contaminated bronchoscopes.[11,13,17,27]

Pseudo-Outbreaks of *Mycobacterium tuberculosis*

Pseudo-outbreaks of tuberculosis (TB) have been associated with false-positive *M tuberculosis* cultures resulting from laboratory errors. Opportunities for laboratory contamination occur during the many steps involved in processing specimens and the prolonged incubation period necessary for isolating *M tuberculosis* from culture. Laboratory contamination of tuberculosis specimens and cultures has been shown to occur during the initial specimen processing, incubation, reading or sampling of the cultures, and susceptibility testing. Cross-contamination has been attributed to a faulty exhaust hood and to instrument or reagent contamination, resulting in carry-over of mycobacteria from one specimen to another, and to the inadvertent inoculation of one patient's culture into another patient's culture during subculturing.[32,35–39] In addition, contamination with low numbers of mycobacteria that may not have been detected in the past is now more easily recognized with newer, more sensitive laboratory equipment and methodologies.[33]

To avoid the misdiagnosis of tuberculosis, false-positive *M tuberculosis* cultures should be suspected when

- a single positive culture occurs in a patient who has multiple negative smears for acid-fast bacilli (AFB)
- a patient's signs, symptoms, and clinical presentation are not consistent with tuberculosis
- another AFB smear-positive and culture-positive specimen was processed the same day as the suspect specimen
- only a few colonies are present on solid growth media or the time for detection in a broth medium is prolonged
- DNA fingerprinting shows the suspect isolate is identical to that of a likely source of contamination
- the patient with the suspect isolate cannot be epidemiologically linked to the patient with the putative source isolate

Measures that can be used to identify clusters and minimize cross-contamination and the occurrence of false-positive cultures have been published by Small et al[39] and by Tokars et al.[40]

A pseudo-outbreak of tuberculosis that was not associated with laboratory contamination occurred among the staff of a county residence for retarded adults (RRA) in New York in 1995.[25] An unexpected cluster of tuberculin skin test conversions among the staff of the residence prompted the county nursing service to conduct an extensive contact investigation to identify the source of infection. Persons with a positive tuberculin skin test were evaluated for signs and symptoms of

TB and received a chest radiograph. Five staff members of the RRA were placed on isoniazid (INH) prophylaxis. The investigation resulted in a considerable amount of anxiety in the staff and the community. Over 100 community members were screened with purified protein derivative (PPD), either as part of the contact investigation or on community members' request because of concern that they were infected. No potential source of infection among staff or clients of the residence or any of their contacts was found. When the state health department was asked to assist in the investigation, its review of the results of the county's findings led to a suspicion that the PPD solution may have been defective or the techniques used to apply or to read the test may have been inappropriate. A careful review of the PPD skin-testing program at the residence revealed that the staff of the facility had been tested with 250 TU (tuberculin units) of PPD rather than with the 5 TU that is recommended for a TB skin-testing program. The newly PPD-positive staff were retested with 5 TU of PPD and were found to be negative, so INH prophylaxis was discontinued. The estimated cost of the investigation was at least $15,000. This included "administration and management salaries, nursing time, staff time for retesting, reading, medical visits, employee overtime for TB training, 5 days of 24-hour RRA coverage for the resident who was hospitalized for bronchoscopy, liver-function tests, prescriptions, eight chest radiographs, and other administrative costs" for the county RRA and costs of the investigation that the local health unit and state health department incurred.[25(p.573)]

Pseudo-outbreaks of tuberculosis have resulted in (1) individuals being misdiagnosed with a disease that carries considerable stigma, (2) extensive contact investigations of personnel, family members, friends, and other contacts of patients with an incorrect diagnosis, (3) needless hospitalization, including respiratory (or airborne) isolation, (4) unnecessary bronchoscopy to confirm the diagnosis, (5) unwarranted treatment and prophylaxis with antituberculous medications, (6) excessive costs to health departments and health care facilities, (7) widespread anxiety and fear of contagion in those affected, and (8) adverse publicity for the facility involved.

Pseudo-Outbreaks of Nontuberculous Mycobacteria

There are many reports in the literature of clusters and pseudo-outbreaks involving nontuberculous mycobacteria (NTM), such as *Mycobacterium chelonei, M xenopi, M marinum, M abscessus, M gordonae, M fortuitum* and *M avium-intracellulare*. These pseudoepidemics have been associated with laboratory processing errors[41,42] and with contaminated laboratory reagents,[11] specimens,[16,43] probes on laboratory instruments,[20] multidose lidocaine sprayers,[23] potable water,[16] and bronchoscopes and bronchoscope cleaner/disinfectors.[11,13,17] In three of these reported outbreak investigations, patients with false-positive NTM cultures were started on antituberculous therapy while identification of the AFB organism was pending— even though the patients had no apparent mycobacterial disease.[11,16,20]

Nontuberculous mycobacteria are commonly found in municipal water supplies. In a 1983 survey of 115 dialysis centers in the United States, NTMs were found in the water supplied to 95 (83 percent) of the centers.[44] Therefore, whenever NTMs are isolated from clinical specimens, the clinician must carefully evaluate the patient's clinical picture to determine if the isolate is causing infection or is a contaminant that was introduced into the specimen during collection (e.g., by a contaminated bronchoscope or by NTMs in the water that may have been used to rinse the patient's mouth) or during specimen processing in the laboratory. When a cluster or an increase in the number of isolates of nontuberculous mycobacteria occurs, a clinical and epidemiologic investigation should be conducted to determine if a true outbreak or a pseudo-outbreak is occurring. The clinical investigation should consist of a review of the medical history and records of each of the patients from whom an NTM is isolated and a determination of whether the organism is causing an infection or is likely to be a contaminant. The epidemiologic investigation should evaluate potential sources for the organisms. If the organisms are judged to be contaminants, then specimen collection and processing methods need to be reviewed and observed. If the organisms are causing disease, then the source may be contaminated water, ice, or solutions used by the patients, or a contaminated medical device such as a bronchoscope.

In one report, a perceived increase in the number of respiratory tract infections caused by acid-fast bacilli prompted an investigation, which found that 16 of 46 bronchoscopies yielded specimens that were positive for AFB.[11] Two of the 16 patients were diagnosed with a mycobacterial infection—an AIDS patient with *Mycobacterium avium-intracellulare* infection and an-

other patient with cavitary tuberculosis. In four patients only the smears were AFB-positive—the cultures were negative. NTMs (*M chelonei* and *M gordonae*) were isolated from the cultures of the other 10 patients; however, none of these had clinical evidence of mycobacterial disease. Despite the lack of evidence for disease, four of the patients were treated with antituberculous medication pending culture results. The investigation led to the discovery of two sources for the NTMs: a contaminated water tank in an automated endoscope washer/disinfector and an antimicrobial culture media additive that was contaminated with *M gordonae*.

PSEUDO-OUTBREAKS OF NONINFECTIOUS ETIOLOGY

Not all pseudo-outbreaks are of an infectious nature. Pseudoepidemics of senile hemangioma have been reported in hospitalized patients and nursing home residents.[9,45,46] One reported pseudo-outbreak occurred in an 800-bed long-term care facility. It began when a health care worker noticed that an elderly resident of a psychogeriatric ward had numerous skin lesions.[9] Since the lesions had not been previously noticed, the floor staff considered them to be of recent onset. Because the lesions were presumed to be of infectious etiology, the staff examined the other residents on the ward and found all 34 of them to have similar lesions. The day after the lesions were noticed on the first resident, a dermatologist diagnosed the lesions on another resident as senile hemangioma. Because the nursing staff were convinced that the lesions had occurred suddenly and had spread among the residents, the public health department and an infectious disease specialist were consulted on day 3 of the outbreak. Based on the lack of clinical and laboratory evidence that either an infectious agent or an environmental toxin was involved, the investigators concluded that the lesions were senile hemangioma. Despite the fact that the investigation was completed by day 4 of the reported outbreak, caregivers (many of whom had little medical training) "were suspicious and fearful of exposure to a pathogen as yet undiscovered by medical science,"[9(p.521)] and continued to be skeptical of the diagnosis. Some of the staff, especially those who were pregnant, requested work schedule revisions. The estimated cost to the long-term care facility for the pseudoepidemic was $10,000. Pseudoepidemics of senile hemangioma have occurred mainly because of the misperception that the lesions had a recent and rapid onset. These pseudo-outbreaks are difficult to control because the caregivers involved must accept the conclusion that the lesions were present long before they were noticed.

RECOGNIZING A PSEUDO-OUTBREAK

It is important that pseudo-outbreaks be recognized promptly because they frequently result in unnecessary diagnostic and treatment procedures, consume valuable infection control and laboratory resources, and cause undue concern of patients, their families, and health care facility staff. Pseudo-outbreaks may be difficult to recognize and may occur for a prolonged period before they are detected. Typically, a pseudo-outbreak is recognized when an unusual organism is isolated from several patients, when there is a sudden increase in the number of isolates of a common pathogen, or when a common pathogen is isolated from several patients who have no signs and symptoms of infection.

Infection control and laboratory personnel and clinicians should routinely review culture results for evidence of clusters or unusual organisms so that outbreaks and pseudo-outbreaks may be quickly recognized. Frequently, the identity of an organism causing a cluster of pseudoinfections, or the types of specimens from which it is isolated, will provide a clue to the source of the organism. In one report, the sudden occurrence of positive cultures of normally sterile bone allograft specimens prompted an epidemiologic investigation.[47] The grafts grew *Pseudomonas cepacia* and *Commomonas acidovorans*. Since these organisms grow well in an aqueous habitat, a water source was suspected. An investigation revealed that a single laboratory technologist had processed all four of the bone allografts that grew gram-negative organisms. A review of her work practices revealed that she had allowed the test tubes containing the bone to float in a sonicator water bath rather than securing them in a test tube rack or beaker. Cultures from the water bath grew the same organisms that were isolated from the bone specimens. The bacterial isolates from the bone allografts had the same antibiogram as those from the water bath, and pulsed-field gel electrophoresis indicated they were the same strains.[47]

Pseudomonas species multiply readily in aqueous solutions and have been implicated in pseudo-outbreaks. Studies have identified this organism in postoperative pseudoinfections associated with a contaminated bottle of sterile saline that was used in the

laboratory to process tissue specimens[18] and with outbreaks of bacteremia, peritonitis, and pseudoinfections that were associated with intrinsically contaminated iodine solutions.[6,10,48] Pseudobacteremia attributed to intrinsic contamination of povidone-iodine was reported by Berkelman et al in 1981.[6] Their investigation was prompted by a New York hospital that reported to the Hospital Infections Branch at the CDC the occurrence of 17 blood cultures positive for *Pseudomonas cepacia* over a 3-month period. A review of the cases revealed that none of the 14 patients had clinical evidence of gram-negative bacteremia. Despite the fact that none of the patients had clinical signs and symptoms of gram-negative sepsis, four of the patients received antimicrobial therapy for possible bacteremia based on the culture results. A telephone survey of other hospitals in the New York City area uncovered three additional hospitals that were experiencing pseudobacteremias with *P cepacia*. *P cepacia* was eventually recovered from 52 patients in four hospitals over a 7-month period. An extensive epidemiologic investigation implicated 10% povidone-iodine solution from one manufacturer as the source of the contamination. The povidone-iodine was used at all four hospitals as a skin preparation for collection of blood cultures. *P cepacia* was also isolated from an abdominal wound that had been packed with povidone-iodine–soaked dressings and from a sputum culture of a patient whose tracheostomy site was cleansed with the implicated povidone-iodine solution.

VERIFYING THE DIAGNOSIS AND VERIFYING THE EXISTENCE OF AN OUTBREAK

The first two steps in the investigation of any epidemic are: (1) verify the diagnosis and (2) verify the existence of an outbreak. Failure to follow these two very important steps before continuing an outbreak investigation may lead the investigator on the proverbial wild-goose chase. At the beginning of an outbreak investigation it is necessary to verify the diagnosis of any reported or suspected cases before proceeding, to avoid wasting time investigating an outbreak that may not exist.

For example, infection control personnel in acute and long-term care facilities occasionally receive calls from personnel reporting an outbreak of methicillin-resistant *Staphylococcus aureus* (MRSA) in a particular unit. When such a call occurs, infection control personnel should first ask for the names of the patients or residents that the health care worker believes are involved in the reported outbreak and then should promptly review the patients' culture reports and medical records. This quick review may reveal that some of the MRSA isolates are actually methicillin-resistant *Staphylococcus epidermidis* (MRSE) or that several of the patients or residents were already culture-positive for MRSA when admitted to the unit. If this is the case, these findings should be promptly reported to the health care worker who expressed concern in order to prevent rumors and fears that the facility is experiencing an outbreak. If clinical features appear to be inconsistent with laboratory results, a pseudoinfection should be suspected. If a cluster or increase in the number of pseudoinfections is detected, than a pseudo-outbreak should be suspected. In this case, the investigator should carefully analyze each step in specimen collection and processing.

Surveillance artefact is a frequent cause of pseudoepidemics, so it is important to verify that an outbreak exists (i.e., that there is an increase in the expected number of nosocomial cases).[1] Surveillance artefact may occur due to (1) failure to properly distinguish community-acquired infections from hospital-acquired infections, (2) a coincidental occurrence of unrelated cases, or (3) a change in the facility's method of conducting surveillance.

Bannatyne et al reported the results of their investigation of an apparent cluster of three MRSA cases in a hospital with a low incidence of MRSA.[21] A review of the culture reports revealed that the three isolates, which appeared over a 16-day period, had different antibiotic susceptibility patterns. Further investigation into the patients' medical histories revealed that two of the patients had prior positive MRSA cultures when at other institutions. Although the three isolates exhibited temporal and geographic clustering, the investigators were able to hypothesize that the organisms were unrelated. When the organisms were typed, they were found to be different phage types, thus confirming the hypothesis that the strains were not related.[21]

Molecular typing methods have greatly facilitated understanding of the epidemiology of nosocomial infections and outbreaks.[49] Personnel responsible for investigating a pseudo-outbreak should consider using molecular typing of isolates in combination with an epidemiologic investigation to identify and confirm the likely source of a pseudoepidemic. As with any laboratory test, care must be taken when evaluating typing results because these results must be combined with a careful epidemiologic study in order to confirm the transmission of a single strain or multiple strains of an organism. Typing methods used for a variety of pathogens implicated in outbreaks and pseudo-outbreaks are discussed in Chapter 11.

PREVENTING PSEUDO-OUTBREAKS

Pseudo-outbreaks can be prevented when laboratory personnel implement and adhere to protocols that reduce the risk of specimen contamination and when clinicians and laboratory and infection control personnel (1) quickly recognize the occurrence of false-positive cultures, (2) are alert to the occurrence of clusters or an increased number of infections/pseudoinfections, (3) use objective criteria for diagnosing the presence of an infection, and (4) use appropriate criteria for categorizing an infection as hospital acquired or community acquired.

Outbreak investigations generally require a large time commitment on the part of the investigators, many of whom are pulled away from their normal job duties. Outbreaks result in a great deal of anxiety and fear in personnel, patients, visitors, and the community. They cause disruption in the lives of patients and personnel and in the provision of health care services. In addition, pseudoinfections or a pseudo-outbreak may result in unnecessary treatment or prophylaxis of patients or staff and the loss of confidence in medical personnel and the laboratory. It is important that pseudoinfections and artefactual clusters of real infections be recognized promptly to avoid these adverse effects.

REFERENCES

1. Weinstein RA, Stamm WE. Pseudoepidemics in hospital. *Lancet.* 1977;2:862–864.

2. Kusek JW. Nosocomial pseudoepidemics and pseudoinfections: an increasing problem. *Am J Infect Control.* 1981;9:70–75.

3. Stamm WE, Weinstein RA, Dixon RE. Comparison of endemic and epidemic nosocomial infections. *Am J Med.* 1981;70:393–397.

4. Jarvis WR. Nosocomial outbreaks: the Centers for Disease Control's Hospital Infections Program experience, 1980–1990. *Am J Med.* 1991;91(suppl 3B):101S–106S.

5. Herwaldt LA, Smith SD, Carter CD. Infection control in the outpatient setting. *Infect Control Hosp Epidemiol.* 1998;19:41–74.

6. Berkelman RL, Lewin S, Allen JR, et al. Pseudobacteremia attributed

to contamination of povidone-iodine with *Pseudomonas cepacia*. *Ann Intern Med*. 1981;95:32–36.

7. Budnick LD, Moll ME, Hull HF, Mann JM, Kendal AP. A pseudo-outbreak of influenza A associated with use of laboratory stock strain. *Am J Public Health*. 1984;76:607–609.

8. Bradley SF, Wilson KH, Rosloniec MA, Kauffman CA. Recurrent pseudobacteremias traced to a radiometric blood culture device. *Infect Control*. 1987;8:281–283.

9. Poulin C, Schlech WF. A pseudo-outbreak in a nursing home. *Infect Control Hosp Epidemiol*. 1991;12:521–522.

10. Panlilio AL, Beck-Sague CM, Siegel JD, et al. Infections and pseudoinfections due to povidone-iodine solution contaminated with *Pseudomonas cepacia*. *Clin Infect Dis*. 1991;14:1078–1083.

11. Gubler JG, Salfinger M, von Graevenitz A. Pseudoepidemic of nontuberculous mycobacteria due to a contaminated bronchoscope cleaning machine: report of an outbreak and review of the literature. *Chest*. 1992;101:1245–1249.

12. Van Horn KG, Tatz JS, Li KI, Newman L, Wormser GP. Copepods associated with a perirectal abscess and copepod pseudo-outbreak in stools for ova and parasite examinations. *Diagn Microbiol Infect Dis*. 1992;15:561–565.

13. Fraser VJ, Jones M, Murray P, Medoff G, Zhang Y, Wallace RJ. Contamination of fiberoptic bronchoscopes with *Mycobacterium chelonae* linked to an automated bronchoscope disinfection machine. *Am Rev Respir Dis*. 1992;145:853–855.

14. Klotz SA, Normand RE, Kalinsky RG. "Through a drinking glass and what was found there": pseudocontamination of a hospital's drinking water. *Infect Control Hosp Epidemiol*. 1992;13:477–481.

15. Pearson ML, Pegues DA, Carson LA, et al. Cluster of *Enterobacter cloacae* pseudobacteremias associated with use of an agar slant blood culturing system. *J Clin Microbiol*. 1993;31:2599–2603.

16. Sniadack DH, Ostroff SM, Karlix MA, et al. A nosocomial pseudo-outbreak of *Mycobacterium xenopi* due to a contaminated potable water supply: lessons in prevention. *Infect Control Hosp Epidemiol*. 1993;14:636–641.

17. Maloney S, Welbel S, Daves B, et al. *Mycobacterium abscessus* pseudoinfection traced to an automated endoscope washer: utility of epidemiologic and laboratory investigation. *J Infect Dis*. 1994;169:1166–1169.

18. Forman W, Axelrod P, St John K, et al. Investigation of a pseudo-outbreak of orthopedic infections caused by *Pseudomonas aeruginosa*. *Infect Control Hosp Epidemiol*. 1994;15:652–657.

19. Hagan ME, Klotz SA, Bartholomew W, Potter L, Nelson M. A pseudoepidemic of *Rhodotorula rubra*: a marker for microbial contamination of the bronchoscope. *Infect Control Hosp Epidemiol*. 1995;16:727–728.

20. Mehta JB, Kefri M, Soike DR. Pseudoepidemic of nontuberculous mycobacteria in a community hospital. *Infect Control Hosp Epidemiol*. 1995;16:633–634.

21. Bannatyne RM, Wells BA, MacMillan SA, Thibault MC. A cluster of MRSA—the little outbreak that wasn't. *Infect Control Hosp Epidemiol*. 1995;16:380.

22. Gravel-Topper D, Sample ML, Oxley C, Toye B, Woods DE, Garber GE. Three-year outbreak of pseudobacteremia with *Burkholderia cepacia* traced to a contaminated blood gas analyzer. *Infect Control Hosp Epidemiol*. 1996;17:737–740.

23. Cox R, deBorja K, Bach MC. A pseudo-outbreak of *Mycobacterium chelonae* infections related to bronchoscopy. *Infect Control Hosp Epidemiol*. 1997;18:136–137.

24. Sule O, Ludlam HA, Walker CW, Brown DFJ, Kauffman ME. A pseudo-outbreak of respiratory infection with *Acinetobacter* species. *Infect Control Hosp Epidemiol*. 1997;18:510–512.

25. Grabau JC, Burrows DJ, Kern ML. A pseudo-outbreak of purified protein derivative skin-test conversions caused by inappropriate testing materials. *Infect Control Hosp Epidemiol*. 1997;18:571–574.

26. Verweij PE, Bilj D, Melchers W, et al. Pseudo-outbreak of multiresistant *Pseudomonas aeruginosa* in a hematology unit. *Infect Control Hosp Epidemiol*. 1997;18:128–131.

27. Agerton T, Valway S, Gore B, et al. Transmission of a highly drug-resistant strain (strain W1) of *Mycobacterium tuberculosis*. *JAMA*. 1997;278:1073–1077.

28. Segal-Maurer S, Kreiswirth BN, Burns JM, et al. *Mycobacterium tuberculosis* specimen contamination revisited: the role of laboratory environmental control in a pseudo-outbreak. *Infect Control Hosp Epidemiol*. 1998;19:101–105.

29. Gravowitz EV, Keenholtz SL. A pseudoepidemic of *Alcaligenes xylosoxidans* attributable to contaminated saline. *Am J Infect Control*. 1998;26:146–148.

30. Ehrenkranz NJ, Richter EI, Phillips PM, Shultz JM. An apparent excess of operative site infections: analyses to evaluate false-positive diagnosis. *Infect Control Hosp Epidemiol*. 1995;16:712–716.

31. Bonten MJM, Gaillard CA, van Tiel FH, van der Geest S, Stobberingh EE. A typical case of cross-acquisition?: the importance of genotypic characterization of bacterial strains. *Infect Control Hosp Epidemiol*. 1995;16:415–416.

32. Centers for Disease Control and Prevention. Multiple misdiagnoses of tuberculosis resulting from laboratory error—Wisconsin, 1996. *MMWR Morb Mortal Wkly Rep*. 1997;46:797–801.

33. Nivin B, Fujiwara PI, Hannifin J, Kreiswirth BN. Cross-contamination with *Mycobacterium tuberculosis*: an epidemiological and laboratory investigation. *Infect Control Hosp Epidemiol*. 1998;19:500–503.

34. Cronin W, Rodriguez E, Valway S, et al. Pseudo-outbreak of tuberculosis in an acute-care general hospital: epidemiology and clinical implications. *Infect Control Hosp Epidemiol*. 1998;19:345–347.

35. Braden CR, Templeton GL, Stead WW, Bates JH, Cave MD, Valway SE. Retrospective detection of laboratory cross-contamination of *Mycobacterium tuberculosis* cultures with use of DNA fingerprint analysis. *Clin Infect Dis*. 1997;24:34–40.

36. Burman WJ, Stone BL, Reeves RR, et al. The incidence of false-positive cultures for *Mycobacterium tuberculosis*. *Am J Respir Crit Care Med*. 1997;155:321–326.

37. Dunlap NE, Harris RH, Benjamin WH Jr, Harden JW, Hafner D. Laboratory contamination of *Mycobacterium tuberculosis* cultures. *Am J Respir Crit Care Med*. 1995;152:1702–1704.

38. Nitta AT, Davidson PT, De Koning ML, Kilman RJ. Misdiagnosis of multidrug-resistant *Mycobacterium tuberculosis* possibly due to laboratory-related errors. *JAMA*. 1996;276:1980–1983.

39. Small PM, McClenny NB, Singh SP, Schoolnik GK, Tompkins LS, Mickelsen PA. Molecular strain typing of *Mycobacterium tuberculosis* to confirm cross-contamination in the mycobacteriology laboratory and modification of procedures to minimize occurrence of false-positive cultures. *J Clin Microbiol*. 1993;31:1677–1682.

40. Tokars JI, Rudnick JR, Kroc K, et al. US hospital mycobacteriology laboratories: status and comparison with state public health department laboratories. *J Clin Microbiol*. 1996;34:680–685.

41. Goodman RA, Smith JD, Kubica GP, Dougherty EM, Sikes RK. Nosocomial mycobacterial pseudoinfection in a Georgia hospital. *Infect Control*. 1984;5:573–576.

42. Jacobson E, Gurevich I, Schoch P, Cunha BA. Pseudoepidemic of nontuberculous mycobacteria in a community hospital. *Infect Control Hosp Epidemiol.* 1996;17:348.

43. Bennett SN, Peterson DE, Johnson DR, Hall WN, Robinson-Dunn B, Dietrich S. Bronchoscopy-associated *Mycobacterium xenopi* pseudoinfections. *Am J Resp Crit Care Med.* 1994;150:245–250.

44. Carson LA, Bland LA, Cusick LB, et al. Prevalence of nontuberculous mycobacteria in water supplies of hemodialysis centers. *Appl Environ Microbiol.* 1988;54:3122–3125.

45. Seville RH, Rao PS, Hutchinson DN, Birchall G. Outbreak of Campbell de Morgan spots. *Br Med J.* 1970;1:408–409.

46. Honish A, Grimsrud K, Miedzinski L, Gold E, Cherry R. Outbreak of Campbell de Morgan spots in a nursing home—Alberta. *Can Dis Wkly Rep.* 1988;14:211–212.

47. Mermel LA, Josephson SL, Giorgio C. A pseudo-epidemic involving bone allografts. *Infect Control Hosp Epidemiol.* 1994;15:757–758.

48. Parrott PL, Terry PM, Whitworth EN, et al. *Pseudomonas aeruginosa* peritonitis associated with contaminated poloxamer-iodine solution. *Lancet.* 1982;2:683–685.

49. Jarvis WR. Usefulness of molecular epidemiology for outbreak investigations. *Infect Control Hosp Epidemiol.* 1994;15:500–503.

CHAPTER 7

Organisms and Diseases Associated with Outbreaks in Various Health Care Settings

Kathleen Meehan Arias

A mighty creature is the germ.

Ogden Nash[1]

INTRODUCTION

The outbreaks discussed in this book have been categorized into the health care setting in which they have most frequently been reported (i.e., acute, long-term, or ambulatory care). It is evident, however, that many agents and disease syndromes, such as diarrhea and respiratory illness, have been associated with endemic and epidemic infections in more than one type of health care setting. Organisms such as methicillin-resistant *Staphylococcus aureus* (MRSA), vancomycin-resistant *Enterococcus* (VRE) species, *Mycobacterium tuberculosis*, *Sarcoptes scabiei*, and *Clostridium difficile* frequently cause nosocomial outbreaks in hospitals and long-term care facilities. *M tuberculosis* has also been responsible for outbreaks in ambulatory care settings such as clinics and emergency rooms. Endemic and epidemic gastrointestinal diseases can occur in many settings and can affect patients, residents, personnel, and visitors. It is important to note that because of the absence of routinely available laboratory tests for some organisms, the etiology of nosocomial epidemics and clusters of infectious gastroenteritis is not always determined, especially if the causative agent is viral.

The purpose of this chapter is to review reported outbreaks caused by MRSA, VRE, *M tuberculosis*, *C difficile*, and parasites and to outline control measures that have been used to prevent and interrupt these outbreaks. Outbreaks of gastrointestinal and respiratory diseases will also be examined. Since nosocomial influenza is more commonly reported in long-term care facilities, this disease is discussed in Chapter 4.

ORGANISMS ASSOCIATED WITH NOSOCOMIAL OUTBREAKS

Methicillin-Resistant *Staphylococcus aureus* in the Acute Care Setting

Epidemiology

Methicillin-resistant *Staphylococcus aureus* (MRSA) emerged as an important clinical problem shortly after the introduction of methicillin and the rise in the percentage of hospital-acquired infections caused by *S aureus* resistant to the beta-lactam antibiotics has been documented by the National Nosocomial Infections Surveillance (NNIS) system.[2,3] The first hospital outbreaks of MRSA in the United States occurred in the late 1960s, and multiple outbreaks have been reported worldwide.[4–11] Initially associated with large tertiary care hospitals, MRSA has become endemic in many institutions.[3] Once considered to be strictly a nosocomial pathogen, MRSA is now prevalent in many communities and has been isolated from patients with no prior history of hospitalization.[12]

Risk factors for acquiring MRSA include previous hospitalization or nursing home stay, length of stay, prior antibiotic therapy, diabetes, an open wound, admission to a critical care or burn unit, surgery, and proximity to a patient with MRSA.[9,12–14] Colonization often precedes infection and one study estimated that between 30 and 60 percent of colonized patients will develop an MRSA infection.[15] It is well-recognized that patients may remain colonized for many months.[7,12,13] Prolonged colonization of hospital personnel also may occur—one study found that several health care workers carried MRSA in their nares for 3 or more months.[16]

Mode of Transmission

In the acute care setting, the mode of transmission of MRSA is person-to-person via direct contact with colonized or infected persons.[15] Direct contact involves body surface–to–body surface contact, such as occurs when a health care worker turns a patient or gives a bath. Although transient contamination of health care worker's hands is considered to be the primary mode of transmission from person to person, infected and colonized personnel have served as reservoirs in common source outbreaks. A physician with a prolonged upper respiratory tract infection and MRSA colonization was the likely source for an outbreak in a surgical intensive care unit,[17] nasal carriers were implicated in an outbreak in a burn unit,[14] and another outbreak was associated with a health care worker who had chronic MRSA sinusitis.[18] Hospital personnel, especially house staff who rotate between facilities, have been found to spread MRSA from hospital to hospital and may be responsible for introducing the organism into a facility.[19-21] Although MRSA can be isolated from the inanimate environment immediately around patients with MRSA, environmental surfaces are not considered to be an important reservoir.[22-24]

Control Measures

Recommendations for preventing the endemic and epidemic transmission of MRSA in the acute care setting have been published by the Centers for Disease Control and Prevention's (CDC) Hospital Infection Control Practices Advisory Committee (HICPAC),[25] the American Hospital Association,[26] many state departments of health,[26] and others.[13,27-30] Guidelines for recognizing, managing, and controlling an MRSA outbreak were published in 1998 by Wenzel et al.[31]

Measures used to control an MRSA outbreak in the hospital include the following:

- hand washing
- laboratory-based surveillance (i.e., the review of positive cultures) to identify cases (both infection and colonization)
- surveillance cultures to detect infected and colonized patients

- surveillance cultures to detect infected and colonized personnel
- contact precautions and use of barriers for infected and colonized patients
- education of health care workers regarding preventing the spread of the organism
- treatment of infected patients or personnel
- decolonization of personnel and patients in certain situations

Hand washing. Good hygiene and proper hand washing, regardless of the use of gloves, is essential to control the person-to-person transmission of MRSA. There is no consensus as to whether or not an antimicrobial soap is more effective than plain soap for limiting the transmission of MRSA. Although the HICPAC Guideline for Isolation Precautions in Hospitals recommends use of an antimicrobial soap or a waterless antiseptic agent for patients on contact precautions,[25] the method for washing, including vigorous rubbing and cleaning of all surfaces of the hands, may very well be more important than the type of soap used.

Laboratory-based surveillance to identify cases. Ongoing surveillance is an essential element of any infection control program and is necessary to establish an endemic or baseline rate of MRSA in order to be able to recognize outbreaks or clusters. Routine surveillance for MRSA is generally conducted by regularly reviewing laboratory reports for *S aureus* isolates that are resistant to methicillin (or nafcillin, oxacillin, etc., depending on which antibiotic is reported by the microbiology laboratory). It should be noted that many patients who are colonized or infected will not be detected by routine cultures obtained for clinical indications. Once MRSA is identified, criteria must be used to determine if the organism is colonizing or infecting the patient and if an infection is community or hospital-acquired. Many hospitals use the criteria developed for the National Nosocomial Infections Surveillance (NNIS) system to categorize a nosocomial infection.[32] However, since patients may be colonized with MRSA for prolonged time periods, it is sometimes difficult to determine if MRSA isolated from a hospitalized patient was present but undetected at the time of admission or was acquired in the hospital. Some infections, by definition, will be categorized as nosocomial even though the causative agent may have been part of the patient's flora at admission. If an outbreak is suspected, laboratory records should be reviewed retrospectively and prospectively to identify both infected and colonized patients and a line-list of nosocomial cases should be maintained as discussed in Chapter 8. Both colonized and infected cases should be identified in order to determine the extent of the outbreak.

Surveillance cultures of patients. Since many patients may be carriers, with no overt signs or symptoms of infection, surveillance cultures are used during an outbreak investigation to detect colonization and to determine the extent of transmission of the organism.[5–7,15,26,31] Since many distinct strains of MRSA may be found in an institution,[5–7,11] surveillance cultures should not be done unless all MRSA isolates are subjected to a discriminatory molecular typing test to provide evidence of strain relatedness. This is especially important if an outbreak is suspected in an area that has a high endemic rate of MRSA. Methods for selecting appropriate culture sites and procedures for collecting specimens are discussed in Chapter 11.

Surveillance cultures of personnel. Since most outbreaks are caused by transmission of MRSA from patient to patient on the hands of personnel, many clusters and outbreaks can be terminated by implementing contact precautions and re-educating all personnel on the importance and use of routine infection control measures, such as standard precautions and proper handwashing techniques. Generally, culturing of personnel is not recommended unless (1) initial control measures, such as contact isolation and the use of barriers and hand washing, fail to terminate the spread of the organism and (2) a thorough epidemiologic investigation links personnel to a cluster of cases (i.e., a common source outbreak is suspected).[26,31] Common source outbreaks are often associated with a personnel carrier and should be suspected if an increase in MRSA cases occurs abruptly, such as when several cases appear in a short time period on a single unit, or when several postoperative wound infections occur in a short time period. When conducting surveillance cultures, it should be remembered that at any given time between 20 and 90 percent of personnel may be nasal carriers of *S aureus* and fewer than 10 percent of healthy carriers disperse the organism into the air.[33] In addition, personnel who are found to be colonized are not necessarily the source of an outbreak as they may have become colonized by contact with the true source or by contact

with colonized or infected patients. Since many strains of MRSA may be circulating in a facility, surveillance cultures should not be done unless all of the MRSA isolates from both personnel and patients involved in an outbreak or cluster are subjected to a discriminatory molecular typing test to confirm that they are the same strain.

Contact precautions and use of barriers. Although much is known about the epidemiology and the mode of transmission of methicillin-resistant *S aureus*, opinions vary considerably on the use and effectiveness of contact isolation precautions and the use of barriers such as gloves, gowns, and/or masks.[5–7,34–37] The routine use of contact isolation for controlling endemic MRSA cross-infection has been debated for many years, especially for institutions with high endemic rates.[7,35,38–40] The HICPAC Guideline for Isolation Precautions in Hospitals recommends that gloves be worn when entering the room of a patient on contact precautions.[25] However, studies on the effectiveness of barrier precautions are conflicting, as some have demonstrated a decreased incidence of MRSA using barrier precautions,[11,15,41] while others have not.[42–45] One carefully conducted study found that contact isolation was effective in controlling the epidemic spread of MRSA in a neonatal intensive care unit.[39] Most authorities recommend the use of some type of contact isolation and barrier precautions to restrict transmission in an outbreak. Each hospital must identify which of these measures are appropriate for its specific situation.[37]

Education of health care workers. Educational programs on the epidemiology and mode of transmission of MRSA and the importance of contact precautions and hand washing should be provided for all members of the health care team, including physicians. An educational program which actively involved staff surgeons and house staff was effective at limiting the spread of MRSA in one hospital.[46]

Treatment of infected or colonized patients. Patients who are either infected or colonized with MRSA may serve as reservoirs. Most patients with infection will be treated with antimicrobials; however, the use of antibiotics to eliminate colonization in patients must be approached with caution since many decolonization regimens have been found to promote the development of resistant organisms.[26,47]

Treatment of infected or colonized personnel. When an outbreak or cluster is detected, the investigator should search for personnel with obvious signs and symptoms of infection or skin breakdown. Personnel with infections should be treated; however, eradication of nasal carriage in personnel is recommended only when there is convincing epidemiologic evidence that a culture-positive health care worker is the source of the epidemic strain.[16,17,26,33,47] Restricting the activities of culture-positive personnel is controversial. If a colonized health care worker is epidemiologically linked to cases and cares for patients who are at a high risk of serious infection (such as in a burn unit or a cardiothoracic intensive care unit), the worker should be restricted from patient care until carriage has been eradicated.[33]

If a health care worker is treated for decolonization, repeat cultures should be done to confirm that the carrier state has been eradicated. Since antimicrobial agents used for decolonizing carriers may promote resistant strains of MRSA, only those personnel who are epidemiologically linked to disease transmission should be treated. Discussions of regimens used for eradicating staphylococcal carriage in health care workers have been published elsewhere.[28,33]

MRSA in the Long-Term Care Setting

Epidemiology

Although the first outbreak of MRSA involving nursing home residents was reported in 1970, reports about the occurrence and epidemiology of MRSA in long-term care (LTC) facilities were scarce until the late 1980s.[48–55] The increase in colonization and infection caused by MRSA in acute care institutions has been paralleled by a similar increase in the long-term care setting.[56–58] Studies have shown varying colonization rates among residents in LTC facilities:[51,54,56,59,60] one found from 4.9 to 15.6 percent on each of eight culture surveys collected over a 15-month period,[59] one detected 8.8 percent of patients colonized at least once over a 1-year period,[56] and a prevalence survey conducted during an outbreak in a Veterans Affairs nursing home indicated that 34 percent of the 114 patients were colonized.[50] Several studies have documented colonization of residents at the time of admission to the facility[50,55,56,60] and several have found that residents may be persistently colonized for months to years.[57] A study by Hsu noted that although a few nursing home residents had persistent colonization, most showed only a temporary or intermittent carriage.[59] There is evidence that transfer of residents and patients between acute care hospitals and long-term care facilities plays a role in maintaining reservoirs of MRSA in each setting.[49,51,59]

Risk factors for acquiring MRSA colonization in the long-term care setting include previous hospitalization, poor functional status, presence of a decubitus ulcer or other wound, underlying diseases and medical conditions that jeopardize skin integrity, use of invasive devices that disrupt the skin barrier (such as gastrostomy tubes), and prior antimicrobial therapy.[50,55,57,59] Risk factors for infection include colonization with MRSA, a debilitated state requiring skilled nursing care, and hemodialysis.[30,52,54] A 1991 report of a 3-year prospective cohort study of 197 patients in a long-term care Veterans Administration Center found that colonization predicted infection, carriage persisted for a median of 118 days, and 8/32 (25 percent) patients with persistent carriage ultimately developed an MRSA infection.[54] Many of these residents had poor functional status and required hemodialysis. In other studies, reported rates of infection varied according to the population studied and ranged from 6 to 25 percent of patients who were colonized with MRSA.[50,54,55,57,58] The risk for serious infection with MRSA appears to be low for most residents of long-term care facilities.[50,55]

Mode of Transmission

The major reservoir of methicillin-resistant *S aureus* in the long-term care setting is colonized and infected residents. The primary mode of transmission is direct contact between residents or from resident to resident via transient carriage on the hands of personnel.[30] Transmission from one roommate to another occurs infrequently and occurs most often in residents who require extensive nursing care.[55] There is little evidence that the environment plays a role in the transmission of MRSA.[55] Studies have documented the existence of several strains of MRSA in a facility that supports the hypothesis that MRSA is introduced and reintroduced into a facility from multiple sources.[57,59]

Control Measures

Recommendations for preventing the endemic and epidemic transmission of MRSA in the long-term care setting have been published by the American Hospital Association,[26] Mulligan et al,[30] Kauffman et al,[52] and Bradley.[57] Measures used to control an MRSA outbreak in the LTC setting include the following:

- hand washing
- laboratory-based surveillance (i.e., the review of positive cultures) to identify cases (both infection and colonization)
- surveillance cultures to detect infected and colonized patients
- surveillance cultures to detect infected and colonized personnel
- cohorting of colonized or infected residents
- contact precautions and use of barriers for infected and colonized residents
- treatment of infected residents or personnel
- education of health care workers regarding preventing the spread of the organism
- decolonization of residents and personnel in certain situations

Hand washing. Good hygiene and proper hand washing, regardless of the use of gloves, is essential to control the person-to-person transmission of MRSA. Either an antimicrobial soap or plain soap may be used; however, the HICPAC Guideline for Isolation Precautions in Hospitals does recommend the use of an antimicrobial soap for patients on contact precautions.[30] Regardless of the type of soap used, personnel should be instructed to vigorously rub and clean all surfaces of their hands and to wash their wrists and forearms.

Laboratory-based surveillance to identify cases. An ongoing surveillance program is necessary to establish the endemic, or baseline, level of MRSA in order to recognize an outbreak or cluster of cases. Laboratory-based surveillance (i.e., the ongoing review of positive cultures on residents) should be routinely conducted in the long-term care setting, even though it is generally less effective for detecting MRSA than in the acute care setting because cultures are less frequently collected. Criteria must be used to determine if a resident is colonized or infected and if an infection is community acquired or nosocomial. Although there is no single widely accepted set of criteria for use in the long-term care setting, many facilities use the nosocomial infection definitions developed by McGeer et al.[61] Surveillance for cases is a critical component of any outbreak investigation because it helps in defining the extent of the problem, the likely mode of transmission, and a possible source. Once an outbreak is suspected, a line-listing of nosocomial cases, both colonized and infected, should be constructed as discussed in Chapter 8.

Surveillance cultures of residents. Studies have shown that many residents of LTC facilities are colonized with MRSA and that routine collection of surveillance cultures is not a cost-effective use of limited infection control resources.[57] Routine prevalence surveys are not recommended for facilities that have endemic colonization and low rates of infection.[30] If an outbreak is suspected, however, surveillance cultures of the nares and wounds may be done to determine the extent of spread. Since many distinct strains of MRSA may be found, surveillance cultures should not be done unless all MRSA isolates are subjected to a discriminatory molecular typing test to provide evidence of strain relatedness. This is especially important if an outbreak is suspected in a facility with a high endemic rate of MRSA. Methods for collecting specimens and typing organisms are discussed in Chapter 11.

Surveillance cultures of personnel. Surveillance cultures of personnel in an LTC facility are rarely warranted because the primary mode of transmission is via transient carriage of MRSA on the hands of health care workers. Culturing of personnel should not be done unless there is epidemiologic evidence that links the cases to a personnel source and unless all of the MRSA isolates from both personnel and residents involved are subjected to a discriminatory molecular typing test to confirm that they are the same strain. Although personnel involved in an outbreak situation may be culture-positive for the epidemic strain, they are not necessarily the source of the outbreak—they may have become colonized by contact with infected or colonized residents.

Cohorting. The practice of cohorting during an outbreak (i.e., separating those who are infected or colonized with MRSA from those who are not, or placing colonized/infected residents in the same room) has been shown to limit the spread of MRSA;[51] however, it is difficult to cohort residents in a long-term care facility in which residents are encouraged to socialize at meals and during daily activities.

Contact precautions and use of barriers. The routine use of contact precautions[25] and barriers such as gloves, gowns, and masks to limit transmission of endemic MRSA in the long-term care setting has been debated—just as it has been debated in the acute care setting.[40,50] The debate notwithstanding, contact isolation has been shown to be useful in preventing the spread of

MRSA in outbreak situations.[49,51] Each facility needs to identify which isolation precautions and types of specific barriers are appropriate for its setting. There are currently no federal guidelines for isolation precautions in the long-term care setting; however, many state health departments have guidelines for controlling MRSA in long-term care facilities.

Treatment of infected or colonized residents. Treatment of infected residents is generally recommended; however, decolonization to eliminate carriage for the purpose of preventing either infection in a colonized resident or transmission to others has not been found to be an effective infection control measure and can lead to development of resistant organisms.[26,57,62] Some investigators have reported recurrent colonization after completion of therapy.[63] Many LTC facilities have attempted to use antimicrobials to eradicate MRSA from their resident population; however, this has met with little success, possibly because of the reintroduction of the organism into the facility through the admission of colonized residents.[51,53,59]

Treatment of colonized or infected personnel. Health care personnel who have a staphylococcal infection should be treated; however, it is not necessary to treat a personnel carrier unless they have been epidemiologically implicated as the source of an outbreak. This is unlikely to occur in the long-term care setting.

Most LTC facilities have limited infection control resources. Because LTC facilities have diverse resident populations and different rates of MRSA colonization and infection, both endemic and epidemic control measures must be tailored to meet the needs and resources of the particular institution.

Education of health care workers. Educational programs on the mode of transmission of MRSA and the importance of contact precautions and hand washing should be provided frequently for caregivers in an LTC facility.

Vancomycin-Resistant *Enterococcus* in the Acute Care Setting

Epidemiology

The incidence of nosocomial infections due to vancomycin-resistant enterococci increased dramatically in U.S. hospitals between 1989 and 1993.[64] Multiple hospital outbreaks and clusters have been reported, and most of these have occurred among critically ill patients in intensive care units and immunosuppressed patients on oncology or transplant units.[65–70] The first community-acquired cases were reported from New York City in 1993.[71] The major reservoir of VRE is infected and colonized patients. There are at least 17 species of enterococci—*Entercoccus faecium* and *Enterococcus faecalis* are the two most commonly encountered in clinical isolates and *E faecium* is inherently more resistant to antibiotics than *E faecalis*. Some outbreaks of VRE appear to involve genetically unrelated strains. This may be because transposons contain the genetic determinants of resistance and transposons can spread easily between different strains of enterococci.[72] The enterococci are less virulent than *Staphylococcus aureus*, usually cause urinary tract infections, and occasionally cause endocarditis and bacteremia. Most serious enterococcal infections have been reported in severely compromised patients.[73–75]

Risk factors for developing VRE infection or colonization include severe underlying disease, intra-abdominal surgery, multiple-antibiotic therapy, vancomycin therapy, sigmoidoscopy and colonoscopy, indwelling urinary or central vascular catheter, and prolonged hospital stay.[65,73,76]

Mode of Transmission

Although the majority of infections are believed to arise from a patient's endogenous flora, VRE can be spread from person to person by direct contact or indirectly via contaminated equipment or environmental surfaces[65,69,77] or transient carriage on health care workers' hands.[78] Since the enterococci are normal inhabitants of the lower intestinal tract, patients may carry VRE asymptomatically in their stool and rectal colonization may persist for months.[72,79,80] The epidemiology of VRE has not been clearly elucidated; however, since VRE can remain viable on inanimate surfaces for prolonged periods,[69,80–83] and one outbreak was associated with use of an electronic thermometer,[77] fomites may play a role in the transmission of VRE.

Control Measures

Guidelines for preventing the spread of vancomycin-resistant enterococci in acute care hospitals were developed by the CDC's Hospital Infection Control Practices Advisory Committee (HICPAC).[76] One of the committee's primary recommendations for preventing the spread of VRE is the prudent use of vancomycin, which has consistently been reported as a major risk factor for colonization and infection with VRE. There is also concern that excessive use of vancomycin will promote the development of vancomycin-resistant *S aureus*. Few studies have been done on the efficacy of control measures used to prevent transmission of VRE. One study found that the use of contact isolation, including gloves, gowns, and a private room, were useful in limiting the spread of VRE in an acute care setting;[69] however, use of gowns and gloves failed to decrease colonization in a hospital in which VRE was endemic.[84]

The following measures have been used to control outbreaks of VRE in the acute care setting:

- hand washing
- laboratory-based surveillance (i.e., the review of positive cultures) to identify cases
- surveillance cultures of patients
- education of personnel
- contact precautions for infected and colonized patients
- cleaning and disinfection of equipment
- cleaning and disinfection of the environment

Hand washing. Proper hand washing, regardless of the use of gloves, is essential to control the person-to-person transmission of VRE. The HICPAC Guideline for Isolation Precautions in Hospitals recommends use of an antimicrobial soap or a waterless antiseptic agent when caring for patients with VRE because *E faecium* has been isolated from hands after they were washed with plain soap.[25,85]

Laboratory-based surveillance to identify cases. Ongoing surveillance should be conducted so that baseline endemic rates can be determined and potential outbreaks and clusters can be identified quickly.[69,76,83] Routine surveillance for VRE is generally conducted by prospective review of laboratory reports for isolates of *Enterococcus* species that are resistant to vancomycin. As is the case with MRSA, not all patients who are colonized or infected will be detected by routine cultures obtained for clinical indications. Once VRE is identified, criteria must be used to determine if the organism is colonizing or infecting the patient and if an infection is community or hospital acquired.[32] The CDC recommends that the laboratory routinely notify patient care and infection control personnel when VRE is isolated so that isolation precautions can be implemented promptly.[76] If an outbreak is suspected, laboratory records should be reviewed retrospectively and prospectively to identify both infected and colonized patients and a line-list of nosocomial cases should be maintained as discussed in Chapter 8. Both colonized and infected cases should be identified in order to determine the extent of the outbreak.

Surveillance cultures of patients. Point-prevalence culture surveys of patients on high-risk wards have been shown to be useful during VRE outbreaks to identify cases not detected by clinical cultures.[69,76] In an outbreak situation, VRE isolates from infected and colonized patients should be identified to the species level, and antimicrobial sensitivity testing should be done to help determine if the organisms may be epidemiologically related. VRE isolates may also be sent to a reference laboratory for strain typing by genotypic methods, as discussed in Chapter 11.

Education of personnel. Personnel involved in caring for patients with VRE should be given information on the extent of the VRE problem, the epidemiology and mode of transmission of VRE, and the importance of adhering to proper infection control practices with an emphasis on hand washing, standard precautions, isolation precautions, and equipment and environmental cleanliness.[76]

Contact precautions for infected and colonized patients. Aggressive infection control measures and strict compliance by hospital personnel are needed to limit the nosocomial spread of VRE and are specified in the HICPAC guidelines:[76]

1. Infected and colonized patients should be placed in a single room or in the same room as other patients with VRE.
2. Gloves should be worn when entering the room because extensive environmental contamination with VRE has been documented in several studies.[65,69,80,82,83]
3. A gown should be worn when entering the room if substantial contact with the patient or environment is anticipated, or if the patient has diarrhea, an ileostomy, a colostomy, or wound drainage not contained by a dressing.

4. Gloves and gowns should be removed before leaving the patient's room.

5. Hands should be washed with an antiseptic soap or cleaned with a waterless antiseptic agent before leaving the patient's room.

6. Noncritical items, such as stethoscopes, sphygmomanometers, and rectal thermometers, should be dedicated to use on patients with VRE; if this is not practical, these items should be cleaned and disinfected before use on other patients.

7. Stool or rectal cultures should be obtained on the roommates of newly identified cases to determine their colonization status and the need for isolation precautions.

If these measures are not effective at limiting nosocomial transmission of VRE, consideration should be given to cohorting patient care personnel to minimize contact of staff with VRE-positive and VRE-negative patients,[66,69,76] personnel should be re-educated on the importance of implementing and adhering to control measures, and verification should be obtained that equipment and environmental surfaces are being adequately cleaned and disinfected. Since personnel carriers have rarely been implicated in the transmission of VRE,[78] culturing of personnel is not generally recommended unless a careful epidemiologic study shows a link between a health care worker and cases.

Cleaning and disinfection of equipment and the environment. Since equipment and the environment may play a role in the transmission of VRE, personnel responsible for cleaning and disinfecting patient care equipment and environmental surfaces should be instructed to adhere to hospital procedures.

As with MRSA, there is little consensus on the measures that should be used to control the spread of VRE and a recent text edited by Pugliese and Weinstein addresses these issues and controversies.[86]

VRE in the Long-Term Care Setting

Epidemiology

Little information has been published to date on the epidemiology of vancomycin-resistant enterococci in the long-term care setting. Brennen et al conducted a two-and-half-year study of vancomycin-resistant *E faecium* (VREF) in a 400-bed long-term care Veterans Administration facility and found 36 patients colonized with VREF.[87] The investigators noted the following: some patients had protracted carriage of VREF; 24 of the 36 patients had VREF at time of transfer from an acute care facility; the risk of VREF infection was low in the population studied; and that patient-to-patient transmission of VREF was infrequent when contact precautions were used. Bonilla et al studied VRE colonization of patients in the medical, intensive care, and long-term care units of a Veterans Affairs Medical Center between December 1994 and August 1996.[80] They found that patients in the long-term care unit were more likely to be colonized than those in the acute care units; seven different strain types were present; transmission from roommate to roommate was uncommon; environmental contamination with VRE was found in the long-term and acute care settings; VRE was isolated from the hands of health care workers in both settings but personnel in the LTC unit were more likely to have VRE on their hands; and the hands of two health care workers remained culture-positive after washing.[80] Studies and clinical experience show that patients in both acute care and long-term care facilities may be colonized with more than one type of resistant organism, such as with MRSA and VRE.[87,88]

Previous hospitalization in an acute care facility is a risk factor for VRE colonization.[79,87] Asymptomatic rectal carriage occurs often among patients in acute and long-term care settings and may persist for months;[69,77,79,89] however, infection occurs only if other risk factors are present (such as multi-antibiotic therapy, severe underlying disease, and immunosuppression).[79] The finding that VRE does not appear to be a frequent cause of infection in residents of LTC facilities may be due to the absence of some of these risk factors.[73,79,87] Although colonization of residents in LTC facilities has frequently been reported, the author was unable to find any published reports of outbreaks of VRE infection in an LTC facility.

The epidemiology of VRE is similar to that of MRSA in that both organisms were initially associated with outbreaks in the acute care setting and both have become endemic in many acute care and long-term care facilities. Both VRE and MRSA can be introduced into an acute care or a long-term care facility by the transfer of colonized or infected patients who serve as reservoirs for transmission between these two settings,[89] and patients and residents can become persistently colonized with VRE or MRSA for many months.

Mode of Transmission

The majority of VRE infections are believed to arise from a patient's endogenous flora. The mode of transmission in the LTC setting has not been well studied. In the acute care setting, VRE can be spread from person to person by direct contact or indirectly via contaminated equipment or environmental surfaces[65,77,83] or by transient carriage on health care workers' hands.[78] Although extensive environmental contamination with VRE can occur, especially when a patient has diarrhea or is incontinent,[69,79] the role of the environment in the transmission of VRE is not clear.

Control Measures

The Long-Term Care Committee of the Society for Healthcare Epidemiology of America (SHEA) developed a position paper that outlines the epidemiology and modes of transmission of VRE and provides guidelines for the control of VRE in the LTC setting.[73] The SHEA guidelines were written to supplement the HICPAC guidelines for acute care facilities,[76] and both should be reviewed before designing an infection control plan for VRE in a long-term care facility. No studies have been published to date on the efficacy of VRE control measures in the long-term care setting.

The following measures, which have been explained in the section on control of VRE in the acute care setting, are recommended to control outbreaks of VRE in the long-term care setting:

- surveillance to identify cases
- laboratory-based surveillance (i.e., the review of positive cultures) to identify cases
- surveillance cultures of residents if an outbreak is suspected
- education of personnel
- contact isolation and barrier precautions for infected and colonized residents
- cleaning and disinfection of equipment
- cleaning and disinfection of the environment

Vancomycin-Intermediate or Vancomycin-Resistant *S aureus*

As of this writing, only a few isolated infections with *S aureus* intermediately resistant to vancomycin (VISA) have been reported.[90,91] Because *S aureus* is one of the most common causes of community- and hospital-ac-

quired infection and is easily transmitted from person to person, the emergence of vancomycin-resistant *S aureus* (VRSA) will pose serious infection control and public health consequences. Guidelines to prevent the spread of *S aureus* with reduced susceptibility to vancomycin have been developed by HICPAC and Edmond et al based on data currently available on the transmission and control of *S aureus*, and these should be used when developing protocols to prevent the spread of VRSA.[92,93]

Since VRSA has not yet been isolated clinically, the occurrence of one case of *S aureus* with reduced susceptibility to vancomycin should be considered an outbreak, and infection control measures should be implemented immediately. The following is a summary of the measures recommended by HICPAC[92] and Edmond et al:[93]

- The laboratory should immediately notify infection control personnel, the clinical unit, and the attending physician of any VISA or VRSA isolates.
- The patient should be placed in a single room and contact precautions should be strictly enforced.
- The number of persons entering the room should be limited to essential personnel—specific health care workers should be dedicated to provide one-on-one care whenever possible.
- Infection control personnel should initiate an epidemiologic investigation in conjunction with the state and local health departments and the CDC.
- Compliance with contact precautions and hand washing should be monitored and strictly enforced.
- All personnel involved in direct patient care should be informed of the epidemiologic implication of VRSA and of the infection control precautions needed to contain it.
- Surveillance cultures should be collected as specified by the CDC.
- The patient should be restricted to the isolation room except for essential medical purposes.
- Horizontal surfaces in the patient's immediate vicinity should be cleaned daily with a quarternary ammonium compound.
- Dedicated equipment, such as stethoscopes, thermometers, and blood pressure cuffs, should be used for the patient.
- All equipment, such as EKG and portable X-ray machines, should be disinfected as soon as tests are complete.

- If transfer is necessary, the receiving unit or institution should be informed of the patient's VRSA status.
- The health department and the CDC should be consulted prior to discharging the patient.

Tuberculosis in the Acute Care and Ambulatory Care Settings

Epidemiology

Outbreaks and nosocomial transmission of *Mycobacterium tuberculosis* have long been recognized in the hospital setting.[94–111] A hospital outbreak that occurred in Texas in 1983–1984 resulted from exposure in the emergency room to a patient with severe cavity tuberculosis (TB).[98] Six employees developed active TB and an immunocompromised patient was also believed to have developed TB as a result of exposure to the patient. An outbreak of multidrug-resistant tuberculosis (MDR-TB) in a hospital in New York occurred despite that fact that the patient was suspected of having pulmonary tuberculosis, was promptly placed in an isolation room, and personnel followed the hospital's TB protocol.[111] An investigation revealed that the ventilation system in some of the isolation rooms was not at negative pressure in relation to the corridor. While many reported nosocomial outbreaks in hospitals have been associated with the close contact of patients and personnel to a person with unrecognized infectious TB, several epidemics have been associated with diagnostic and therapeutic procedures such as bronchoscopy,[96] endotracheal intubation and suctioning,[97] irrigation of an open abscess,[99] autopsy,[100–102] and sputum induction and aerosol treatments.[104]

An outbreak in a Florida primary care health clinic was associated with sputum induction and aerosolized treatment of human immunodeficiency virus (HIV)-infected patients.[103] This outbreak most likely could have been avoided if cough-inducing procedures such as aerosolized pentamidine and sputum induction had been carried out using either local exhaust ventilation, such as a booth or special enclosure, or a room meeting the ventilation requirements for TB isolation.[112] An outbreak in a drug treatment center was associated with a client with unrecognized pulmonary disease even though the client had a history of tuberculosis when admitted to the facility. Because the treatment center had no health screening program in place, no precautions were taken to prevent the transmission of *M tuberculosis* from the new client.[110]

Several well-publicized hospital outbreaks of MDR-TB occurred among HIV-infected patients and health care workers in the early 1990s.[94,95,103,108] These outbreaks reflected the increased incidence of tuberculosis that occurred in many communities from 1988 through 1992. Factors that contributed to these outbreaks of MDR-TB included the following factors:[94]

- delayed identification of patients with MDR-TB
- delayed treatment of patients with MDR-TB
- lack of proper isolation of patients with infectious MDR-TB
- failure to keep patients in their isolation room
- failure of patients to wear a mask when they were outside of their isolation room
- inadequate respiratory protection for health care workers
- inadequate environmental controls such as negative air pressure rooms

Since 1993, the incidence of tuberculosis in the United States has been declining and in 1997 it reached the lowest number and rate of reported TB cases since measurement began in 1953.[113]

Mode of Transmission

M tuberculosis is spread via the airborne route by droplet nuclei, particles that are produced when persons with pulmonary or laryngeal TB sneeze, cough, speak, or sing. Droplet nuclei are approximately 1–5 μm in size, have the ability to remain suspended in air for prolonged periods, and can be carried through a building on air currents.[112] Infection occurs when a susceptible person inhales these particles into the lungs.

Control Measures

Control measures to prevent the transmission of tuberculosis in a variety of health care settings were published by the CDC in 1994; that document provides a detailed discussion of tuberculosis in acute care and ambulatory care facilities.[112] The CDC guidelines focus on measures that have been shown to interrupt outbreaks and to prevent nosocomial transmission. Exhibit 7–1, from the CDC guidelines, outlines the characteristics of an effective tuberculosis infection control program for a health care facility in which there is a high risk for transmission of *M tuberculosis*. The elements that should be chosen for inclusion in a health care facility's infection control program will depend on the

Exhibit 7–1 Characteristics of an Effective Tuberculosis (TB) Infection Control Program*

I. Assignment of responsibility

A. Assign responsibility for the TB infection-control program to qualified person(s).

B. Ensure that persons with expertise in infection control, occupational health, and engineering are identified and included.

II. Risk assessment, TB infection-control plan, and periodic reassessment

A. Initial risk assessments
1. Obtain information concerning TB in the community.
2. Evaluate data concerning TB patients in the facility.
3. Evaluate data concerning purified protein derivative (PPD)-tuberculin skin-test conversions among health care workers (HCWs) in the facility.
4. Rule out evidence of person-to-person transmission.

B. Written TB infection-control program
1. Select initial risk protocol(s).
2. Develop written TB infection-control protocols.

C. Repeat risk assessment at appropriate intervals.
1. Review current community and facility surveillance data and PPD-tuberculin skin-test results.
2. Review records of TB patients.
3. Observe HCW infection-control practices.
4. Evaluate maintenance of engineering controls.

III. Identification, evaluation, and treatment of patients who have TB

A. Screen patients for signs and symptoms of active TB:
1. On initial encounter in emergency department or ambulatory-care setting.
2. Before or at the time of admission.

B. Perform radiologic and bacteriologic evaluation of patients who have signs and symptoms suggestive of TB.

C. Promptly initiate treatment.

IV. Managing outpatients who have possible infectious TB

A. Promptly initiate TB precautions.

B. Place patients in separate waiting areas or TB isolation rooms.

C. Give patients a surgical mask, a box of tissues, and instructions regarding the use of these items.

V. Managing inpatients who have possible infectious TB

A. Promptly isolate patients who have suspected or known infectious TB.

B. Monitor the response to treatment.

C. Follow appropriate criteria for discontinuing isolation.

VI. Engineering recommendations

A. Design local exhaust and general ventilation in collaboration with persons who have expertise in ventilation engineering.

B. Use a single-pass air system or air recirculation after high-efficiency particulate air (HEPA) filtration in areas where infectious TB patients receive care.

C. Use additional measures, if needed, in areas where TB patients may receive care.

D. Design TB isolation rooms in health-care facilities to achieve ≥6 air changes per hour (ACH) for existing facilities and ≥12 ACH for new or renovated facilities.

E. Regularly monitor and maintain engineering controls.

F. TB isolation rooms that are being used should be monitored daily to ensure they maintain negative pressure relative to the hallway and all surrounding areas.

G. Exhaust TB isolation room air to outside or, if absolutely unavoidable, recirculate after HEPA filtration.

VII. Respiratory protection

A. Respiratory protective devices should meet recommended performance criteria.

B. Respiratory protection should be used by persons entering rooms in which patients with known or suspected infectious TB are being isolated, by HCWs when performing cough-inducing or aerosol-generating procedures on such patients, and by persons in other settings where administrative and engineering controls are not likely to protect them from inhaling infectious airborne droplet nuclei.

C. A respiratory protection program is required at all facilities in which respiratory protection is used.

VIII. Cough-inducing procedures

A. Do not perform such procedures on TB patients unless absolutely necessary.

B. Perform such procedures in areas that have local exhaust ventilation devices (e.g., booths or special enclosures) or, if this is not feasible, in a room that meets the ventilation requirements for TB isolation.

C. After completion of procedures, TB patients should remain in the booth or special enclosure until their coughing subsides.

IX. HCW TB training and education

A. All HCWs should receive periodic TB education appropriate for their work responsibilities and duties.

B. Training should include the epidemiology of TB in the facility.

C. TB education should emphasize concepts of the pathogenesis of and occupational risk for TB.

D. Training should describe work practices that reduce the likelihood of transmitting *M tuberculosis*.

X. HCW counseling and screening

A. Counsel all HCWs regarding TB and TB infection.

B. Counsel all HCWs about the increased risk to immunocompromised persons for developing active TB.

C. Perform PPD skin tests on HCWs at the beginning of their employment, and repeat PPD tests at periodic intervals.

D. Evaluate symptomatic HCWs for active TB.

XI. Evaluate HCW PPD test conversions and possible nosocomial transmission of *M tuberculosis*

XII. Coordinate efforts with public health department(s)

*A program such as this is appropriate for health care facilities in which there is a high risk for transmission of *Mycobacterium tuberculosis*.
Source: Reprinted from Guidelines for Preventing the Transmission of *Mycobacterium Tuberculosis* in Health-Care Facilities, *Morbidity and Mortality Weekly Report,* Vol. 43, No. RR-13, pp. 20–21, 1994, Centers for Disease Control and Prevention.

risk of transmission of *M tuberculosis* in that setting. An algorithm for assessing that risk is shown in Figure 7–1, and methods for identifying the risk of transmission in a health care setting are discussed in the CDC guidelines.[112] Because epidemics of TB, especially those caused by MDR-TB, can result in significant morbidity and mortality, acute care and ambulatory care facilities should implement those sections of the CDC guidelines that are relevant for their practice setting. Regardless of the setting or the risk of transmission for *M tuberculosis*, the most important measures for controlling the spread of TB are prompt identification and adequate treatment of persons with TB.

The elements that health care facilities should consider for inclusion in a TB prevention and control program are as follows:[112]

- a training program for health care workers that includes information on the epidemiology, mode of transmission, signs and symptoms, occupational risk, and control measures used to prevent the spread of TB
- a mechanism for screening patients with signs and symptoms suggestive of pulmonary tuberculosis
- early identification of persons (patients, personnel, and visitors) with pulmonary TB
- prompt radiologic and bacteriologic evaluation of persons who have signs and symptoms consistent with TB
- prompt and appropriate isolation of persons with known or suspected TB (NOTE: In the outpatient setting, patients with known or suspected TB should be placed in a separate waiting area if no isolation room is available. They should be given a surgical mask and a box of tissues and should be instructed how to wear the mask and to use the tissues when coughing or sneezing. Since covering the mouth while coughing can reduce the number of tubercle bacilli expelled into the air, this simple intervention should not be overlooked.)
- patient adherence to isolation precautions, including the use of masks when leaving the isolation room
- personnel adherence to isolation precautions, including the use of respirators
- prompt and effective treatment of persons who have active TB (NOTE: There is no consensus on how long a patient who is smear-positive for acid-fast bacilli should remain in isolation after treatment has begun. Two recent articles discuss the contagiousness of persons with active pulmonary tuberculosis;[114,115] however relatively little is

known about how long tubercle bacilli in the sputum remain infectious after effective therapy has been started. After reviewing the literature, Menzies concluded that "after initiation of therapy, patients who are still smear-positive should be considered still contagious."[114(p.585)])

- a purified protein derivative (PPD) skin-testing program for personnel with occupational exposure to *M tuberculosis*
- a management program for health care workers inadvertently exposed to *M tuberculosis*[116]
- provision of preventive therapy to health care workers who convert their PPD
- a PPD screening program for patients and clients at risk for TB (e.g., intravenous drug users and clients in drug treatment programs)

If tuberculosis is present in the community served, a PPD screening program for personnel and patients is an integral part of a facility's overall infection control program and is essential for detecting unrecognized infection with *M tuberculosis* and preventing the development of disease.[112]

Tuberculosis in Long-Term Care Facilities

Epidemiology

The endemic and epidemic transmission of *M tuberculosis* among residents in long-term care facilities has long been recognized.[117–125] A study conducted by the CDC in 1984–1985 found that elderly nursing home residents were at greater risk for tuberculosis than elderly persons living in the community.[126] Outbreaks of TB in nursing homes have affected both residents and staff.[118,122–125] In one outbreak a highly infectious resident with unrecognized cavitary tuberculosis infected 30 percent (49/161) of previously tuberculin-negative residents, eight of whom developed pulmonary tuberculosis, and 15 percent (21/138) of tuberculin-negative employees, one of whom developed tuberculosis.[118] The outbreak investigation revealed that the resident was an outgoing man who participated in social activities at the nursing home and he had probably been infectious for close to a year. In most of the outbreaks reported in the literature the source for nosocomial transmission in long-term care facilities is a resident with unrecognized pulmonary tuberculosis.

Mode of Transmission

The mode of transmission of *M tuberculosis* is via the airborne route as described in the previous section.

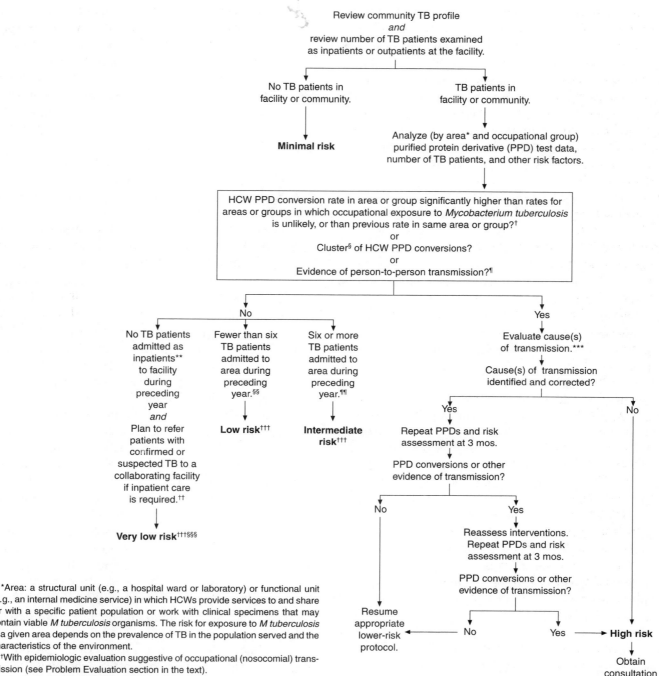

*Area: a structural unit (e.g., a hospital ward or laboratory) or functional unit (e.g., an internal medicine service) in which HCWs provide services to and share air with a specific patient population or work with clinical specimens that may contain viable *M tuberculosis* organisms. The risk for exposure to *M tuberculosis* in a given area depends on the prevalence of TB in the population served and the characteristics of the environment.

†With epidemiologic evaluation suggestive of occupational (nosocomial) transmission (see Problem Evaluation section in the text).

§Cluster: two or more PPD skin-test conversions occurring within a 3-month period among HCWs in a specific area or occupational group, and epidemiologic evidence suggests occupational (nosocomial) transmission.

¶For example, clusters of *M tuberculosis* isolates with identical DNA fingerprint (RFLP) patterns or drug-resistance patterns, with epidemiologic evaluation suggestive of nosocomial transmission (see Problem Evaluation section in the text).

**Does not include patients identified in triage system and referred to a collaborating facility or patients being managed in outpatient areas.

††To prevent inappropriate management and potential loss to follow-up of patients identified in the triage system of a very low-risk facility as having suspected TB, an agreement should exist for referral between the referring and receiving facilities.

§§Or, for occupational groups, exposure to fewer than six TB patients for HCWs in the particular occupational group during the preceding year.

¶¶Or, for occupational groups, exposure to six or more TB patients for HCWs in the particular occupational group during the preceding year.

***See Problem Evaluation section in the text.

†††Occurrence of drug-resistant TB in the facility or community, or a relatively high prevalence of HIV infection among patients or HCWs in the area, may warrant a higher risk rating.

§§§For outpatient facilities, if TB cases have been documented in the community but no TB patients have been examined in the outpatient area during the preceding year, the area can be designated as very low risk.

Figure 7–1 Protocol for Conducting a Tuberculosis (TB) Risk Assessment in a Health Care Facility. *Source:* Reprinted from Guidelines for Preventing the Transmission of *Mycobacterium Tuberculosis* in Health-Care Facilities, *Morbidity and Mortality Weekly Report,* Vol. 43, No. RR-13, pp. 10–11, 1994, Centers for Disease Control and Prevention.

Control Measures

In addition to its 1994 guidelines for preventing the transmission of *M tuberculosis* in health care facilities, in 1990 the CDC published recommendations for prevention and control of tuberculosis in facilities providing long-term care to the elderly in 1990.[112,126] The guidelines state that each long-term care facility should have a TB prevention and control program that addresses surveillance, containment, assessment, and education. The CDC guidelines can be downloaded from the MMWR Reports and Recommendations section of the CDC Web site at http://www.cdc.gov.

Surveillance. There should be a surveillance mechanism in place for identifying and reporting all cases of tuberculosis in the facility. All cases of tuberculosis should be reported to the local health department. There should also be a PPD skin-testing program for identifying all infected residents and staff. A PPD skin-testing program for residents should include administration and reading of a PPD skin test at the time of admission to the facility and periodically thereafter, depending on the facility's risk assessment. The CDC recommends a two-step procedure for baseline testing.[112,126] Staff and volunteers should have a baseline PPD test done at the time they begin work unless they have documentation of a previous positive reaction. The CDC recommends periodic repeat skin testing for skin test–negative employees and volunteers who have 10 or more hours of contact per week with elderly residents. Care must be taken to ensure that PPD tests are placed and read properly. A study by Naglie et al found that less than 30 percent of the long-term care facilities surveyed correctly defined a positive skin test.[127] Guidelines for interpreting PPD skin test results are shown in Exhibit 7–2.

The results of all skin testing should be recorded in millimeters of induration and documented. A sample form that can be used to record PPD testing and follow-up is shown in Exhibit 7–3.

Residents and staff who convert from PPD-negative to PPD-positive should have a chest radiograph and should be given prophylaxis if the radiograph is negative. If the radiograph is suggestive for tuberculosis a medical evaluation, including sputum smear and culture for acid-fast bacilli (AFB), must be done.

Studies have shown that many long-term care facilities lack an adequate surveillance program.[121,127] The mere existence of a PPD skin-testing program will not prevent TB outbreaks.[124] In order for a skin-testing program to be effective, action must be taken based on the results of screening. This means that those who are found to be newly infected should be medically evaluated and given appropriate prophylactic therapy, when indicated, to prevent the development of disease, and a search for the index case (i.e., the source of infection) should be conducted to prevent further transmission.

Containment. The CDC guidelines for long-term care facilities state that "persons with suspected or confirmed tuberculosis can remain in their usual environment provided (1) chemotherapy is promptly instituted at the time the diagnosis is suspected or confirmed, (2) recent and current contacts are evaluated and placed on appropriate therapy, and (3) new contacts can be prevented for a one to two week period."[126(p.10)] If these conditions cannot be met, the resident should be placed in airborne precautions as specified in the CDC guidelines for preventing the transmission of tuberculosis in health care facilities.[112]

Treatment for clinical disease should be given in accordance with the latest public health service recommendations. Residents who are given antituberculosis medications should be observed swallowing each dose to ensure that they are complying with therapy.

Whenever a person is diagnosed with infectious pulmonary tuberculosis (e.g., the person is coughing or has positive AFB smears and an abnormal chest radiography compatible with TB) a contact investigation should be conducted. All close contacts, including those who sleep, live, work, or share a common ventilation system for prolonged periods, should be skin tested for evidence of infection. Guidelines for investigating contacts have been published by the CDC;[112,126] however, the local health department should be consulted for guidance.

Unless medically contraindicated, preventive therapy should be given to contacts who have a documented skin test conversion, no clinical signs or symptoms of TB, and a negative chest radiograph.[112,116,126] Persons who refuse preventive therapy should be instructed to promptly seek medical evaluation if they develop signs or symptoms compatible with tuberculosis, such as a persistent cough, weight loss, fatigue, anorexia, or night sweats. Residents who are close contacts of an infectious person but who are not given prophylaxis should be carefully observed for the devel-

Exhibit 7–2 Summary of Interpretation of Purified Protein Derivative (PPD) Tuberculin Skin Test Results

1. An induration of ≥5 mm is classified as positive in
   - persons who have human immunodeficiency virus (HIV) infection or risk factors for HIV infection but unknown HIV status;
   - persons who have had recent close contact* with persons who have active tuberculosis (TB);
   - persons who have fibrotic chest radiographs (consistent with healed TB).
2. An induration of ≥10 mm is classified as positive in all persons who do not meet any of the criteria above but who have other risk factors for TB, including
   High-risk groups—
   - injecting-drug users known to be HIV seronegative;
   - persons who have other medical conditions that reportedly increase the risk for progressing from latent TB infection to active TB (e.g., silicosis; gastrectomy or jejuno-ileal bypass; being ≥10% below ideal body weight; chronic renal failure with renal dialysis; diabetes mellitus; high-dose corticosteroid or other immunosuppressive therapy; some hematologic disorders, including malignancies such as leukemias and lymphomas; and other malignancies);
   - children <4 years of age.
   High-prevalence groups—
   - persons born in countries in Asia, Africa, the Caribbean, and Latin America that have high prevalence of TB;
   - persons from medically underserved, low-income populations;
   - residents of long-term care facilities (e.g., correctional institutions and nursing homes);
   - persons from high-risk populations in their communities, as determined by local public health authorities.
3. An induration of ≥15 mm is classified as positive in persons who do not meet any of the above criteria.
4. Recent converters are defined on the basis of both size of induration and age of the person being tested:
   - ≥10 mm increase within a 2-year period is classified as a recent conversion for persons <35 years of age;
   - ≥15 mm increase within a 2-year period is classified as a recent conversion for persons ≥35 years of age.
5. PPD skin-test results in health-care workers (HCWs)
   - In general, the recommendations in sections 1, 2, and 3 of this exhibit should be followed when interpreting skin-test results in HCWs; however, the prevalence of TB in the facility should be considered when choosing the appropriate cut-point for defining a positive PPD reaction. In facilities where there is essentially no risk for exposure to *Mycobacterium tuberculosis* (i.e., minimal- or very low-risk facilities), an induration ≥15 mm may be a suitable cut-point for HCWs who have no other risk factors. In facilities where TB patients receive care, the cut-point for HCWs with no other risk factors may be ≥10 mm.
   - A recent conversion in an HCW should be defined generally as a ≥10 mm increase in size of induration within a 2-year period. For HCWs who work in facilities where exposure to TB is very unlikely (e.g., minimal-risk facilities), an increase of ≥15 mm within a 2-year period may be more appropriate for defining a recent conversion because of the lower positive-predictive value of the test in such groups.

*Recent close contact implies either household or social contact or unprotected occupational exposure similar in intensity and duration to household contact.

Source: Reprinted from Guidelines for Preventing the Transmission of *Mycobacterium Tuberculosis* in Health-Care Facilities, *Morbidity and Mortality Weekly Report*, Vol. 43, No. RR-13, pp. 62–63, 1994, Centers for Disease Control and Prevention.

opment of symptoms consistent with tuberculosis. TB can cause significant morbidity and mortality in the long-term care setting. Because health care workers and residents with exposure and documented PPD conversion have developed clinical disease, it is important that preventive therapy be taken.[118,124] The author is personally aware of a nurse who converted from PPD-negative to PPD-positive following inadvertent occupational exposure to a patient with TB and who refused isoniazid prophylaxis. Six months later, the nurse developed infectious pulmonary tuberculosis and exposed family, friends, co-workers, and patients to *M tuberculosis*.

Assessment. A record-keeping system should be developed to track and assess the facility's experience regarding TB infection and TB disease.[126] This will allow the facility to evaluate the effectiveness of its surveillance and containment practices.

Education. Regardless of the facility's risk for transmission of tuberculosis, health care workers should be educated about the signs and symptoms of tuberculosis and the control measures that should implemented for suspected or known cases. The medical staff should be alert for typical and atypical presentation of clinical disease, especially in the elderly, so that evaluation and treatment can be promptly initiated.

Clostridium difficile Infection

Epidemiology

Clostridium difficile has emerged as a major nosocomial pathogen that can cause antibiotic-associated diar-

Exhibit 7–3 Prototype Tuberculosis Summary Record for Facilities Providing Long-Term Care to the Elderly

NAME: Last   First   Middle   Room Number or Work Location: SS or ID Number: Date of Admission/Employment: Mo   Day   Yr

DOB: Mo   Day   Yr   RACE: ☐ White   ☐ Amer. Ind. or Alaskan Native   ☐ Black   ☐ Asian or Pacific Islander   ETHNIC ORIGIN: ☐ Hispanic   ☐ Non-Hispanic   ☐ Employee   ☐ Resident

BASELINE TESTING

INITIAL SKIN TEST: (or Documented History of Positive Mantoux)   Date Given: Mo Day Yr   Date Read: Mo Day Yr   Size: ___ mm   Was Therapy Recommended: ☐ Yes ☐ No

SECOND SKIN TEST: (In approximately 1 week if initial test is negative)   Date Given: Mo Day Yr   Date Read: Mo Day Yr   Size: ___ mm   Was Therapy Recommended: ☐ Yes ☐ No

Skin Test Date	Size	Skin Test Date	Size	Skin Test Date	Size	Skin Test Date	Size	Skin Test Date	Size
	mm		mm		mm		mm		mm
	mm		mm		mm		mm		mm
	mm		mm		mm		mm		mm

X-RAY: Date: Mo Day Yr   ☐ Normal   ☐ Abnormal   IF ABNORMAL: ☐ Cavitary   ☐ Non-Cavitary   ☐ Stable   ☐ Worsening   HISTORY OF PREVIOUS TB TREATMENT: ☐ Infection ___   ☐ TB Disease ___   Dates

BACTERIOLOGY FOR *M. TUBERCULOSIS:*   Microscopy ☐ Pos ☐ Neg   Culture ☐ Pos ☐ Neg   Date Collected ___   Source ___

DIAGNOSIS DATE: Mo Day Yr   ☐ Active TB   ☐ TB Infection w/o disease

CHEMOTHERAPY FOR INFECTION OR DISEASE:

Drugs Recommended: _____

Date Drugs Started: Mo Day Yr

Date Drugs Stopped: Mo Day Yr   Reason Stopped _____

Supervised by: _____

If Not Started, Give Reason: _____

FOR ACTIVE TB:

Major Site of Disease   ☐ Pulmonary   ☐ Other (Specify _____)

Case reported to Health Department?   ☐ Yes ☐ No

Date of Report: Mo Day Yr

Contact Investigation Done?   ☐ Yes ☐ No

HIV TEST: Date: Mo Day Yr

If Not Done, Give Reason: _____

Date	Event/Comment:	Date	Event/Comment:

Source: Reprinted from Prevention and Control of Tuberculosis in Facilities Providing Long-Term Care to the Elderly: Recommendations of the Advisory Committee for Elimination of Tuberculosis, *Morbidity and Mortality Weekly Report,* Vol. 39, No. RR-10, p. 17, 1990, Centers for Disease Control and Prevention.

rhea, antibiotic-associated colitis, and pseudomembranous colitis in hospitalized patients and residents of long-term care facilities. A small percentage of healthy adults carry *C difficile* in their gastrointestinal tract.[128] Neonates and infants are frequently asymptomatically colonized with *C difficile*. Colonization rates in hospitalized adults and residents of long-term care facilities vary widely[128,129] and reported incidence rates of diarrhea caused by *C difficile* in hospitals vary from 1 to 30 cases per 1,000 discharges.[130] Nosocomial *C difficile*-associated disease (CDAD) in adults is responsible for significant morbidity, increased length of stay, and rare fatalities in the acute and long-term care settings.[131,132] Diarrhea can lead to volume depletion and wound infection and can significantly increase medical costs. Although the major risk factor for nosocomial CDAD is previous antibiotic therapy, gastrointestinal surgery and older age have also been found to increase the risk of disease.[128]

Once thought to arise solely from endogenous flora, it is now clear that nosocomial acquisition of *C difficile* can occur, and outbreaks and clusters of CDAD have been reported in hospitals[129,130,132] and long-term care facilities.[133] When determining if a cluster or an outbreak exists in a health care facility, one of the first steps in the investigation is the development of a clear case definition. In reviewing the literature it is clear that not all investigators use the same criteria for defining a case of *C difficile*-associated diarrhea. Case definitions that would be useful for surveillance of nosocomial CDAD have been published by Olson et al[131] and Gerding et al.[128]

Mode of Transmission

Nosocomial acquisition and transmission via cross-infection has been demonstrated by molecular typing and fingerprinting.[128,130,132] The major reservoir for *C difficile* is infected and colonized patients and residents, and newly admitted colonized patients have been responsible for introducing the organism into a hospital.[134] The mode of transmission is thought to be via the hands of personnel or contaminated equipment or devices.[128] Environmental contamination of the area surrounding *C difficile*-infected patients and residents has long been recognized,[128–130] however, the role of environmental contamination and contaminated items, such as commodes and electronic thermometers, in outbreaks has been poorly defined as multiple strains may be isolated from the environment.[128,129]

Control Measures

Control measures that can be used to prevent endemic and epidemic transmission of *C difficile* have been analyzed by Gerding et al in a position paper of the Society for Healthcare Epidemiology of America (SHEA).[128] There are two approaches for preventing nosocomial *C difficile*-associated disease: (1) interrupting the transmission of *C difficile* and thus preventing the patient or resident from acquiring the organism and (2) reducing an individual's risk of developing disease.

Control measures that have been used to prevent nosocomial acquisition and to interrupt outbreaks include:[128]

- use of barrier precautions for infected persons, especially the use of gloves for handling feces and fecally contaminated items[135]
- either cohorting or providing a private room for persons with CDAD (especially for incontinent patients)
- hand washing
- environmental cleaning
- use of disposable rectal thermometers (Several studies have shown that eliminating the use of electronic thermometers can reduce the incidence of CDAD.[136–138])

Since prior exposure to antibiotics is the major risk factor for disease, the most important control measure that can be used to reduce the risk of CDAD is the restriction of antimicrobial agents.[128,139]

An active surveillance program must be in place in order to recognize clusters or outbreaks of CDAD. Mylotte described an easily conducted laboratory surveillance method that is based on the review of *C difficile* stool toxin assays and is similar to the surveillance method that is used at the author's institution.[140]

Parasitic Diseases

Introduction

Parasites that have the potential to cause nosocomial outbreaks fall into three broad categories: (1) enteric parasites, such as *Giardia lamblia*, *Entamoeba histolytica*, and *Cryptosporidium* species, (2) blood and tissue parasites, such as *Pneumocystis carinii*, and (3) ectoparasites, such as *Sarcoptes scabiei*. Although nosocomial transmission of parasitic and ectoparasitic diseases has been well-documented, reports of outbreaks caused by nosocomially acquired parasites are rare, except for those caused by *Sarcoptes scabiei*, the scabies mite.[141–143] Outbreaks of scabies in health care facilities, especially in long-term care facilities, have long been recognized.[142,144] Despite the excessive fear that many health care workers have of catching head or body lice from an infested patient or resident, outbreaks caused by lice have not been reported in the health care setting. In the past two decades, *Cryptosporidium parvum* and *Pneumocystis carinii* have emerged as important human pathogens, especially in persons with impaired natural host defense mechanisms, such as those with acquired immune deficiency syndrome or those undergoing immunosuppressive therapy. Only recently has nosocomial transmission and suspected outbreaks of these two organisms been reported.[141,142,145–153] Parasites that have been reported to cause outbreaks in the health care setting are listed in Table 7–1.[143,150,153–156]

Only those parasites that have been reported to cause outbreaks in health care facilities will be discussed in this section. For further information on the nosocomial transmission of parasites, the reader is referred to the series of articles by Lettau who reviewed published reports of nosocomial transmission and outbreaks of parasitic diseases in hospitals, research laboratories, and institutions for the mentally ill.[141–143]

Sarcoptes scabiei *(Scabies)*

Scabies is caused by an itch mite, *Sarcoptes scabiei*, which is transmitted from person to person by direct skin-to-skin contact and can sometimes be spread via contact with underclothes and bedding that were recently contaminated.[143] The female mite burrows into the skin to lay her eggs and this causes a reaction that is usually manifested as an intense pruritis but varies considerably, depending on the immune status of the host. The eggs hatch and mature into adults in 10 to 14 days.[157] The incubation period (time from infestation to observance of itching and rash) can be from several days to several weeks. Therefore, a person can transmit the organism to others before the symptoms are recognized. Most persons with scabies are said to harbor an average of 5 to 15 mites,[157,158] however, patients with

Table 7–1 Parasites with Potential for Causing Outbreaks in Health Care Facilities

Organism	Disease	Usual Mode of Transmission	Example of a Nosocomial Outbreak	Reference (Year)
Cryptosporidium species	Diarrhea	Person to person via fecal-oral route; waterborne	Patient to patient in pediatric hospital in Mexico	150 (1990)
Dermanyssus gallinae; Ornithonyssus sylvarium (avian mites)	Mite infestation; dermatitis	Birds to human	Mites entered crevices in wall and infected patients in a surgical intensive care unit; source was pigeon roosts on roof	154 (1983)
Entamoeba histolytica	Diarrhea	Person to person via fecal-oral route	Contaminated colonic irrigation equipment used in a chiropractic clinic	155 (1982)
Giardia lamblia	Diarrhea	Person to person via fecal-oral route; waterborne	Foodborne and person-to-person outbreak in a nursing home	156 (1989)
Pneumocystis carinii	Lower respiratory tract	Probably by inhalation of organism; possibly from person to person by droplet spread	Cluster of infections in pediatric hospital thought to be acquired by person-to-person spread	153 (1985)
Sarcoptes scabiei	Dermatitis	Person to person by skin-to-skin contact	Multiple outbreaks in hospitals and long-term care facilities	143 (1991)

compromised immune defenses can develop Norwegian, or crusted, scabies in which thousands of mites may be present. An adult mite can survive off the host and remain infective for only 24 to 36 hours at room temperature.[159] Fomites are not usually important modes of transmission, however, they have played a role in outbreaks when patients or residents had Norwegian scabies.[144,160] Mites have been found to survive in mineral oil for up to seven days;[157] therefore, oil-based ointments and creams could possibly serve as a reservoir. Because the appearance of the rash is so variable, a diagnosis of suspected scabies should routinely be confirmed by taking skin scrapings of the suspicious lesions and viewing them under a microscope.[144] The diagnosis can be confirmed if the adult mites, eggs, or scybala can be seen. Diagnosis should be relatively easy in a case of Norwegian scabies because of the large number of mites present; however, several scrapings may have to be done to confirm scabies infestation in a normal host because only a few mites may be present.

There are many published reports of scabies outbreaks in acute care[143,160–166] and long-term care settings.[144,161,167–172] Most of these occurred after contact with a patient or resident with Norwegian scabies as this presentation is often unrecognized or misdiagnosed and is highly contagious due to the large number of mites on the body. Scabies is particularly problematic in the in the long-term care setting where residents often have direct contact with each other and many require extensive hands-on care.

Outbreaks in both acute and long-term care facilities are difficult to control since continued spread frequently occurs due to (1) misdiagnoses and unrecognized cases among patients, residents, or personnel and (2) ineffective or improperly applied treatment.[168,170] Continued exposure to unrecognized or inadequately treated cases can lead to prolongation of an outbreak. Treatment failures due to resistance to scabicides are well recognized.[164,169,171,172] Guidelines for managing outbreaks in acute and long-term care settings have been published by several authors and include the following:[144,172–175]

- education of personnel on recognizing signs and symptoms of typical and atypical scabies
- education of personnel on measures used to prevent the transmission of scabies, especially on the importance of thorough application of scabicides
- development and implementation of a plan to evaluate and categorize patients, residents, personnel, and their contacts according to their probability of infestation[144]
- identification of symptomatic patients, residents, and personnel
- use of contact precautions for symptomatic patients and residents until 24 hours after treatment is applied
- identification of symptomatic household contacts, significant others, and visitors of patients and residents
- identification of symptomatic household contacts and significant others of personnel
- effective treatment of symptomatic persons (NOTE: It is important that the directions for scabicides are followed carefully and that treatment is applied to the entire body from the neck down including under the fingernails. For persons with Norwegian scabies, some scabicides should be reapplied 7 days after the initial treatment. Instructions on the package insert for the medication used should be carefully followed.)
- application of treatment to all identified persons within the same 24- to 48-hour period whenever possible
- restriction of infested personnel from work until initial treatment is completed (after overnight application of scabicide)
- re-examination of confirmed or suspected scabies cases at 14 and 28 days after initial treatment to evaluate treatment success
- careful identification and surveillance of exposed patients and personnel who are asymptomatic
- for continuing outbreak, prophylaxis for exposed patients and personnel who are asymptomatic (Mass prophylaxis of asymptomatic contacts is generally not recommended.)
- development of an ongoing surveillance program[170]

The Maryland Department of Health and Mental Hygiene *Guidelines for Control of Scabies in Long-Term Care Facilities* are reprinted in the appendix. These guidelines contain information on recognizing and diagnosing scabies, a procedure for performing skin scrapings, a protocol for the assessment and control of scabies outbreaks in LTC facilities, a line-list for scabies cases, and a scabies fact sheet.

Scabies outbreaks are extremely disruptive when they occur in health care facilities. They frequently result in adverse publicity and media coverage, overuse of prophylactic medication, and much fear and stress in personnel due to the stigma attached to having the disease and to the fact that their family members and significant others are frequently affected.[144,160,164,170,172] Once a scabies outbreak is confirmed (i.e., scabies has been diagnosed by skin scrapings), a carefully coordinated infection control plan must be implemented. This plan must be a multidisciplinary effort involving those responsible for infection control and employee health in the facility, the physicians caring for the residents or patients, all affected personnel, the household contacts of affected personnel, residents, or patients, the pharmacy, and the facility's administration and public relations departments. It is important that information on the extent of the outbreak and the control measures being taken be communicated consistently and frequently to personnel to avoid panic and misconceptions, especially if the outbreak is extensive or prolonged. It is useful to appoint a single spokesperson for the facility so that conflicting information is not provided to personnel and the community.

The most important measures that can be taken to prevent a scabies epidemic in any health care setting is the prompt recognition and treatment of infested persons.

Cryptosporidium *Species*

Cryptosporidium parvum is an intestinal protozoan that causes diarrhea in humans and is spread directly from person to person via the fecal-oral route or indirectly via contaminated water or food.[141] Several highly publicized waterborne[176] and foodborne outbreaks[177,178] of *Cryptosporidium* have occurred in the United States, calling attention to the enteric parasites. In 1993, *Cryptosporidium* caused the largest waterborne disease outbreak ever documented in the United States when the municipal water in Milwaukee became contaminated with *Cryptosporidium* oocysts—an estimated 403,000 persons were infected.[176] *Cryptosporidium* has recently been recognized as a cause of nosocomial diarrhea in immunosuppressed patients and possibly in the elderly.[145–150] A few hospital outbreaks of cryptosporidiosis have been reported to date.[145,148,150] An outbreak of cryptosporidiosis has also been reported in a day care center associated with a hospital.[180] Outbreaks caused by this organism may be missed because many laboratories do not routinely test for *Cryptosporidium*. Since infectious oocysts may be excreted in the stool of symptomatic and asymptomatic persons, control measures to prevent person-to-person transmission in the health care setting include standard precautions, hand washing, and careful handling of feces and fecally contaminated items. Contact precautions and use of a private room are recommended for hospitalized children less than 6 years of age who are diapered or incontinent.[25]

Giardia lamblia

Giardia lamblia is a common intestinal parasite in humans that can be transmitted via direct person-to-person contact or via contaminated water or food.[156] Although *G lamblia* is a common cause of day care center epidemics[181] and waterborne outbreaks,[179] there is only one reported outbreak associated with nosocomial acquisition and this occurred in residents and employees of a long-term care facility and in children and staff of a day care center at the facility.[156] The outbreak investigation in this nursing home revealed that transmission probably occurred via two routes: (1) by direct transmission between the children in the day care center and from the children to the day care center staff and the nursing home residents who participated in an "adopted grandparents" program and (2) by uncooked food prepared by infected food handlers (one of whom was the mother of an infected child in the day care center). Control measures used to terminate the outbreak included the following:[156]

- education for employees regarding hand washing
- instructions to the day care center staff to wash their hands after changing diapers and before preparing food
- instructions to the nursing home staff to wash hands after caring for nursing home residents
- treatment of symptomatic and asymptomatic persons who had *G lamblia* in their stool
- removal of infected food handlers until after they were treated and their symptoms resolved

Pneumocystis carinii

Pneumocystis carinii is a protozoan parasite that genetically resembles a fungus. It is an opportunistic pathogen that causes lower respiratory tract infection in immunocompromised patients. Studies suggest that *P carinii* can be transmitted from patient to patient in hospitals[148,182] and there are several reports of nosocomial infection clusters.[151,153] All of these reports involved immunosuppressed patients. Although little is known about the epidemiology and mode of transmission of nosocomial pneumocystis, acquisition of *P carinii* is believed to occur via inhalation.[142] The CDC guidelines for isolation precautions in hospitals currently recommend that patients with *P carinii* pneumonia not be placed in the same room with an immunocompromised patient.[25]

Ectoparasites Other Than Scabies

Several outbreaks of human infestation with avian mites have been reported in hospitals.[154,183] The source of these mites was pigeon roosts in close proximity to patient rooms. Since avian mites (*Ornithonyssus sylviarum* and *Dermanyssus gallinae*) can cause pruritic rashes in humans, health care personnel should be aware of the possible presence of these mites in the vicinity of areas used by nesting pigeons. These mites are larger than *Sarcoptes scabiei* and, unlike *S scabiei*, they can be seen by the naked eye and do not burrow under the skin. It should be noted that *D gallinae* is not affected by treatment with 1% gamma benzene hexachloride (Kwell).[183]

DISEASE SYNDROMES— GASTROINTESTINAL ILLNESS

Epidemiology

Nosocomial diarrhea commonly occurs in hospitalized patients and residents of long-term care facilities and may be caused by a variety of intrinsic and extrinsic factors: underlying diseases, gastric acidity, tube feedings, antacids, laxatives, antibiotics and other medications, and infectious agents. Gastrointestinal infections are caused by a variety of bacterial, viral, parasitic, and fungal agents; however, only a few of these agents have been involved in reported nosocomial outbreaks, and these are listed in Exhibit 7–4. A detailed discussion of each of these agents is beyond the scope of this chapter. For additional information on agents causing gastrointestinal illness in health care facilities, the reader is referred to the chapters on infectious gastroenteritis that appear in each of the infection control textbooks listed in the Suggested Reading section at the end of Chapter 5.

There is little data on the incidence of nosocomial gastroenteritis. Hospitals participating in the housewide surveillance component of the CDC National Nosocomial Infections Surveillance (NNIS) system from 1985 to 1991 reported nosocomial gastroenteritis rates from 7.8 to 14.2 infections per 10,000 discharges, depending on the type and size of hospital.[184] Nicolle and Garibaldi reported the incidence of gastrointestinal infection in nursing homes to be from 0 to 2.5 infections per 1,000 resident-days.[185] *Salmonella*, *Clostridium difficile*, and the caliciviruses (Norwalk-like agents or small round structured viruses [SRSVs]) are among the most commonly reported causes of outbreaks of nosocomial gastrointestinal infections in hospitals and long-term care facilities. Because the etiology for diarrhea is frequently not determined, it is likely that many outbreaks in health care facilities are not recognized—especially if they are caused by viral agents, as clinical microbiology laboratories do not routinely screen for viruses. Rotaviruses are among the most important causes of infectious diarrhea in infants, young children, and the elderly and are responsible for causing both sporadic and epidemic gastroenteritis in acute and LTC facilities.

Exhibit 7–4 Etiologic Agents Involved in Outbreaks of Gastrointestinal Illness in Health Care Facilities

Bacterial	*Viral*	*Parasitic*
Aeromonas hydrophilia	Adenovirus	*Cryptosporidium*
Campylobacter species	Astrovirus	*Entamoeba histolytica*
Clostridium botulinum	Calicivirus (Norwalk and Norwalk-like viruses	*Giardia lamblia*
Clostridium difficile	or small round structured viruses [SRSVs])	
Clostridium perfringens	Coxsackievirus	
Escherichia coli O157:H7	Rotavirus	
Listeria monocytogenes		
Salmonella species		
Shigella species		
Staphylococcus aureus		
Yersinia enterocolitica		

Mode of Transmission

Agents causing infectious gastroenteritis may be transmitted in the health care setting by contact with an infected individual[128,129,156,186–189] or a contaminated object[136,155,189,190] or by consuming contaminated food, water, or other beverages.[156,186,188,190] Examples of nosocomial outbreaks of gastrointestinal illness that have occurred in hospitals and long-term care facilities, including the causative agent, the implicated source, and the probable mode of transmission, are shown in Table 7–2.[129,133,156,187,189,192–206] Once introduced into a health care facility, many of these agents can readily be spread from person to person, and outbreaks frequently involve both patients or residents and personnel[156,186,187,189,192,196–198,203,205,206] with occasional secondary spread to the household contacts of personnel.[196,197] Attack rates in the 50 percent range are frequently reported for the small round structured viruses.[187,197] In 1994, 62 of 121 residents (51 percent) and 64 of 136 staff (47 percent) of a Maryland nursing home developed vomiting and diarrhea that was subsequently determined to be caused by a SRSV.[187] The index case was a nurse who became ill at work and continued to work for 3 days (three 12-hour shifts) although she was ill with explosive diarrhea. A nurse aide who worked with the nurse subsequently developed nausea, vomiting, and diarrhea and continued to work. Both of these personnel were thought to be responsible for introducing the agent into the wards. The outbreak had an overall attack rate (staff and residents) of 50 percent and resulted in three hospitalizations and two deaths among the 121 residents.[187] The investigators highlighted the importance of having a sick leave policy that encourages personnel to report gastrointestinal illnesses immediately and cease work until 48 hours after the resolution of vomiting and diarrhea.

Community outbreaks of rotavirus in temperate climates generally occur during the winter months and can result in nosocomial transmission via person-to-person spread.[206] Although the primary mode of transmission of the agents causing infectious gastroenteritis is fecal-oral, there is some evidence that the Norwalk-like viruses and rotavirus can be transmitted via aerosolization of feces or vomitus, such as may occur when a person handles contaminated laundry or has explosive vomiting or diarrhea.[190,207,208] Gastroenteritis caused by rotavirus can be characterized by severe diarrhea, vomiting, fever, and respiratory symptoms, how-ever, there is little evidence that rotavirus is spread via respiratory secretions. Since rotavirus is fairly resistant to disinfectants and germicides and can survive on environmental surfaces for prolonged periods, fomites probably play a role in the transmission of this agent.[206]

Foodborne Outbreaks

Food and waterborne outbreaks may be caused by a variety of agents: bacteria, viruses, parasites, natural toxins, and chemicals.[190,207–215] The characteristics of foodborne agents that cause gastrointestinal disease are shown in Table 7–3. Many recognized causes of foodborne outbreaks are emerging or re-emerging infectious agents (i.e., they have emerged in the United States as pathogens within the past two decades): *Campylobacter*, *Escherichia coli* O157:H7, *Helicobacter pylori*, *Listeria monocytogenes*, *Vibrio cholerae* and *vulnificus*, group A beta-hemolytic streptococcus, Norwalk and Norwalk-like agents, *Anisakis*, *Cryptosporidium*, *Giardia lamblia*, microsporidia, *Toxoplasma gondii*, and cyclospora. To date, only those agents listed in Exhibit 7–4 have been associated with nosocomial outbreaks. Information on foodborne pathogens and toxins can be obtained from the U.S. Food and Drug Administration (FDA) Web site at http://www.fda.gov. The FDA's *Foodborne Pathogenic Microorganisms and Natural Toxins Handbook* (also known as the "Bad Bug Book") can be viewed and downloaded from http://vm.cfsan.fda.gov. This handbook provides useful facts on organisms and toxins, foods associated with outbreaks, characteristic disease symptoms, and recent outbreaks. It also provides hypertext links to recent articles from the *Morbidity and Mortality Weekly Reports* on foodborne disease outbreaks and to educational information on preventing foodborne infections.

Several large, highly publicized community outbreaks caused by food and waterborne agents occurred in the 1990s. In 1993, over 400,000 people developed diarrhea after drinking the Milwaukee municipal water that was contaminated with *Cryptosporidium* oocysts.[176] That same year, a large multistate outbreak of *E coli* O157:H57 in the Pacific Northwest was linked to hamburgers served by a fast-food chain.[216] In 1997, several outbreaks of cyclosporiasis were associated with commercially distributed fresh raspberries, mesclun lettuce, and basil.[217] These outbreaks call attention to the fact that contaminated water or commer-

Table 7–2 Selected Outbreaks of Nosocomial Gastrointestinal Illness

Agent	Implicated Source	Probable Mode of Transmission	Health Care Setting	Comments	Reference (Year Reported)
Salmonella species	Chicken liver	Foodborne*	LTC	Affected residents and personnel	192 (1997)
	Eggs, chicken, turkey, pureed food	Foodborne	LTC	Multiple outbreaks reported	193 (1991)
	Soiled linen and asymptomatic cook	Foodborne, contact with laundry, person to person	LTC	Affected residents, laundry workers, and nurses	189 (1991)
	Unknown—probable chronic carrier	Foodborne, person to person	Hospital	Cases occurred over a 5-year period	194 (1985)
	Eggs	Foodborne	Hospital	Multiple outbreaks reported	195 (1998)
Staphylococcus aureus	Egg salad, chicken salad, potato salad, chicken, chopped beef livers	Foodborne	LTC	Multiple outbreaks reported	193 (1991)
Clostridium difficile	Infected residents	Person to person	LTC	Primary risk factor is prior antimicrobials	133 (1990)
	Infected patients	Person to person	Hospital	Primary risk factor is prior antimicrobials	129 (1989)
Caliciviruses (Norwalk-like)	Unknown	Person to person	LTC	Affected personnel and residents; was also transmitted to families of personnel	196 (1993)
	Ill nurse and nurse's aide	Person to person	LTC	Index case was ill nurse who worked while symptomatic; affected residents and personnel	187 (1996)
	Unknown	Person to person	LTC	Affected personnel and residents; was also transmitted to families of personnel	197 (1990)
	Ill nurse	Person to person	Hospital	Index case was hospitalized nurse; affected personnel and patients	198 (1998)
Clostridium perfringens	Meatloaf, split pea soup, roast beef, shepherd's pie, turkey	Foodborne	LTC	Multiple outbreaks	193 (1991)
	Canned tuna	Foodborne	Hospital	Affected personnel	199 (1994)
Listeria monocytogenes	Raw vegetables	Foodborne	Hospital	Involved 20 patients in 8 hospitals	200 (1986)
Bacillus cereus	Beef stew	Foodborne	LTC	Affected residents and personnel	201 (1988)
Aeromonas hydrophilia	Unknown	Unknown	LTC	Affected residents	202 (1990)
Campylobacter jejuni	Chicken liver	Foodborne	LTC	Affected residents and personnel	192 (1997)
Escherichia coli O157:H7	Sandwiches	Foodborne and person to person	LTC	Affected residents and personnel	203 (1987)
	Hamburger	Foodborne	LTC	Affected residents	204 (1986)

continues

Table 7–2 continued

Agent	Implicated Source	Probable Mode of Transmission	Health Care Setting	Comments	Reference (Year Reported)
Giardia lamblia	Children and sandwiches	Person to person and foodborne	LTC and associated child day care center	Affected children, personnel, and residents	156 (1989)
Rotavirus	Not identified	Person to person	LTC	Affected residents and personnel	205 (1980)
	Pediatric patients with community-acquired infection	Person to person	Hospital	Nosocomial transmission occurred in patients during community outbreak	206 (1990)
Niacin intoxication	Cornmeal	Foodborne	LTC	Oversupplementation of cornmeal with vitamins and minerals	193 (1991)

*LTC = long-term care facility.

cially available products could affect health care workers through community exposure or could be served and consumed in a health care facility, thus infecting patients, residents, personnel, and visitors.

In 1995, the CDC, the U.S. Department of Agriculture (USDA), the Food and Drug Administration, and the California, Connecticut, Georgia, Minnesota, and Oregon health departments initiated the Foodborne Disease Active Surveillance Network (FoodNet) to monitor the incidence of foodborne diseases.[212] Maryland and New York joined FoodNet in 1997. The primary goals of FoodNet are to characterize, understand, and respond to foodborne illnesses in the United States. FoodNet conducts active surveillance for laboratory confirmed cases of *Campylobacter*, *E coli* O157:H7, *Listeria*, *Salmonella*, *Shigella*, *Vibrio*, *Yersinia*, *Cryptosporidium*, and *Cyclospora*. In 1997, *Campylobacter* was the most commonly isolated of these nine pathogens, followed by *Salmonella*, *Shigella*, *Cryptosporidium*, and *E coli* O157:H7.[212] Additional information about FoodNet is available on the World Wide Web at http://www.cdc.gov/nciod/dbmd/foodnet.

Nosocomial outbreaks of foodborne pathogens have long been recognized.[188,193,195,209,210] Outbreaks in hospitals and nursing homes accounted for 3.3 percent of the foodborne outbreaks and 28.9 percent of the related deaths reported to the CDC from 1975 to 1992.[195] A confirmed causative agent was determined in 67 of 123 reported hospital outbreaks and 92 of 168 reported nursing home outbreaks. In hospitals, *Salmonella* was the most commonly reported agent (52 percent) followed by scombroid fish poisoning (12 percent), *Clostridium perfringens* (11 percent), and *Staphylococcus aureus* (8 percent). In nursing homes, the most common agent was also *Salmonella* (66 percent) followed by *Staphylococcus aureus* (15 percent), *Clostridium perfringens* (9 percent), and *Campylobacter jejuni* (3 percent).

Control Measures

Control measures for preventing the spread of agents that cause gastrointestinal infections depend on the mode of transmission and reservoir for the organism. It is important to remember that many of these agents have several modes of transmission (many can be spread by both the contact and foodborne routes).[156,186,189,194,203] When an outbreak is first identified or suspected, neither the agent nor the mode of transmission may be known, so control measures should be implemented based on the most likely agent, reservoir, and mode(s) of transmission. This can be determined by evaluating the characteristic signs and symptoms of those affected and conducting an initial, quick epidemiologic study (identifying persons, place, time of onset, and incubation period). Table 7–3 can be used to help identify possible foodborne agents. Foods

Table 7–3 Characteristics of Agents Causing Foodborne Diseases

I. Disease typified by vomiting (and little or no fever) after a short incubation fever

Agent	Incubation Period Usual (Range)	Symptoms*	Characteristic Foods
Bacillus cereus	2–4 hours (1–6 hours)	N, V, D	Fried rice
Heavy metals (cadmium, copper, tin, zinc)	5–15 minutes (5 minutes to 8 hours)	N, V, C, D	Foods and beverages prepared, stored, or cooked in containers coated, lined, or contaminated with offending metal
Staphylococcus aureus	2–4 hours (1/2–8 hours)	N, C, V; D, F may be present	Sliced/chopped ham and meats, custards, cream fillings

II. Diseases typified by diarrhea (often with fever) after a moderate to long incubation period

Agent	Incubation Period Usual (Range)	Symptoms*	Characteristic Foods
Bacillus cereus	8–16 hours (6–24 hours)	C, D	Custards, cereals, puddings, sauces, meat loaf
Campylobacter jejuni	2–5 days (2–10 days)	C, D, B, F	Raw milk, poultry, water
Clostridium perfringens	10–12 Hours	C, D (V, F rare)	Meat, poultry
Cyclospora species	1 week (1–11 days)	D, N, V, C	Berries, lettuce
Escherichia coli enterotoxigenic	6–48 hours	D, C	Uncooked vegetables, salads, water, cheese
Escherichia coli enteroinvasive	Variable	C, D, F, H	Same
Escherichia coli enterohemorrhagic (*E coli* O157:H7 and others)	72–96 hours (1–10 days)	B, C, D, H, F infrequent	Beef, raw milk, water
Norwalk-like agents (Norwalk, Hawaii, Snow Mountain)	16–48 hours (15–77 hours)	N, V, C, D	Shellfish, water
Rotavirus	24–72 hours	N, V, C, D	Foodborne transmission not well documented
Salmonella (nontyphoid)	6–48 hours (6 hours to 10 days)	D, C, F, V, H Septicemia or enteric fever	Poultry, eggs, milk, meat (cross-contamination important)
Shigella	24–48 hours (12 hours to 6 days)	C, F, D, B, H, N, V	Foods contaminated by infected food handler; usually not foodborne

continues

Table 7–3 continued

II. Diseases typified by diarrhea (often with fever) after a moderate to long incubation period (continued)

Agent	Incubation Period Usual (Range)	Symptoms*	Characteristic Foods
Vibrio cholerae non-O1	1–5 days	D, V	Shellfish
Vibrio cholerae O1	1–5 days	D, V	Shellfish, water, or foods contaminated by infected person or obtained from contaminated environmental source
Vibrio parahaemolyticus	4–30 hours	C, D N, V, F, H, B	Seafood
Yersinia enterocolitica	4–6 days usual (1–10 days)	F, D, C, V, H	Pork products, foods contaminated by infected human or animal

III. Botulism

Agent	Incubation Period Usual (Range)	Symptoms*	Characteristic Foods
Clostridium botulinum	12–48 hours (2 hours to 8 days)	V, D Descending paralysis	Improperly canned or preserved foods that provide anaerobic conditions

IV. Diseases most readily diagnosed from the history of eating a particular type of food

Agent	Incubation Period Usual (Range)	Symptoms*	Characteristic Foods
Ciguatera poisoning	2–8 hours	D,N,V, paresthesias, reversal of temperature sensation	Large ocean fish (i.e., barracuda, snapper)
Scombroid fish poisoning	usually <1 hour (1 minute to 3 hours)	N,C,D,H, flushing, urticaria	Mishandled fish (i.e., tuna)

*B, bloody stools; C, cramps; D, diarrhea; F, fever; H, headache; N, nausea; V, vomiting.
Source: Adapted from Epidemiology Program Office, *Principles of Epidemiology: An Introduction to Applied Epidemiology and Biostatistics,* 2nd ed., pp. 493–497, 1992, Centers for Disease Control and Prevention.

that require handling and no subsequent cooking constitute the greatest risk of serving as vehicles for foodborne outbreaks. Many gastroenteritis outbreaks in health care facilities are caused by the Norwalk-like agents, even though confirmation is frequently not made. These agents generally cause a mild to moderate, self-limited disease characterized by nausea, vomiting, diarrhea, and abdominal pain with one or more of these symptoms lasting from 24 to 48 hours. The incubation period is usually from 24 to 48 hours and can be as short as 15 hours.[215]

Preventing Person-to-Person Transmission of Enteric Agents

The following control measures have been recommended to prevent the spread of enteric pathogens by direct person-to-person contact or indirect contact with contaminated items:[25,33,187,190]

- Instruct personnel, patients, residents, and visitors to practice careful hand washing; hand washing is the single most important measure for preventing the person-to-person transmission of enteric pathogens.

- Exclude ill personnel from patient care and food handling for at least 2 days after resolution of illness.
- Ensure that personnel adhere to standard and contact precautions, including the use of gloves when handling feces or fecally soiled articles or equipment.[25]
- Institute contact precautions for diapered or incontinent patients who have an acute diarrheal disease of suspected infectious etiology.[25]
- Instruct personnel to carefully handle feces and fecally contaminated items (especially bedpans and soiled laundry) to avoid aerosolization.
- Use appropriate cleansers/disinfectants to clean and disinfectant soiled environmental surfaces, articles, and equipment; some disinfectants are not active against rotavirus.[218]

During an outbreak, the following additional measures are recommended:

- Determine the likely causative agent, source, and mode of transmission so that appropriate measures can be identified and implemented, i.e., conduct an epidemiologic study by collecting information on the identity of affected persons, their characteristic symptoms, unit(s) affected, date and time of onset; determine the incubation period by drawing an epidemic curve.
- The absence of routinely available laboratory tests for viral agents make it difficult to confirm the etiology of many outbreaks; consult with the laboratory regarding the collection of stool specimens.[190,219]
- Conduct active surveillance to identify new cases among patients, residents, personnel, and visitors.
- Isolate or cohort ill patients and residents.
- Ensure that ill personnel are reassigned to non-patient care and non-food handling duties or are restricted from work until at least 2 days after resolution of vomiting and/or diarrhea. (NOTE: Many states have specific regulations regarding work restrictions for food handlers and health care personnel and when they can return to work after salmonellosis or shigellosis is diagnosed.)
- Minimize contact between well and ill persons as much as possible (cohort personnel and patients/residents whenever possible).

- Alert visitors to wash their hands carefully if visiting an affected patient or resident.
- In long-term care facilities: (1) restrict ill residents from group activities, including meals, until 2 days after resolution of vomiting and/or diarrhea and (2) depending on the organism involved and the extent of the outbreak, close the ward to new admissions.
- In pediatric settings: (1) close the playroom, (2) identify patients exposed to the index case and avoid placing them with unexposed patients for the duration of the incubation period, (3) depending on the organism involved and the extent of the outbreak, close the ward to new admissions, and (4) instruct parents and other household contacts in the use of proper hand washing and handling of feces and diapers.
- Emphasize careful handling of soiled linen, clothing, and diapers to avoid aerosolization of feces and contamination of the environment.
- If a Norwalk-like agent is the likely cause of the outbreak, instruct personnel to wear masks when cleaning areas grossly soiled with feces or vomitus.

Many states have guidelines for investigating and controlling gastroenteritis outbreaks in long-term care facilities and these should be followed when available. The Maryland Department of Health and Mental Hygiene Guidelines for the Epidemiological Investigation of Gastroenteritis Outbreaks in Long-Term Care Facilities can be found in Appendix I.

Preventing Foodborne Transmission of Enteric Agents

The control measures for preventing the foodborne transmission of pathogens depends on the agent involved. For instance, since viral agents cannot multiply outside the host, the initial innoculum in the food source determines infectivity and food storage is not as critical as if the contaminating agent were *Staphylococcus aureus,* which will readily multiply in food held at room temperature. Control measures for preventing and investigating foodborne outbreaks have been published by the CDC and state health departments:[187,190,211]

- Exclude ill personnel from handling food for at least 2 days after resolution of diarrhea and vomiting.
- Emphasize the importance of proper hand washing for all personnel who handle food.

- Train food handlers in food safety practices (i.e., the proper handling, storage, preparation, and cooking of food—especially the handling of eggs and the importance of maintaining proper temperatures for hot or cold foods and avoiding cross-contamination between cooked and uncooked foods).
- Follow state regulations, as appropriate, for food handlers with infectious gastroenteritis.

Control measures for interrupting and investigating a foodborne outbreak include the following:

- Exclude ill personnel from handling food for at least 2 days after resolution of diarrhea and vomiting.
- Consult with the laboratory regarding the collection of stool specimens.[190,219]
- Conduct active surveillance to identify new cases among patients, residents, personnel, and visitors.
- Isolate or cohort ill patients and residents.

- Ensure that ill personnel are reassigned to non-patient care and non-food handling duties or are restricted from work until at least 2 days after resolution of vomiting and/or diarrhea. (NOTE: Many states have specific regulations regarding work restrictions for food handlers and health care personnel and when they can return to work after salmonellosis or shigellosis is diagnosed.)

Pathogens introduced into a facility via food can be further transmitted from person to person by direct contact with an infected person or a contaminated item;[156,186,189,194,203] therefore, measures to prevent person-to-person transmission, as noted above, should also be considered.

Although most cases of foodborne disease are caused by infectious agents, it is important to remember that pesticides and other chemicals have been responsible for outbreaks involving gastrointestinal and neurologic illness.[215,220]

REFERENCES

1. Nash O. *Selected Poems of Ogden Nash.* Smith L, Eberstadt I, eds. New York: Little Brown & Company; 1975:59.

2. Jevons MP. "Celbenin"-resistant staphylococci. *Br Med J.* 1961;1: 124–125.

3. Panlilo AL, Culver DH, Gaynes RP, et al. Methicillin-resistant *Staphylococcus aureus* in US hospitals, 1975–1991. *Infect Control Hosp Epidemiol.* 1992;13:582–586.

4. Barrett FF, McGehee RP Jr, Finland M. Methicillin-resistant *Staphylococcus aureus* at Boston City Hospital. *N Engl J Med.* 1968;279: 441–448.

5. Wenzel RP, Nettleman MD, Jones RN, et al. Methicillin-resistant *Staphylococcus aureus*: implications for the 1990s and effective control measures. *Am J Med.* 1991;91:3B-221S–3B-227S.

6. Harstein AI, LeMonte AM, Iwamoto PKL. DNA typing and control of methicillin-resistant *Staphylococcus aureus* at two affiliated hospitals. *Infect Control Hosp Epidemiol.* 1997;18:42–48.

7. Lugeon C, Blanc DS, Wenger A, et al. Molecular epidemiology of methicillin-resistant *Staphylococcus aureus* at a low-incidence hospital over a 4-year period. *Infect Control Hosp Epidemiol.* 1995;16:260–267.

8. Embil J, Ramotar K, Romance L, et al. Methicillin-resistant *Staphylococcus aureus* in tertiary care institutions on the Canadian prairies 1990–1992. *Infect Control Hosp Epidemiol.* 1994;15:646–651.

9. Layton MC, Hierholzer WJ, Patterson JE. The evolving epidemiology of methicillin-resistant *Staphylococcus aureus* at a university hospital. *Infect Control Hosp Epidemiol.* 1995;16:12–17.

10. Harstein AI, Denny MA, Morthland VH, et al. Control of methicillin-resistant *Staphylococcus aureus* in a hospital and an intensive care unit. *Infect Control Hosp Epidemiol.* 1995;16:405–411.

11. Linnemann CC Jr, Moore P, Staneck JL, et al. Reemergence of epidemic methicillin-resistant *Staphylococcus aureus* in a general hospital associated with changing staphylococcal strains. *Am J Med.* 1991;91:3B-238S–3B-244S.

12. Troilett N, Carmeli Y, Samore MH, et al. Carriage of methicillin-resistant *Staphylococcus aureus* at hospital admission. *Infect Control Hosp Epidemiol.* 1998;19:181–185.

13. Boyce JM. Methicillin-resistant *Staphylococcus aureus* in hospitals and long-term care facilities: microbiology, epidemiology, and preventive measures. *Infect Control Hosp Epidemiol.* 1992;13:725–737.

14. Meier PA, Carter CC, Wallace SE, et al. A prolonged outbreak of methicillin-resistant *Staphylococcus aureus* in the burn center of a tertiary medical center. *Infect Control Hosp Epidemiol.* 1996;17:798–802.

15. Thompson RL, Cabezudo I, Wenzel RP. Epidemiology of nosocomial infections caused by methicillin-resistant *Staphylococcus aureus*. *Ann Intern Med.* 1982;97:309–317.

16. Boyce JM, Landry M, Deetz TR, et al. Epidemiologic studies of an outbreak of methicillin-resistant *Staphylococcus aureus* infections. *Infect Control.* 1981;2:110–116.

17. Sheretz RJ, Reagan DR, Hampton KD, et al. A cloud adult: the *Staphylococcus aureus* virus interaction revisited. *Ann Intern Med.* 1996;124:539–547.

18. Boyce JM, Opal SM, Potter-Bynoe G, et al. Spread of methicillin-resistant *Staphylococcus aureus* in a hospital after exposure to a health care worker with chronic sinusitis. *Clin Infect Dis.* 1993;17:496–504.

19. Haley RW, Hightower AW, Khabbaz RF, et al. The emergence of methicillin-resistant *Staphylococcus aureus* in United States hospitals: the possible role of the house-staff patient transfer circuit. *Ann Intern Med.* 1982;97:297–308.

20. Ward TT, Winn RE, Harstein AI, et al. Observations relating to an inter-hospital outbreak of methicillin-resistant *Staphylococcus aureus*: role of antimicrobial therapy in infection control. *Infect Control.* 1981;2:453–459.

21. Reboli AC, John JF Jr, Platt CG, et al. Methicillin-resistant *Staphylococcus aureus* outbreak at a Veterans Affairs medical center: importance of carriage of the organism by hospital personnel. *Infect Control Hosp Epidemiol.* 1990;11:291–296.

22. Layton MC, Perez M, Heald P, et al. An outbreak of mupirocin-resistant *Staphylococcus aureus* on a dermatology ward with an environmental reservoir. *Infect Control Hosp Epidemiol.* 1993;14:369–375.

23. Barg NL. Environmental contamination with *Staphylococcus aureus* and outbreaks: the cause or the effect? *Infect Control Hosp Epidemiol.* 1993;14:367–368.

24. Boyce JM, Potter-Bynoe G, Chenevert C, et al. Environmental contamination due to methicillin-resistant *Staphylococcus aureus*: possible infection control implications. *Infect Control Hosp Epidemiol.* 1997;18:622–627.

25. Garner JS, and the Hospital Infection Control Practices Advisory Committee, Centers for Disease Control and Prevention (CDC). Guideline for isolation precautions in hospitals. *Infect Control Hosp Epidemiol.* 1996;17:53–80.

26. Boyce JM, Jackson MM, Pugliese G, et al. Methicillin-resistant *Staphylococcus aureus* (MRSA): a briefing for acute care hospitals and nursing facilities. *Infect Control Hosp Epidemiol.* 1994;15:105–115.

27. Bennett ME, Thurn JR, Klicker R, et al. Recommendations from a Minnesota task force for the management of persons with methicillin-resistant *Staphylococcus aureus*. *Am J Infect Control.* 1992;20:42–48.

28. Duckworth G. Report of a combined working party of the Hospital Infections Society and the British Society for Antimicrobial Chemotherapy. Revised guidelines for the control of epidemic methicillin-resistant *Staphylococcus aureus*. *J Hosp Infect.* 1990;16:351–377.

29. Goldmann DA, Weinstein RA, Wenzel RP, et al. Strategies to prevent and control the emergence and spread of antimicrobial-resistant microorganisms in hospitals: a challenge to hospital leadership. *JAMA.* 1996;275:234–240.

30. Mulligan ME, Murray-Leisure KA, Ribner BS, et al. Methicillin-resistant *Staphylococcus aureus*: a consensus review of the microbiology, pathogenesis, and epidemiology with implications for prevention and management. *Am J Med.* 1993;94:313–328.

31. Wenzel RP, Reagan DR, Bertino JS, et al. Methicillin-resistant *Staphylococcus aureus* outbreak: a consensus panel's definition and management guidelines. *Am J Infect Control.* 1998;26:102–110.

32. Garner JS, Jarvis WR, Emori TG, Horan JM. CDC definitions for nosocomial infections, 1988. *Am J Infect Control.* 1991;19:19–35.

33. Bolyard EA, Tablan OC, Williams WW, et al. Guideline for infection control in health care personnel, 1998. *Am J Infect Control.* 1998;26:289–354.

34. Guiguet M, Rekacewicz C, Leciercq B, et al. Effectiveness of simple measures to control an outbreak of nosocomial methicillin-resistant *Staphylococcus aureus* infections in an intensive care unit. *Infect Control Hosp Epidemiol.* 1990;11:23–26.

35. Harstein AI. Improved understanding and control of nosocomial methicillin-resistant *Staphylococcus aureus*: Are we overdoing it? *Infect Control Hosp Epidemiol.* 1995;16:257–259.

36. Strausbaugh L. Antimicrobial resistance: problems, laments, and hopes. *Am J Infect Control.* 1997;25:294–296.

37. Goetz AM, Muder RR. The problem of methicillin-resistant *Staphylococcus aureus*: a critical appraisal of the efficacy of infection control procedures with a suggested approach for infection control programs. *Am J Infect Control.* 1992;20:80–84.

38. Boyce JM. Should we vigorously try to contain and control methicillin-resistant *Staphylococcus aureus*? *Infect Control Hosp Epidemiol.* 1991;12:46–54.

39. Jernigan JA, Titus M, Groschel DHM, et al. Effectiveness of contact isolation during a hospital outbreak of methicillin-resistant *Staphylococcus aureus*. *Am J Epidemiol.* 1996;143:496–504.

40. Mylotte JM. Control of methicillin-resistant *Staphylococcus aureus*: the ambivalence persists. *Infect Control Hosp Epidemiol.* 1994;15:73–77.

41. Cohen SH, Morita MM, Bradford M. A seven-year experience with methicillin-resistant *Staphylococcus aureus*. *Am J Med.* 1991;91:3B-233S–3B-237S.

42. Murray-Leisure KA, Geib S, Graceley D, et al. Control of epidemic methicillin-resistant *Staphylococcus aureus*. *Infect Control Hosp Epidemiol.* 1990;11:343–350.

43. Rao N, Jacobs S, Joyce L. Cost-effective eradication of an outbreak of methicillin-resistant *Staphylococcus aureus* in a community teaching hospital. *Infect Control Hosp Epidemiol.* 1988;9:255–260.

44. Reboli AC, John JF, Levkoff AH. Epidemic methicillin-gentamycin-resistant *Staphylococcus aureus* in a neonatal intensive care unit. *Am J Dis Control* 1989;143:34–39.

45. Fazal BA, Telzak TE, Blum S, et al. Trends in the prevalence of methicillin-resistant *Staphylococcus aureus* associated with discontinuation of an isolation policy. *Infect Control Hosp Epidemiol.* 1996;17:372–374.

46. Nettleman MD, Trilla A, Fredrickson M, et al. Assigning responsibility: using feedback to achieve sustained control of methicillin-resistant *Staphylococcus aureus*. *Am J Med.* 1991;91:3B-228S–3B-232S.

47. Boyce JM. Preventing staphylococcal infections by eradicating nasal carriage of *Staphylococcus aureus*: proceeding with caution. *Infect Control Hosp Epidemiol.* 1996;17:775–779.

48. O'Toole RD, Drew WL, Dahlgren BJ, et al. An outbreak of methicillin-resistant *Staphylococcus aureus*. Observations in hospital and nursing home. *JAMA.* 1970;213:257–263.

49. Storch GA, Radcliff JL, Meyer PL, et al. Methicillin-resistant *Staphylococcus aureus* in a nursing home. *Infect Control.* 1987;8:24–29.

50. Strausbaugh LJ, Jacobson C, Sewell DL, et al. Methicillin-resistant *Staphylococcus aureus* in extended-care facilities: experiences in a Veterans' Affairs nursing home and a review of the literature. *Infect Control Hosp Epidemiol.* 1991;12:36–45.

51. Thomas JC, Bridge J, Waterman S, et al. Transmission and control of methicillin-resistant *Staphylococcus aureus* in a skilled nursing facility. *Infect Control Hosp Epidemiol.* 1989;10:106–110.

52. Kauffman CA, Bradley SF, Terpenning MS. Methicillin-resistant *Staphylococcus aureus* in long-term care facilities. *Infect Control Hosp Epidemiol.* 1990;11:600–603.

53. Mylotte JM, Karuza J, Bentley DW. Methicillin-resistant *Staphylococcus aureus*: a questionnaire survey of 75 long-term care facilities in western New York. *Infect Control Hosp Epidemiol.* 1992;13:711–718.

54. Muder RR, Brennen C, Wagener MW, et al. Methicillin-resistant staphylococcal colonization and infection in a long-term care facility. *Ann Intern Med.* 1991;114:107–112.

55. Bradley SF, Terpenning MS, Ramsey MA, et al. Methicillin-resistant *Staphylococcus aureus*: colonization and infection in a long-term care facility. *Ann Intern Med.* 1991;115:417–422.

56. Lee Y, Cesario T, Gupta G, et al. Surveillance of colonization and infection with *Staphylococcus aureus* susceptible or resistant to methicillin in a community skilled-nursing facility. *Am J Infect Control.* 1997;25:312–321.

57. Bradley SF. Methicillin-resistant *Staphylococcus aureus* in nursing homes. Epidemiology, prevention and management. *Drugs Aging.* 1997;10:185–198.

58. Mulhausen PL, Harrell LJ, Weinberger M, et al. Contrasting methicillin-resistant *Staphylococcus aureus* colonization in Veterans Affairs and community nursing homes. *Am J Med.* 1996;100:24–31.

59. Hsu CCS. Serial survey of methicillin-resistant *Staphylococcus aureus* nasal carriage among residents in a nursing home. *Infect Control Hosp Epidemiol.* 1991;12:416–421.

60. Lee YL, Gupta G, Cesario T, et al. Colonization by *Staphylococcus aureus* resistant to methicillin and ciprofloxacin during 20 months' surveillance in a private skilled nursing facility. *Infect Control Hosp Epidemiol.* 1996;649–653.

61. McGeer A, Campbell B, Emori TG, et al. Definitions of infection for surveillance in long-term care facilities. *Am J Infect Control.* 1991;19:1–7.

62. Kauffman CA, Terpenning MS, Xiaogong H, et al. Attempts to eradicate methicillin-resistant *Staphylococcus aureus* from a long-term care facility with the use of mupirocin ointment. *Am J Med.* 1993;94:371–378.

63. Strausbaugh LJ, Jacobson C, Sewell DL, et al. Antimicrobial therapy for methicillin-resistant *Staphylococcus aureus* colonization in residents and staff of a Veterans Affairs nursing home care unit. *Infect Control Hosp Epidemiol.* 1993;13:151–159.

64. CDC. Nosocomial enterococci resistant to vancomycin—United States, 1989–1993. *MMWR.* 1993;42:597–599.

65. Karanfil LV, Murphy M, Josephson A, et al. A cluster of vancomycin-resistant *Enterococcus faecium* in an intensive care unit. *Infect Control Hosp Epidemiol.* 1992;13:195–200.

66. Handwerger S, Raucher B, Altarac D, et al. Nosocomial outbreak due to *Enterococcus faecium* highly resistant to vancomycin, penicillin, and gentamicin. *Clin Infect Dis.*1993;16:750–755.

67. Boyle JF, Soumakis SA, Rendo A, et al. Epidemiologic analysis and genotypic characterization of a nosocomial outbreak of vancomycin-resistant enterococci. *J Clin Micro.* 1993;31:1280–1285.

68. Montecalvo MA, Horowitz H, Gedris C, et al. Outbreak of vancomycin-, ampicillin-, and aminoglycoside-resistant *Enterococcus faecium* bacteremia in an adult oncology unit. *Antimicrob Agents Chemother.* 1994;38:1363–1367.

69. Boyce JM, Opal SM, Chow JW, et al. Outbreak of multidrug-resistant *Enterococcus faecium* with transferable vanB class vancomycin resistance. *J Clin Microbiol.* 1994;32:1148–1153.

70. Quale J, Landman D, Atwood E, et al. Experience with a hospital-wide outbreak of vancomycin-resistant enterococci. *Am J Infect Control.* 1996;24:372–379.

71. Frieden TR, Munsiff SS, Low DE, et al. Emergence of vancomycin-resistant enterococci in New York City. *Lancet.* 1993;342:76–79.

72. Morris JT Jr, Shay DK, Hebden J, et al. Enterococci resistant to multiple antimicrobial agents, including vancomycin. Establishment of endemicity in a university medical center. *Ann Intern Med.* 1995;123:250–259.

73. Crossley K, and the Long-Term Care Committee of the Society for Healthcare Epidemiology of America. Vancomycin-resistant enterococci in long-term care facilities. *Infect Control Hosp Epidemiol.* 1998;19:521–525.

74. Edmond MB, Ober JF, Weinbaum DL, et al. Vancomycin-resistant *Enterococcus faecium* bacteremia; risk factors for infection. *Clin Infect Dis.* 1995;20:1126–1133.

75. Bonten MJM, Hayden MK, Nathan C, et al. Epidemiology of colonization of patients and environment with vancomycin-resistant enterococci. *Lancet.* 1996;348:1615–1619.

76. The Hospital Infection Control Practices Advisory Committee. Recommendations for preventing the spread of vancomycin resistance: recommendations of the Hospital Infection Control Practices Advisory Committee (HICPAC). *Am J Infect Control.* 1995;23:87–94.

77. Livornese LL, Dias S, Samel C, et al. Hospital-acquired infection with vancomycin-resistant *Enterococcus faecium* transmitted by electronic thermometer. *Ann Intern Med.* 1992;117:112–114.

78. Rhinehart E, Smith NE, Wennersten C. Rapid dissemination of beta-lactamase producing, aminoglycoside-resistant *Enterococcus faecalis* among patients and staff in an infant-toddler surgical ward. *N Engl J Med.* 323:1814–1818.

79. Montecalvo MA, deLencastre H, Carraher M, et al. Natural history of colonization with vancomycin-resistant *Enterococcus faecium.* *Infect Control Hosp Epidemiol.* 1995;16:680–685.

80. Bonilla HF, Zervos MA, Lyons MJ, et al. Colonization with vancomycin-resistant *Enterococcus faecium*: comparison of a long-term care unit with an acute-care hospital. *Infect Control Hosp Epidemiol.* 1997;18:333–339.

81. Noskin GA, Stosor V, Cooper I, et al. Recovery of vancomycin-resistant enterococci on fingertips and environmental surfaces. *Infect Control Hosp Epidemiol.* 1995;16:577–581.

82. Bonilla HF, Zervos MJ, Kauffman CA. Long-term survival of vancomycin-resistant *Enterococcus faecium* on a contaminated surface. *Infect Control Hosp Epidemiol.* 1996;17:770–772 (letter and comments).

83. Boyce JM, Mermel LA, Zervos MJ, et al. Controlling vancomycin-resistant enterococci. *Infect Control Hosp Epidemiol.* 1995;16:634–637.

84. Slaughter S, Hayden MK, Nathan C, et al. A comparison of the effect of universal use of gloves and gowns with that of glove use alone on acquisition of vancomycin-resistant enterococci in a medical intensive care unit. *Ann Intern Med.* 1996;125:448–456.

85. Wade JJ, Desai N, Casewell MW. Hygienic hand disinfection for the removal of epidemic vancomycin-resistant *Enterococcus faecium* and gentamicin-resistant *Enterobacter cloacae.* *J Hosp Infect.* 1991;18:211–218.

86. Pugliese G, Weinstein RA. *Issues and Controversies in Prevention and Control of VRE, Vancomycin-Resistant Enterococci.* Chicago: Etna Communications; 1998.

87. Brennen C, Wagener MM, Muder RR. Vancomycin-resistant *Enterococcus faecium* in a long-term care facility. *J Am Geriatr Soc.* 1998;46:157–160.

88. Terpenning MS, Bradley SF, Wan JY, et al. Colonization and infection with antibiotic resistant bacteria in a long-term care facility. *J Am Geriatr Soc.* 1994;42:1062–1069.

89. Revuelta MP, Nord JA, Yarrish RL, et al. Recycling of hospital-acquired colonization with vancomycin resistant enterococci via nursing home residents. *Clin Infect Dis.* 1995;21:730. Abstract.

90. CDC. Update: *Staphylococcus aureus* with reduced susceptibility to vancomycin—United States, 1997. *MMWR.* 1997;46:813–815.

91. Ploy MC, Grelaud C, Martin C, et al. First clinical isolate of vancomycin-intermediate *Staphylococcus aureus* in a French hospital. *Lancet.* 1998;351:1212.

92. CDC. Interim guidelines for prevention and control of staphylococcal infection associated with reduced susceptibility to vancomycin. *MMWR.* 1997;46:626–628,635.

93. Edmond MB, Wenzel RP, Pasculle W. Vancomycin-resistant *Staphylococcus aureus*: perspectives on measures needed for control. *Ann Intern Med.* 1996;124:329–334.

94. Jarvis WR. Nosocomial transmission of multidrug-resistant *Mycobacterium tuberculosis.* *Am J Infect Control.* 1995;23:146–151.

95. Edlin BR, Tokars JI, Garieco MH, et al. An outbreak of multidrug-resistant tuberculosis among hospitalized patients with the acquired immunodeficiency syndrome. *N Engl J Med.* 1992;326:1514–1521.

96. Catanzaro A. Nosocomial tuberculosis. *Am Rev Respir Dis.* 1982;125:559–562.

97. Ehrenkranz NJ, Kicklighter JL. Tuberculosis outbreak in a general hospital: evidence of airborne spread of infection. *Ann Intern Med.* 1972;77:377–382.

98. Haley CE, McDonald RC, Rossi L, et al. Tuberculosis epidemic among hospital personnel. *Infect Control Hosp Epidemiol.* 1989; 10:204–210.

99. Hutton MD, Stead WW, Cauthen GM, et al. Nosocomial transmission of tuberculosis associated with a draining tuberculous abscess. *J Infect Dis.* 1990; 161:286–295.

100. Kantor HS, Poblete R, Pusateri SL. Nosocomial transmission of tuberculosis from unsuspected disease. *Am J Med.* 1988;84:833–838.

101. Lundgren R, Norman E, Asberg I. Tuberculous infection transmitted at autopsy. *Tubercle.* 1987;68:147–150.

102. Templeton GL, Illing LA, Young L, et al. Comparing the risk for transmission of *Mycobacterium tuberculosis* at the bedside and during autopsy. *Ann Intern Med.* 1995;122:922–925.

103. CDC. *Mycobacterium tuberculosis* transmission in a health clinic—Florida, 1988. *MMWR.* 1989; 38:256–258,263–264.

104. Beck-Sague C, Dooley SW, Hutton MD, et al. Outbreak of multidrug-resistant *Mycobacterium tuberculosis* infections in a hospital: transmission to patients with HIV infection and staff. *JAMA.* 1992; 268:1280–1286.

105. CDC. Nosocomial transmission of multidrug-resistant tuberculosis to health care workers and HIV-infected patients in an urban hospital—Florida. *MMWR.* 1990;39:718–722.

106. CDC. Nosocomial transmission of multidrug-resistant tuberculosis among HIV-infected persons—Florida and New York, 1988–1991. *MMWR.* 1991;40:585–591.

107. Pearson ML, Jereb JA, Frieden TR, et al. Nosocomial transmission of multidrug-resistant *Mycobacterium tuberculosis*: a risk to patients and health care workers. *Ann Intern Med.* 1992;117:191–196.

108. Dooley SW, Jarvis WR, Martone WJ, et al. Multidrug-resistant tuberculosis (editorial). *Ann Intern Med.* 1992;117:257–258.

109. Dooley SW, Villarino ME, Lawrence M, et al. Nosocomial transmission of tuberculosis in a hospital unit for HIV-infected patients. *JAMA.* 1992;267:2632–2634.

110. CDC. Transmission of multidrug-resistant tuberculosis from an HIV-positive client in a residential substance-abuse treatment facility—Michigan. *MMWR.* 1991;40:129–131.

111. Ikeda RM, Birkhead GS, DiFerdinando GT Jr, et al. Nosocomial tuberculosis: an outbreak of a strain resistant to seven drugs. *Infect Control Hosp Epidemiol.* 1995;16:152–159.

112. CDC. Guidelines for preventing the transmission of *Mycobacterium tuberculosis* in heath-care facilities, 1994. *MMWR.* 1994;43(no. RR-13):1–132.

113. CDC. Tuberculosis morbidity—United States, 1997. *MMWR.* 1998;47:253–257.

114. Menzies D. Effect of treatment on contagiousness of patients with active pulmonary tuberculosis. *Infect Control Hosp Epidemiol.* 1997;18:582–586.

115. Sepkowitz K. How contagious is tuberculosis? *Clin Infect Dis.* 1996;23:954–962.

116. Stead WW. Management of health care workers after inadvertent exposure to tuberculosis: a guide for the use of preventive therapy. *Ann Intern Med.* 1995;122:906–912.

117. Brennen C, Muder RR, Muraca PW. Occult endemic tuberculosis in a chronic care facility. *Infect Control Hosp Epidemiol.* 1988;9:548–552.

118. Stead WW. Tuberculosis among elderly persons: an outbreak in a nursing home. *Ann Intern Med.* 1981;94:606–610.

119. Stead WW. Special problems in tuberculosis. Tuberculosis in the elderly and in residents of nursing homes, correctional facilities, long-term care hospitals, mental hospitals, shelters for the homeless, and jails. *Clin Chest Med.* 1989;10:397–405.

120. Bentley DW. Tuberculosis in long-term care facilities. *Infect Control Hosp Epidemiol.* 1990.11:42–46.

121. Steimke EH, Tenholder MF, McCormick MI, et al. Tuberculosis surveillance: lessons from a cluster of skin test conversions. *Am J Infect Control.* 1994;22:236–241.

122. CDC. Tuberculosis—North Dakota. *MMWR.* 1979;27:523–525.

123. CDC. Tuberculosis in a nursing home—Oklahoma. *MMWR.* 1980:29:465–467.

124. CDC. Tuberculosis in a nursing care facility—Washington. *MMWR.* 1983;32:121–122,128.

125. Stead WW, Lofgren JP, Warren E, et al. Tuberculosis as an endemic and nosocomial infection among the elderly in nursing homes. *N Engl J Med.* 1985;312:1483–1487.

126. CDC. Prevention and control of tuberculosis in facilities providing long-term care to the elderly: recommendations of the Advisory Committee for Elimination of Tuberculosis. *MMWR.* 1990;39(RR-10):7–20.

127. Naglie G, McArthur M, Simor A, et al. Tuberculosis surveillance practices in long-term care institutions. *Infect Control Hosp Epidemiol.* 1995;16:148–151.

128. Gerding DN, Johnson S, Peterson LR, et al. *Clostridium difficile*-associated diarrhea and colitis. *Infect Control Hosp Epidemiol.* 1995;16:459–477.

129. McFarland LV, Mulligan ME, Kwok RYY, et al. Nosocomial acquisition of *Clostridium difficile* infection. *N Engl J Med.* 1989;320:204–210.

130. Samore MH, Venkataraman L, DeGirolami PC, et al. Clinical and molecular epidemiology of clustered cases of nosocomial *Clostridium difficile* diarrhea. *Am J Med.* 1996;110:32-40.

131. Olson MM, Stanholtzer CJ, Lee JT, et al. Ten years of prospective *Clostridium difficile*-associated disease surveillance and treatment at the Minneapolis VA Medical Center, 1982–1991. *Infect Control Hosp Epidemiol.* 1994;15:371–381.

132. Nath SK, Thornley JH, Kelly M, et al. A sustained outbreak of *Clostridium difficile* in a general hospital: persistence of a toxigenic clone in four units. *Infect Control Hosp Epidemiol.* 1994;15:382–389.

133. Bentley DW. *Clostridium difficile*-associated disease in long-term care facilities. *Infect Control Hosp Epidemiol.* 1990;11:434–438.

134. Clabots CR, Johnson S, Olson MM, et al. Acquisition of *Clostridium difficile* by hospitalized patients: evidence for colonized new admissions as a source of infection. *J Infect Dis.* 1992;166:561–567.

135. Johnson S, Gerding DN, Olson MM, et al. Prospective controlled study of vinyl glove use to interrupt *Clostridium difficile* nosocomial transmission. *Am J Med.* 1990;88:137–140.

136. Brooks SE, Veal RO, Kramer M, et al. Reduction in the incidence of *Clostridium difficile*-associated diarrhea in an acute care hospital and a skilled nursing facility following replacement of electronic thermometers with single-use disposables. *Infect Control Hosp Epidemiol.* 1992;13:98–103.

137. Brooks SE, Khan A, Stoica D, et al. Reduction in vancomycin-resistant enterococcus and *Clostridium difficile* infections following

change to tympanic thermometers. *Infect Control Hosp Epidemiol.* 1998;19:333–336.

138. Jernigan JA, Siegman-Igra Y, Guerrant RC, et al. A randomized cross-over study of disposable thermometers for prevention of *Clostridium difficile* and other nosocomial infections. *Infect Control Hosp Epidemiol.* 1998;19:494–499.

139. Brown E, Talbot GM, Axelrod P, et al. Risk factors for *Clostridium difficile* toxin-associated diarrhea. *Infect Control Hosp Epidemiol.* 1990;11:283–290.

140. Mylotte JM. Laboratory surveillance method for nosocomial *Clostridium difficile* diarrhea. *Am J Infect Control.* 1998;26:16–23.

141. Lettau LA. Nosocomial transmission and infection control aspects of parasitic and ectoparasitic diseases: part I. Introduction/enteric parasites. *Infect Control Hosp Epidemiol.* 1991;12:59–65.

142. Lettau LA. Nosocomial transmission and infection control aspects of parasitic and ectoparasitic diseases: part II. Blood and tissue parasites. *Infect Control Hosp Epidemiol.* 1991;12:111–121.

143. Lettau LA. Nosocomial transmission and infection control aspects of parasitic and ectoparasitic diseases: part III. Ectoparasites/summary and conclusions. *Infect Control Hosp Epidemiol.* 1991;12:179–185.

144. Degelau J. Scabies in long-term care facilities. *Infect Control Hosp Epidemiol.* 1992;13:421–425.

145. Roncoroni AJ, Gomez MA, Mera J, et al. *Cryptosporidium* infection in renal transplant patients. *J Infect Dis.* 1989;160:559.

146. Sarabia-Arce S, Salazar-Lindo E, Gilman RH, et al. Case-control study of *Cryptosporidium parvum* infection in Peruvian children hospitalized for diarrhea: possible association with malnutrition and nosocomial infection. *Ped Infect Dis J.* 1990;9:627–631.

147. Neill MA, Rice SK, Ahmad NV, et al. Cryptosporidiosis: an unrecognized cause of diarrhea in elderly hospitalized patients. *Clin Infect Dis.* 1996;22:168–170.

148. Craven DE, Steger KA, Hirschorn LR. Nosocomial colonization and infection in persons infected with human immunodeficiency virus. *Infect Control Hosp Epidemiol.* 1996;17:304–318.

149. Gardner C. An outbreak of hospital-acquired cryptosporidiosis. *Brit J Nurs.* 1994;3:152,154–158.

150. Navarrete S, Stetler HC, Avila C, et al. An outbreak of *Cryptosporidium* diarrhea in a pediatric hospital. *Ped Infect Dis J.* 1991;10:248–250.

151. Perera DR, Western KA, Johnson HD, et al. *Pneumocystis carinii* pneumonia in a hospital for children. Epidemiologic aspects. *JAMA.* 1970;214:1074–1078.

152. Hennequin C, Page B, Roux P, et al. Outbreak of *Pneumocystis carinii* pneumonia in a renal transplant unit. *Eur J Clin Microbiol Infect Dis.* 1995;14:122–126.

153. Fenelon LE, Keane CT, Bakir M, et al. A cluster of *Pneumocystis carinii* infections in children. *Br Med J.* 1985;291:1683.

154. Vargo JA, Ginsberg MM, Mizrahi M. Human infestations by the pigeon mite: a case report. *Am J Infect Control.* 1983;11:24–25.

155. Istre GR, Hreiss K, Hopkins RS, et al. An outbreak of amebiasis spread by colonic irrigation at a chiropractic clinic. *N Engl J Med.* 1982;307:339–342.

156. White KE, Hedberg CW, Edmonson LM, et al. An outbreak of giardiasis in a nursing home with evidence for multiple modes of transmission. *J Infect Dis.* 1989;160:298–304.

157. Burkhart CG. Scabies: an epidemiologic reassessment. *Ann Intern Med.* 1983;98:498–503.

158. Green MS. Epidemiology of scabies. *Epidemiol Rev.* 1989;11:126–150.

159. Arlian LG, Runyan RA, Achar S, et al. Survival and infectivity of *Sarcoptes scabiei* var *canis* and var *hominis. J Am Acad Dermatol.* 1984;11(2 Pt 1):210–215.

160. Paternak J, Richtman R, Ganme APP, et al. Scabies epidemic: price and prejudice. *Infect Control Hosp Epidemiol.* 1994;15:540–542.

161. Estes SA, Estes J. Therapy of scabies: nursing homes, hospitals, and the homeless. *Semin Dermatol.* 1993;12:26–33.

162. Sirera G, Rius F, Romeu J, et al. Hospital outbreak of scabies stemming from two AIDS patients with Norwegian scabies. *Lancet.* 1990;335:1227.

163. Purvis RS, Tyring SK. An outbreak of lindane-resistant scabies treated successfully with permethrin 5% cream. *J Am Acad Dermatol.* 1991;25(6 Pt 1):1015–1016.

164. Clark J, Friesen DL, Williams WA. Management of an outbreak of Norwegian scabies. *Am J Infect Control.* 1992;20:217–220.

165. Boix V, Sanchez-Paya J, Portilla J, et al. Nosocomial outbreak of scabies clinically resistant to lindane. *Infect Control Hosp Epidemiol.* 1997;18:677.

166. Bannatyne RM, Patterson TA, Wells BA, et al. Hospital outbreak traced to a case of Norwegian scabies. *Can J Infect Control.* 1992;7:111–113.

167. Holness DL, DeKoven JG, Nethercott JR. Scabies in chronic health care institutions. *Arch Dermatol.* 1992;128:1257–1260.

168. Yokonsky D, Ladi L, Gackenheimer L, et al. Scabies in nursing homes: an eradication program with permethrin 5% cream. *J Am Acad Dermatol.* 1990;23(6 Pt 1):1133–1136.

169. Haag ML, Brozena SJ, Fenske NA. Attack of the scabies: what to do when an outbreak occurs. *Geriatrics.* 1993;48:45–46,51–53.

170. Jimenez-Lucho VE, Fallon F, Caputo C, et al. Role of prolonged surveillance in the eradication of nosocomial scabies in an extended care Veterans Affairs medical center. *Am J Infect Control.* 1995;23:44–49.

171. Paules SJ, Levisohn D, Heffron W. Persistent scabies in nursing home patients. *J Family Pract.* 1993;37:82–86.

172. CDC. Scabies in health-care facilities—Iowa. *MMWR.* 1988;37:178–179.

173. Bolyard EA, Tablan OC, Williams WW, et al. CDC Guideline for infection control in health care personnel, 1998. *Am J Infect Control.* 1998;26:289–354.

174. Juranek DD, Currier RW, Millikan LE. Scabies control in institutions. In: Orkin M, Mailback HI, eds. *Cutaneous Infestations and Insect Bites.* New York: Dekker; 1985:139–156.

175. Sargent SJ. Ectoparasites. In: Mayhall CG, ed. *Hospital Epidemiology and Infection Control.* Baltimore, MD: Williams & Wilkins; 1996:465–472.

176. MacKenzie WR, Hoxie NJ, Proctor ME, et al. A massive outbreak in Milwaukee of *Cryptosporidium* infection transmitted through the public water supply. *N Engl J Med.* 1994;331:161–167.

177. CDC. Foodborne outbreak of cryptosporidiosis—Spokane, Washington, 1997. *MMWR.* 1998;47:565–567.

178. Millard PS, Gensheimer KF, Addiss DG, et al. An outbreak of cryptosporidiosis from fresh-pressed apple cider. *JAMA.* 1994;272:1592–1596.

179. Kramer MH, Herwaldt BL, Calderon RL, Juranek DD. Surveillance for waterborne disease outbreaks—United States, 1993–1994. In: CDC Surveillance Summaries. *MMWR.* 1996;45:1–33.

180. Combee CL, Collinge ML, Britt EM. Cryptosporidiosis in a hospital-associated day care center. *Pediatr Infect Dis.* 1986;5:528–532.

181. Black RE, Dykes AC, Sinclair SP, et al. Giardiasis in daycare centers: evidence of person-to-person transmission. *Pediatrics.* 1977;60:486–491.

182. Haron E, Bodey GP, Luna MA, et al. Has the incidence of *Pneumocystis carinii* pneumonia in cancer center patients increased with the AIDS epidemic? *Lancet.* 1988;2:904–905.

183. Regan AM, Metersky ML, Craven DE. Nosocomial dermatitis and pruritis caused by pigeon mite infestation. *Arch Intern Med.* 1987;147:2185–2187.

184. Jarvis WR, Hughes JM. Nosocomial gastrointestinal infections. In: Wenzel RP, ed. *Prevention and Control of Nosocomial Infections.* 2nd ed. Baltimore: Williams & Wilkins; 1992:708–745.

185. Nicolle LE, Garibaldi RA. Infection control in long-term care facilities. *Infect Control Hosp Epidemiol.* 1995;16:348–353.

186. Steere AC, Craven PJ, Hall WJ 3rd, et al. Person-to-person spread of *Salmonella* after a hospital common-source outbreak. *Lancet.* 1975;1:319–322.

187. Rodriquez EM, Parrott C, Rolka H, et al. An outbreak of viral gastroenteritis in a nursing home: importance of excluding ill employees. *Infect Control Hosp Epidemiol.* 1996;17:587–592.

188. Schroeder SA, Askeroff, Brachman PS. Epidemic Salmonellosis in hospitals and institutions: public health importance and outbreak management. *N Engl J Med.* 1968;279:674–678.

189. Standaert SM, Hutcheson RH, Schaffner W. Nosocomial transmission of *Salmonella* gastroenteritis to laundry workers in a nursing home. *Infect Control Hosp Epidemiol.* 1994;15:22–26.

190. CDC. Viral agents of gastroenteritis. Public health importance and outbreak management. *MMWR.* 1990;39(RR-5):1–24.

191. Khuri-Bulos NA, Abu Khalaf M, Shehabi A, et al. Foodhandler-associated *Salmonella* outbreak in a university hospital despite routine surveillance cultures of kitchen employees. *Infect Control Hosp Epidemiol.* 1994;15:311–314.

192. Layton MC, Calliste SG, Gomez TM, et al. A mixed foodborne outbreak with *Salmonella heidelberg* and *Campylobacter jejuni* in a nursing home. *Infect Control Hosp Epidemiol.* 1997;18:115–121.

193. Levine WC, Smart JF, Archer DL, et al. Foodborne disease outbreaks in nursing homes, 1975 through 1987. *JAMA.* 1991;266:2105–2109.

194. Linnemann CC Jr, Cannon CG, Stancek JL, et al. Prolonged hospital epidemic of salmonellosis: use of trimethoprim-sulfamethoxazole for control. *Infect Control Hosp Epidemiol.* 1985;6:221–225.

195. Slutsker L, Villarino ME, Jarvis WR, et al. Foodborne disease prevention in healthcare facilities. In: Bennett JV, Brachman PS, eds. *Hospital Infections.* 4th ed. Philadelphia: Lippincott-Raven; 1998:22–341.

196. Pegues DA, Woernle CH. An outbreak of acute nonbacterial gastroenteritis in a nursing home. *Infect Control Hosp Epidemiol.* 1993;14:87–94.

197. Gellert GA, Waterman SH, Ewert D, et al. An outbreak of acute gastroenteritis caused by a small round structured virus in a geriatric convalescent facility. *Infect Control Hosp Epidemiol.* 1990;11:459–464.

198. Caceres VM, Kim DK, Bresee JS, et al. A viral gastroenteritis outbreak associated with person-to-person spread among hospital staff. *Infect Control Hosp Epidemiol.* 1998;19:162–167.

199. Khatib R, Naber M, Shellum N, et al. A common source outbreak of gastroenteritis in a teaching hospital. *Infect Control Hosp Epidemiol.* 1994;15:534–535.

200. Ho JL, Shands, KN, Fredland G, et al. A outbreak of type 4b *Listeria monocytogenes* infection involving patients from eight Boston hospitals. *Arch Intern Med.* 1986;146:520–524.

201. DeBuono BA, Brondum J, Kramer JM, et al. Plasmid, serotype and enterotoxin analysis of *Bacillus cereus* in an outbreak setting. *J Clin Microbiol.* 1988;26:1571–1574.

202. Bloom HG, Bottone EJ. *Aeromonas hydrophilia* diarrhea in a long-term care setting. *J Am Geriatr Soc.* 1990;38:804–806.

203. Carter AO, Birczyk AA, Carlson JA, et al. A severe outbreak of *Escherichia coli* O157:H7—associated hemorrhagic colitis in a nursing home. *N Engl J Med.* 1987;317:1496–1500.

204. Ryan CA, Tauxe RV, Hosek GW, et al. *Escherichia coli* O157:H7 in a nursing home: clinical epidemiological, and pathological findings. *J Infect Dis.* 1986;154:631–638.

205. Halvorsrud J, Orstavik I. An epidemic of rotavirus-associated gastroenteritis in a nursing home for the elderly. *Scand J Infect Dis.* 1980;12:161–164.

206. Raad I, Sheretz RJ, Russell BA, et al. Uncontrolled nosocomial rotavirus transmission during a community outbreak. *Am J Infect Control.* 1990;18:24–28.

207. Emont SL, Cote TR, Dwyer DM, et al. Gastroenteritis outbreak in a Maryland nursing home. *Maryland Med J.* 1993;42:1099–1103.

208. Sawyer LA, Murphy JJ, Kaplan JE, et al. 25- to 30-nm virus particle associated with a hospital outbreak of acute gastroenteritis with evidence for airborne transmission. *Am J Epidemiol.* 1988;127:1261–1271.

209. Wall PG, Ryan MJ, Ward LR, et al. Outbreaks of salmonellosis in hospitals in England and Wales: 1992–1994. *J Hosp Infect.* 1996;33:181–190.

210. Collier PW, Sharp JC, MacLeod AF, et al. Food poisoning in hospitals in Scotland, 1978–1987. *Epidemiol Infect.* 1988;101:661–667.

211. Hedberg CW, Osterholm MT. Outbreaks of foodborne and waterborne viral gastroenteritis. *Clin Microbiol Rev.* 1993;6:199–210.

212. CDC. Incidence of foodborne illnesses—FoodNet, 1997. *MMWR.* 1998;47:782–786.

213. Steiner TS, Theilman NM, Guerrant RL. Protozoal agents: what are the dangers for the public water supply? *Annual Rev Med.* 1997;48:329–340.

214. US Food and Drug Administration. Center for Food Safety and Applied Nutrition. *Foodborne Pathogenic Microorganisms and Natural Toxins Handbook.* Washington, DC: Center for Food Safety and Applied Nutrition; 1992.

215. Bean NH, Goulding JS, Lao C, Angulo FJ. Surveillance for foodborne-disease outbreaks—United States, 1988–1992. In: CDC surveillance summaries, October 25, 1996. *MMWR.* 1996;45:1–67.

216. Bell BP, Goldoft M, Griffin PM, et al. A multistate outbreak of *Escherichia coli* O157:H7-associated bloody diarrhea and hemolytic uremia syndrome from hamburgers: the Washington experience. *JAMA.* 1994;272:1349–1353.

217. CDC. Outbreak of cyclosporiasis—Northern Virginia–Washington, DC–Baltimore, Maryland, Metropolitan Area, 1997. *MMWR.* 1997;46:689–691.

218. Sattar SA, Jacobsen H, Rahman H, et al. Interruption of rotavirus spread through chemical disinfection. *Infect Control Hosp Epidemiol.* 1994;15:751–756.

219. Lew JF, LeBaron CW, Glass RI, et al. Recommendations for collection of laboratory specimens associated with outbreaks of gastroenteritis. *MMWR.* 1990;39(RR-14):1–13.

220. CDC. Aldicarb as a cause of food poisoning—Louisiana, 1998. *MMWR.* 1999;48:269–271.

CHAPTER 8

Investigation and Control of Outbreaks in the Health Care Setting

Kathleen Meehan Arias

Sickness is catching.
> William Shakespeare, *A Midsummer*
> *Night's Dream*—I, i, 186

Although outbreaks in health care facilities account for only a small proportion of nosocomial infections,[1-3] they can result in significant morbidity and mortality, disruption of services, and fear and anxiety among personnel, patients, residents, and the community. Chapters 3–7 describe outbreaks that have been reported in various health care settings and that have been associated with a variety of diseases, health-related conditions, organisms, products, procedures, devices, and technical errors. The investigations of these outbreaks have been instrumental in defining the sources, modes of transmission, and measures used to prevent and control the spread of nosocomial infections and in defining noninfectious risks associated with health care.

While most people associate the word "outbreak" with an infectious disease, it can also be used to describe an excess of noninfectious diseases, conditions, and health-related events. The epidemiologic methods used to identify and investigate outbreaks caused by infectious agents can also be applied to study outbreaks of noninfectious etiology.[4-9] Personnel who are responsible for the quality management, performance improvement, and infection surveillance, prevention, and control programs in health care facilities can gain a valuable perspective from studying the findings of outbreak investigations because this knowledge can help them to identify potential risk factors and effective control measures if a similar outbreak occurs in their facility. The purpose of this chapter is to discuss practical methods that can be used to recognize, investigate, and control an outbreak in a health care facility.

RECOGNIZING A POTENTIAL OUTBREAK

An outbreak is the occurrence of more cases of a disease or event than expected during a specified period of time in a given area or among a specific group of people. In a health care facility, an outbreak may be suspected when routine surveillance activities detect an unusual microbial isolate, a cluster of cases, or an apparent increase in the usual number or incidence of cases; when a clinician diagnoses an uncommon disease; or when an alert physician, nurse, or laboratory worker notices a cluster of cases. A cluster is a group of cases of a disease or other health-related event that occurs closely related in time and place. In a cluster, the number of cases may or may not exceed the expected number—frequently the expected number is not known.

Because the endemic rates for nosocomial diseases, injuries, and other adverse events are different for each health care facility, few definitive criteria exist for determining when to evaluate a potential problem or initiate an investigation. The following questions may be asked to help decide what action needs to be taken:

- Is there a documented increase in the number or incidence of observed cases? Is it unlikely that the increase is due to normal statistical variation? Is the increase significant? If the answers are yes, then an evaluation should be done to determine if an investigation should be initiated.

- Are there published criteria for evaluating the occurrence of the particular disease or event? The Centers for Disease Control and Prevention (CDC) National Nosocomial Infections Surveillance System (NNIS) rates[10] can be used as a benchmark for endemic infections but are not particularly useful for evaluating an outbreak. However, there are published thresholds for evaluating cases of measles, staphylococcal infections in the nursery, tuberculosis in long-term care facilities, and nosocomial infections caused by group A streptococci, *Legionella* species, and methicillin-resistant *Staphylococcus aureus* as shown in Table 8–1.[11–16] If these thresholds are reached or exceeded, enhanced surveillance and an investigation may be recommended, as noted. In addition, some state health departments have threshold criteria for investigating certain diseases. For instance, the Maryland Department of Health and Mental Hygiene provides guidelines for investigating, preventing, and controlling acute respiratory illnesses, gastroenteritis, and scabies in long-term care facilities. These guidelines, which are printed in their entirety in the appendix, provide criteria for defining an outbreak.
- Is the reported case an unusual disease or event? Even one case of an unusual disease or event should trigger an investigation. For instance, one case of nosocomial *Citrobacter koseri* meningitis in a nursery should prompt a limited investigation, which includes enhanced surveillance for additional cases, a retrospective review of laboratory records to identify any previous isolates of *C koseri* from any body sites in infants, and a request that the laboratory save all *C koseri* isolated from infants or postpartum patients. Certain adverse drug reactions and adverse events related to commercially available medical products and devices (for example, renal insufficiency[17] and endotoxin-like reactions[18]) should also prompt an investigation and, when appropriate, should be reported to the proper authorities (e.g., the Food and Drug Administration's MedWatch Program at 800-322-1088 or http://www.fda.gov/medwatch, the CDC's Hospital Infections Program at 404-639-6413, and the local or state health department) and to the manufacturer. Adverse events such as clusters of excessive bleeding after surgery,[19] pyrogenic reactions after hemodialysis,[20] and unexplained deaths[7,9] should also be investigated.

INITIATING AN OUTBREAK INVESTIGATION

A full-scale outbreak investigation generally requires expert assistance (such as from the health department or the CDC) and consumes valuable time and resources. R.E. Dixon has described a systematic approach to a hospital outbreak investigation that includes an initial evaluation of a suspected outbreak followed by a decision to conduct either a basic outbreak investigation or a major (full-scale) epidemiologic investigation.[21] This approach works well in a variety of health care settings and has been used successfully for many years. In many health care facility clusters and outbreaks, an initial evaluation followed by a carefully conducted literature search and a basic investigation (i.e., a descriptive epidemiologic study which characterizes the cases by person, place, and time) will be sufficient to verify the existence of an outbreak, identify the most likely causal factor(s), and identify control measures that have been shown to be effective in similar circumstances. Once these control measures are implemented, prospective (ongoing) surveillance will allow the investigator to determine if they are effective at preventing new cases. If these empirically applied measures are effective at interrupting the outbreak, then no further investigation is needed. A basic investigation is all that may be needed if the only objective is to control the outbreak and the investigators do not wish to publish their findings or identify the most likely causal factor by statistically demonstrating differences in exposures between the cases and a control population.

A full-scale investigation is warranted if a suspected outbreak is facility-wide, appears to be associated with a commercially available product or medical device, involves a disease or condition which causes considerable morbidity or mortality, or appears to be unique in that it has not been previously reported and there are no control measures which have previously been shown to be effective. A full-scale investigation consists of the steps conducted in a basic investigation plus a statistical (comparative) study of the proposed causal factors (i.e., formulation and testing of hypotheses to explain the observed disease pattern) as described in Chapter 10. Case-control or cohort studies are most commonly used to test associations between risk factors and disease in outbreak investigations in the health care setting.

It is important to keep in mind the objectives of an outbreak investigation:

Table 8–1 Suggested Thresholds for Investigating a Potential Outbreak

Disease or Condition	Threshold	Recommended Action(s)	Reference
Group A streptococci	One patient with GAS postoperative or postpartum infection	Review medical and laboratory records to identify other cases; heighten surveillance to identify additional episodes; save isolates from infected patients.	CDC[11]
Measles	One case of confirmed measles	Rapidly investigate all reports of suspected measles; identify contacts and promptly vaccinate susceptible persons; all persons who cannot provide proof of immunity should be vaccinated or excluded from the setting (e.g., health care facility, school, day care center).	CDC[12]
Staphylococcus aureus in a nursery	Two or more concurrent cases of staphylococcal disease related to a nursery	Investigate possibility of an outbreak; culture all lesions; examine health care personnel for draining lesions; save clinically important isolates for 6 months; institute isolation precautions for cases.	Benenson[13]
Methicillin-resistant *Staphylococcus aureus*	An increase in the rate of MRSA cases or a clustering of new cases. Several definitions of increased case rate proposed: 1. A statistically significant increase in the incidence or incidence density ratio 2. Monthly case rate increase of 25% above the baseline 3. Increased number of new nosocomial cases compared with a hospital of a similar size (see reference for details) 4. One case per month in ICU, NICU, burn unit, or dialysis unit	Use a four-phase approach to conduct and manage an outbreak investigation: I. Conduct basic epidemiologic study and compile a line list; isolate cases; promote routine infection control practices such as handwashing. II. Generate initial hypothesis (probable source, reservoir, and mode of transmission); save isolates; notify management of potential problem. III. Conduct standard epidemiologic study including hypothesis testing and culturing of select persons; search for cases in other areas. IV. Type isolates; arrange meeting to review data.	Wenzel et al.[14]
Legionnaires' disease	One patient with definite nosocomial LD or two persons with possible nosocomial LD within 6 months	Initiate an epidemiologic investigation; heighten prospective surveillance for additional cases; conduct retrospective review of serologic, microbiologic, and postmortem data to identify previously unrecognized cases.	CDC[15]
Tuberculosis	One case of infectious TB in a long-term care facility	Report case to health department; do contact tracing; skin test (PPD) contacts; provide preventive therapy for contacts who have documented skin test conversion; provide treatment for those with TB disease.	CDC[16]

GAS, Group A streptococci; MSRA, methicillin-resistant *S aureus*; ICU, intensive care unit; NICU, neonatal intensive care unit; LD, Legionnaires' disease; TB, tuberculosis.

- to describe the situation and occurrence of cases
- to determine the most likely etiologic agent, source, and method of spread
- to interrupt the outbreak
- to prevent the recurrence of a similar episode

STEPS IN CONDUCTING AN OUTBREAK INVESTIGATION

Many of the steps in an outbreak investigation will occur simultaneously; however, whenever an outbreak or a cluster is suspected, the investigator must first conduct an initial evaluation of the reported cases to confirm that a potential epidemic exists, and then decide whether to initiate a basic or a full-scale investigation. Exhibit 8–1 is an outline for investigating an outbreak.

Exhibit 8–1 Outline for Investigating an Outbreak*

The Initial Evaluation

Verify the diagnosis of reported cases before initiating an outbreak investigation.

Evaluate the severity of the problem.

Conduct a retrospective review to identify other cases.

Develop a line-listing of cases.

Review the existing data; determine if a potential problem exists.

The Outbreak Investigation

Identify and verify the diagnosis of new cases.

Develop a case definition.

Review clinical and laboratory findings.

Document and organize findings at each step in the investigation.

Confirm the existence of an epidemic.

Conduct a literature search.

Consult with the laboratory.

Notify those who need to know.

Assemble a team.

Appoint a spokesperson to ensure that consistent information is disseminated; be prepared to answer questions and address the concerns of the community and personnel, patients or residents, and their families.

Record actions taken (keep records of communications such as memos, letters, and e-mails).

Decide if outside assistance is needed (consult with outside agencies and experts, as needed).

Communicate findings and recommendations frequently; distribute written reports.

Institute early control measures.

Seek additional cases; create a data collection form.

Orient the data as to person, place, and time.

Evaluate the problem; observe practices that are potentially related to the occurrence of the outbreak.

Determine the need for additional cultures or other diagnostic testing.

Formulate a tentative hypothesis.

Institute control measures.

Evaluate efficiency of control measures.

Test the hypotheses; consult a statistician to ensure use of appropriate study method and statistical tests.

Conduct further analysis and investigation.

Prepare and Distribute a Written Report

*Many of these steps will occur simultaneously.

Initial Evaluation

The purpose of the initial evaluation is to provide a quick analysis of the likelihood that an important excess of cases has occurred and to determine if a potential problem exists.[22] The steps in the initial evaluation are as follows:

1. Verify the diagnosis of the reported cases. The diagnosis should be verified by reviewing laboratory reports and medical records. In addition, clinical findings can be discussed with the attending health care providers—especially when there appears to be a discrepancy between the clinical findings and the laboratory findings. If the clinical findings do not support the laboratory findings, then a pseudoinfection or a misdiagnosis should be suspected.

   Note: Rule number one in outbreak investigation is to verify the diagnosis of the initial case(s) before any further steps are taken. Many investigators have started off on the proverbial wild goose chase only to discover later that the clinical or laboratory findings of the cases did not match the reported diagnoses. Much time and effort can be wasted investigating an outbreak that does not exist if the reported diagnoses are not verified before proceeding. For instance, several years ago *Pseudomonas* (now *Ralstonia*) *pickettii* was isolated from blood cultures of several infants in the neonatal intensive care unit (NICU) at Hahnemann University Hospital. A review of the cases revealed that none of the infants had signs or symptoms consistent with *Pseudomonas* bacteremia and the investigators suspected specimen or laboratory contamination. Serendipitously, one of the infection control practitioners (ICPs) worked part-time in the microbiology laboratory of a local hospital and discovered that the other hospital had also experienced a recent cluster of *P pickettii*-positive blood cultures. A little shoe leather epidemiology revealed that both hospitals used the same type of broth culture media and both had used the same lot number. The outbreak was actually a pseudo-outbreak that was attributable to intrinsically contaminated culture media.

2. Evaluate the severity of the problem. For example, is the disease or condition likely to affect many people or only a few? Is it associated with

significant morbidity or mortality, or is it mild and inconsequential? If the condition is severe, a full-scale investigation may be needed. If it is mild or affects only a few people, then a basic investigation may be all that is needed.

3. Conduct a retrospective review of surveillance records, laboratory reports, and clinical records to identify other cases.

4. Develop a line-listing of cases. A line-listing may be created on a computer or by hand. Each row in a line-listing represents one case and each column represents an important characteristic that may aid in the investigation, for example, name, record number, age, sex, unit(s), or ward(s), date of admission, date of onset, service, signs and symptoms, types of therapy, surgery, and dates and results of laboratory tests. When a line-listing is created in a computer database program, the cases can be sorted by specified characteristics—this makes it easier to detect common risk factors. Exhibit 8–2 is an example of a line-listing developed to study a suspected increase in the incidence of surgical site infections following coronary artery bypass graft surgery.

5. Review the existing information and determine if a potential problem exists (i.e., does the incidence rate appear to be greater than expected).

6. If a potential outbreak exists, decide whether to begin a basic or a full-scale outbreak investigation. Because the initial steps for both investigations are similar, no time will be lost if the investigator decides to begin a basic investigation and subsequently finds that a full-scale study is warranted.

Outbreak Investigation

Identifying and Verifying the Diagnosis of Newly Reported Cases

Conduct prospective surveillance for new cases by monitoring laboratory results, clinical records, and reports from attending health care providers. Add any new cases to the line-listing.

Developing a Case Definition

One of the first steps in an outbreak investigation is to develop a case definition that will be used to identify affected persons. A case definition uses epidemiologic, clinical, and laboratory criteria to define and classify cases and usually restricts cases to a specific time,

place, and person. The definition may categorize cases as possible, probable, and definite. At the beginning of an investigation, the case definition should be broad to ensure that all those who have the disease or condition are included in the study. An example of a preliminary case definition for an outbreak of gastrointestinal illness in a long-term care facility may be "all residents and personnel in Greentree Nursing Home with onset of vomiting or diarrhea (i.e., two or more loose stools per day or an unexplained increase in the number of bowel movements) during the month of April." The case definition can be refined and narrowed as the investigation progresses. Appendix C contains the CDC definitions for infectious conditions that are reportable to local and state health departments. These may be useful for developing a case definition for an outbreak in a health care facility.

Reviewing Clinical and Laboratory Findings

If the outbreak is of infectious etiology, clinical and laboratory findings should be reviewed early in the investigation to determine if the cases are infected or colonized or if they represent pseudoinfection (i.e., the cultures are false-positives). It is important to recognize pseudoinfections promptly because they may lead to an incorrect diagnosis and unnecessary treatment and control measures.

Confirming the Existence of an Epidemic

Rule number two in outbreak investigation is to confirm the existence of an epidemic. This is done by determining if the incidence rate or the number of cases is above the endemic, or expected, rate. This may be relatively easy if the disease or condition is unusual or serious, such as *Pseudomonas cepacia* bacteremia or pyrogenic reactions after hemodialysis. If, however, cases occur at low levels over a prolonged period or if an outbreak is caused by a relatively common organism, such as *Escherichia coli*, then recognition will be more difficult. Frequently, the baseline or background rate of a disease or condition is not known and it is difficult to determine if an outbreak truly exists. Many authors have described methods that can be used to identify significant increases.[1,11–16,23–34] Unfortunately, there is no standard method for determining statistically if an outbreak exists in a health care facility. In practice, many outbreaks are recognized when personnel detect an increase in the number of cases of a disease or health-related event—even without calculating rates.

Exhibit 8–2 Sample Line-Listing Form

SSI FOLLOWING CABG

Name	Record #	Date CABG	Surgeon	Date SSI Onset	Chest SSI (Note Type)*	Leg SSI (note type)*	Date of Culture	Organism

SSI, surgical site infection; CABG, coronary artery bypass graft.
*TYPE: S/I, superficial/incisional; DI, deep infection; O/S, organ/space infection.

Some questions should be answered before a decision is made to conduct a full-scale investigation:

- Is there a possibility that the perceived increase is due to surveillance artifact? It is important to recognize that a change in surveillance techniques, which may occur if there is a change in personnel in the infection control or quality management departments or a change in criteria used to define a particular disease, may produce artifactual changes that are perceived as increases or decreases in the incidence of a disease or event. It is also important to ensure that infections that were present at admission are not categorized as nosocomial. For instance, a cluster of methicillin-resistant *Staphylococcus aureus* (MRSA) in a health care facility may be due to the coincidental admission of several patients who had MRSA at the time of admission.
- If the suspected outbreak is of infectious etiology, have there been any changes in the way specimens are collected, transported, or processed? It is important to determine if (1) there has been any change in the way specimens are collected or (2) there has been any change in the laboratory procedures used to process specimens or identify the suspect agent. Changes in the way specimens are collected or processed may produce a change in the incidence of an organism and have been responsible for many reported pseudo-outbreaks as discussed in Chapter 6. For instance, a pseudo-outbreak of *Pseudomonas aeruginsoa* in neutropenic patients in a hematology unit occurred when some personnel collected stool cultures by sampling feces from the toilet. The toilet water contaminated the specimens.[35] Once the personnel were instructed how to properly collect the stool cultures, the outbreak subsided.

Conducting a Literature Search

A literature search should be conducted early in the investigation, as discussed in Chapter 9, to determine if other health care facilities have had a similar experience and have identified risk factors, sources, reservoirs, modes of transmission, and effective control measures. When conducting a literature search for outbreaks caused by a specific organism, the investigator should keep in mind that the nomenclature of some microorganisms changes frequently, as shown in Table 8–2, and older articles may use a prior name.

Consulting with the Laboratory

If the outbreak is of infectious etiology, laboratory personnel should be notified as soon as possible about the likelihood of an outbreak and they should be instructed to save sera and all isolates of the suspected agent, as appropriate, for possible future study (e.g., molecular typing of bacterial isolates to determine strain relatedness). Chapter 11 provides a complete discussion of the laboratory's role in outbreak investigation.

Notifying Essential Personnel

The facility's administrative staff should be notified as soon as possible of the likelihood of an outbreak—especially if the epidemic involves considerable morbidity or mortality. If the suspected outbreak involves a disease, such as Legionnaires' disease, scabies, salmonellosis, or meningitis, that is likely to attract media attention then the public relations department should also be notified. It would be unfortunate if either of these were to first learn about an outbreak in their facility through a reporter calling to request information.

Personnel in affected departments should be alerted as soon as the existence of an outbreak is confirmed. If likely prevention and control measures, such as hand washing or contact isolation, can be identified then personnel should be instructed to take those precautions. The local health department should be notified if a reportable disease is involved or if local regulations require that outbreaks in health care facilities be reported. Risk management personnel should also be notified because outbreaks frequently result in lawsuits being filed against a facility.

Assembling a Team

An investigative team should be assembled and a member of the team should be appointed to be the primary contact person who will answer questions and communicate findings and recommendations. The team may be composed of personnel from infection control, infectious disease, quality management, risk management, laboratory, pharmacy, employee health, patient/resident care services and administration, as needed. If the outbreak is covered by the media, it is helpful to have a spokesperson for the facility who is not actively involved in the investigation so that a person is not pulled away from the investigation to do interviews.

Outbreaks usually generate much fear and anxiety in personnel, patients or residents, and their families and

Table 8–2 Changing Nomenclature of Selected Organisms Associated with Outbreaks in the Health Care Setting

Bacteria

Current Name	Other Names
Acinetobacter baumanii	Acinetobacter anitratus
Burkholderia cepacia	Pseudomonas cepacia
Citrobacter koseri	Citrobacter diversus
Enterococcus faecalis	Streptococcus faecalis (Group D enterococcus)
Enterococcus faecium	Streptococcus faecium (Group D enterococcus)
Ralstonia pickettii	Pseudomonas pickettii, Burkholderia pickettii
Stenotrophomonas maltophilia	Pseudomonas maltophilia, Xanthomonas maltophilia
Streptococcus agalactiae	Group B streptococcus
Streptococcus pyogenes	Group A streptococcus
Xanthomonas maltophilia	Pseudomonas maltophilia

Fungi

Current Name	Other Names
Candida albicans	Candida stellatoidea, Monilia albicans
Candida glabrata	Torulopsis glabrata
Malassezia furfur	Cladosporium mansonii, Pityrosporum orbiculare, Pityrosporum ovale
Malassezia pachydermatis	Pityrosporum pachydermatis

Viruses

Genus Name	Other Names
Calicivirus	Norwalk and Norwalk-like viruses, small round structured viruses
Rhinovirus	Common cold virus

the team should anticipate overreaction, and possibly panic, and should be prepared to answer many questions. For instance, in the early 1980s, Frankford Hospital experienced an outbreak of *Citrobacter diversus* (now *koseri*) meningitis in neonates in the normal newborn nursery. The local health department and the CDC participated in the outbreak investigation, which attracted extensive media coverage. An employee who did not work in patient care and did not work in the nursery asked "to be tested for meningitis" because she was "afraid of bringing meningitis home" to her family. In addition, one of the investigators was pregnant and experienced pressure from her family to "let someone else" work on the investigation so she would not "catch something."

Determining the Need for Outside Assistance

The investigative team should decide if outside assistance is needed. When conducting an extensive investigation that involves a case control or cohort study, the investigators should seek the assistance of a trained statistician. Local and state health departments can arrange for assistance in conducting an outbreak investigation and in many localities disease outbreaks of known or unknown etiology are reportable to the health department. A health department will frequently call the Hospital Infections Program (HIP) of the CDC if an outbreak involves an unusual condition, a disease with high morbidity or mortality, or a common source outbreak linked to a commercially available product (such as food or medication). The HIP personnel provide epidemiologic, laboratory, statistical, and technical (computer) assistance.

In addition, if a full-scale investigation is conducted, it will be necessary to arrange secretarial, clerical, technical, and laboratory support for the investigative team.

Instituting Early Control Measures

Since the major objective of an outbreak investigation is to interrupt the outbreak, control measures should be identified and instituted as soon as possible. These should be based on the magnitude and nature of the problem and relevant findings from the literature search.

Seeking Additional Cases

A thorough retrospective and concurrent search should be conducted to detect additional cases. This can be done by reviewing laboratory reports, surveillance records, medical records, and health department reports; calling area facilities to determine if they have detected cases; and encouraging personnel and physicians to report new cases. If the disease or condition has a long incubation period and it is likely that patients may be discharged before symptoms develop, then active surveillance for new cases can be conducted by calling physicians' offices to uncover additional cases. If the illness can be asymptomatic, it may be necessary to test for infection in order to detect cases (e.g., if a resident in a long-term care facility is diagnosed with infectious tuberculosis, then PPD skin testing must be done to detect *M tuberculosis* infection in the resident's contacts).

Create a data collection form. The investigators should create a data collection form to collect information on each case. The data elements to be included on the form will depend on the disease, condition, or event being studied. This form must be designed carefully to (1) include the information needed to determine if a case fits the case definition, (2) avoid wasting time collecting too much information, and (3) avoid missing data that are later found to be needed.

If data will be entered into a computer database, it is helpful to design the form so that the data elements are in the same order as they are entered into the computer. As noted, the information that should be collected depends on the disease being studied. Data elements may include the following:

- identification information, such as name, record number, unit or ward, address, phone, and admission date
- demographic information such as age, sex, and race
- clinical information such as date of onset, signs and symptoms, underlying diseases, dates of collection and types of specimens, laboratory results, radiology results, and outcome
- name and service of attending physician or surgeon
- risk factors that are relevant to the disease or condition being studied (e.g., food and date/time eaten, medications and date/time given, therapeutic and diagnostic procedures and dates done, exposures to personnel, types of intravascular devices used and dates/time inserted, and presence of urinary catheters and dates used). Information collected during the literature search should be used to identify potential risk factors.

Investigators should take care to avoid collecting data that will not be used because this is a waste of time and resources. For example, a patient's address and phone number would not be needed unless the patient must be contacted for follow-up or the outbreak involves a reportable disease and this information is needed to complete a communicable disease report form.

Selected information is then abstracted from each data collection form and recorded on the line-listing. Examples of a line-listing form and its corresponding data collection tool are shown in Exhibits 12–1 and 12–2 in Chapter 12. Additional examples of line-listing and data collection forms can be found in Appendix B.

Describing the Epidemic: Person, Place, and Time

Once data are collected, the investigators can conduct the descriptive phase of the investigation by characterizing the outbreak with respect to person, place, and time. For instance, did the cases occur in one area of a facility or during a short period of time?

Person. Cases should be identified and entered on the line-listing so that risk factors common to the affected persons can be identified. The population at risk should then be determined and, when possible, attack rates should be calculated. The formula for calculating an attack rate is the same as that for an incidence rate except an attack rate is always expressed as the number of cases per 100 population (i.e., as a percentage):

$$\text{Attack rate (\%)} = \frac{\begin{array}{c}\text{number of new cases of a disease}\\\text{or condition in a specified}\\\text{period of time}\end{array}}{\begin{array}{c}\text{population at risk for the same}\\\text{period of time}\end{array}} \times 100$$

$$\text{Example:} \quad \frac{\begin{array}{c}\text{3 surgical site infections}\\\text{following total hip surgery}\\\text{in January}\end{array}}{\begin{array}{c}\text{35 total hip arthroplasties}\\\text{done in January}\end{array}} \times 100 = \begin{array}{c}\text{8.6 percent}\\\text{attack rate}\end{array}$$

It is not always possible to calculate an attack rate because the denominator (the population at risk) cannot always be quantitated. The use and calculation of rates are discussed in Chapter 10.

Place. The location of the cases, such as hospital unit, ward in a long-term care facility, or an ambulatory care center should be identified. It may be helpful to construct a spot map to illustrate the location of cases in a facility. By showing the distribution of cases, it may be possible to formulate a hypothesis on the mode of transmission or a potential source. Figure 12–12 in Chapter 12 is an example of a spot map. It illustrates the occurrence of mumps cases in the trading pits of exchange A in Chicago, Illinois, from August 18, 1987, to December 25, 1987.

Time. The date of onset should be recorded for each case. Both date and time of onset should be determined for acute diseases, such as gastroenteritis, which have an abrupt onset and a short incubation period (i.e., the period between which exposure occurs and symptoms develop). Both date and time of occurrence should be recorded for adverse events such as falls and other injuries because if adverse events are found to occur on a particular shift, then attention can be focused on identifying risk factors that exist on that shift but not on another. Several investigations have implicated personnel as the cause of an outbreak because data on the shifts on which the events occurred were recorded and analyzed. For example, an investigation of cardiac arrests in an intensive care unit revealed that the patients of a particular nurse on the evening shift were 47.5 times more likely to experience a cardiac arrest than were the other nurses' patients.[7] Many of the implicated nurse's patients were found to have unexplained hyperkalemia and unexpected cardiac arrests. The outbreak ended when the nurse stopped working in the ICU.

For some infectious diseases, once the causative agent is identified and the incubation period is determined, the probable period of exposure can be postulated. The incubation periods of selected foodborne gastrointestinal diseases are listed in Table 7–3 in Chapter 7.

Outbreaks may involve cases that are not temporally related (do not occur closely spaced in time). There are several reported nursery outbreaks of *C koseri* meningitis in which the cases were separated by many months.[36,37] In an unpublished outbreak that occurred at one hospital, the cases occurred in May, September, and the following February.

Drawing an Epidemic Curve

An epidemic curve is a graph (a histogram) that is constructed by plotting the number of cases on the y-axis and the date of onset on the x-axis as shown in Chapter 12. A properly constructed epidemic curve can often be used to distinguish between a common source and a propagated outbreak.

In a common source outbreak, the cases are exposed to a common noxious influence. If this exposure is brief and essentially simultaneous, then disease develops within one incubation period and the outbreak is called a point source outbreak. Examples of a point source outbreak would be food poisoning caused by consumption of contaminated food at a single meal, gastrointestinal illness associated with a recreational water activity,[38] and the 1976 Legionnaires' disease outbreak among the attendees of the American Legion Convention. Figure 8–1 shows the epidemic curve for a point source outbreak of cryptosporidiosis associated with a water sprinkler fountain.[38] A common source outbreak may occur over a wide geographic area (e.g., multistate outbreaks have occurred when a widely distributed food or medical product from a single source is contaminated) or may extend over a prolonged period, as may occur if Legionnaires' disease occurs sporadically in persons exposed to a contaminated air conditioning unit but the cases are not readily detected and the outbreak is not recognized for many months.

Some outbreaks will originate from a common source and then spread further via person-to-person contact. This often occurs in outbreaks of diseases that have several modes of transmission, such as salmonellosis or hepatitis A, as these can be introduced into a population through contaminated food and then spread to others by direct person-to-person contact and by contact with feces.[39]

In a propagated or progressive outbreak, the disease is transmitted from person-to-person such as during an outbreak of chickenpox, measles, or influenza. Figure 8–2 shows the epidemic curve for a propagated outbreak of measles.[40] The case shown on August 10 was the index case (the first case), a visitor from another country, who introduced the disease into the population.

Evaluating the Problem

Existing data should be reviewed to determine the nature of the disease or event. If the outbreak is of in-

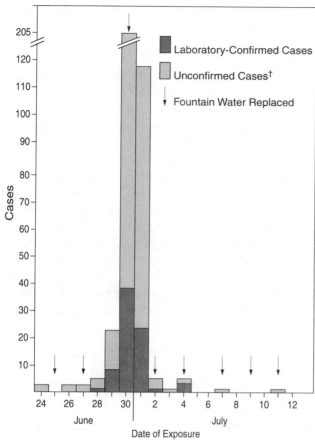

* n=369.

† Defined as vomiting or three or more loose stools within a 24-hour period, with onset 3–15 days after fountain exposure of at least 3 days.

Figure 8–1 Epidemic Curve for a Point-Source Outbreak: Reported Cases of Cryptosporidiosis Associated with a Water Sprinkler Fountain, by Date of Exposure—Minnesota, 1997 (*n* = 369). *Source:* Reprinted from Outbreak of Cryptosporidiosis Associated with a Water Sprinkler Fountain—Minnesota, 1997, *MMWR,* 1998;47:856–860, Centers for Disease Control and Prevention.

fectious etiology, the identity and characteristics of the infecting organism will often indicate where to look further. For instance, *S aureus* outbreaks are spread by person-to-person contact and the reservoir is an infected or colonized person. If an outbreak occurs among postoperative patients or is clustered on a single unit and occurs abruptly, a potential source would be an infected or colonized health care worker, and therefore personnel should be evaluated for signs and symptoms of infection, such as a lesion.[41] If the outbreak spreads slowly, it may be the result of a breakdown in proper infection control practices, such as hand washing and aseptic technique.[42]

Group A streptococci outbreaks in health care facilities are invariably associated with a health care worker who is infected or is an asymptomatic carrier.[43–45] Environmental reservoirs have not been implicated in group A streptococcal outbreaks; however, there have been foodborne outbreaks of group A streptococcal pharyngitis in which the source was an infected food handler who contaminated the food while preparing it.[46]

Outbreaks caused by certain organisms, such as *Pseudomonas* or nontuberculous *Mycobacterium* species, are frequently associated with contaminated water or solutions, and this information can guide the investigators to look for aqueous reservoirs by evaluating common risk factors such as medications and solutions diluted with water or procedures involving fluid.[47]

If the outbreak involves postoperative infections, the investigator needs to determine if a personnel carrier or an environmental source is most likely by reviewing the characteristics of the infecting organism. This information can usually be found by conducting a careful literature search. For example, outbreaks of postoperative infections caused by group A streptococcus are generally associated with a human carrier[45] and those caused by gram negative rods are frequently associated with an environmental reservoir.[48]

Data should be reviewed for evidence of person-to-person spread or a common source reservoir. For instance, if all of the infected and colonized patients had the same procedure (such as bronchoscopy) or therapy (such as mechanical ventilation),[47] or all of the ill persons ate the same meal, then the investigator could hypothesize that the disease occurred as a result of this common exposure.

The investigators should observe practices that may possibly contribute to the occurrence of the outbreak. These practices could involve patient care, resident care, preparation of food, or cleaning, disinfection, and sterilization of equipment and medical devices—depending on the circumstances of the outbreak.

Note: Rule number 3 in outbreak investigation is to observe the practices being reviewed. Although policies and procedures may reflect appropriate infection control techniques, personnel frequently do not adhere to written protocols. Personnel will often state the proper method that should be used; however, one should not assume that personnel are actually practicing what they say. Careful observation, done in a nonthreatening manner, will sometimes discover unrecognized breaks in proper technique. If an outbreak

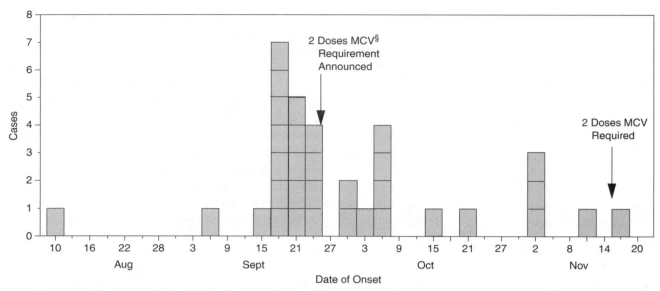

* A confirmed case was laboratory confirmed or met the clinical case definition and was epidemologically linked to a confirmed case. A clinical case was defined as an illness characterized by generalized rash lasting ≥3 days; temperature ≥101°F (≥38.3°C); and either cough, coryza, or conjunctivitis; n=33.

† n=33.

§ Measles-containing vaccine.

Figure 8–2 Epidemic Curve for a Propagated Outbreak: Number of Confirmed* Measles Cases, by Date of Rash Onset, by 3-Day Interval—Anchorage, Alaska, August 10–November 23, 1998.† *Source:* Reprinted from Transmission of Measles Among a Highly Vaccinated School Population—Anchorage, Alaska, 1998, *MMWR,* 1999;47:1109–1111, Centers for Disease Control and Prevention.

involves postoperative infections, it is particularly important to observe operating room and instrument and equipment processing practices.

Two cases illustrate the importance of observing practices. The first case involved an investigation of an outbreak of *Burkholderia cepacia* lower respiratory tract infection and colonization that occurred in the ICUs of a large tertiary care hospital.[47] Since 38 of the 44 case patients were on mechanical ventilators, respiratory therapy was thought to play a role in the outbreak. A literature search revealed a report of an outbreak of *B cepacia* respiratory tract infections that was associated with nebulized albuterol. A review of the cases in the tertiary care hospital found that all 44 patients had received albuterol bronchodilator therapy.[47] *B cepacia* was isolated from an opened in-use multidose vial of albuterol and polymerase chain reaction ribotyping showed that the albuterol isolate and 12 patient isolates had identical banding patterns. Observation of the practices of the respiratory therapists revealed that the albuterol was dispensed from a multidose vial via a plastic eyedropper. The personnel

would frequently touch the tip of the eyedropper to the side of the nebulizer reservoir and then insert the eyedropper back into the vial, which they placed in their pockets for use on the next patient. After aseptic technique and proper nebulization practices were reviewed with the respiratory therapy staff, no new cases occurred. The most likely source of the *B cepacia* was determined to be extrinsically contaminated albuterol.

The second case involved an outbreak of gram-negative bacteremia in open-heart surgery patients that was traced to probable contamination of pressure-monitoring equipment.[48] The equipment (disposable transducers, intravenous extension tubing, heparinized saline, and stopcocks) was frequently set up at the end of the day for possible emergency use during the evening or night shifts. If it was not used overnight, it was used for the first case of the day. The equipment was not covered. When housekeeping practices were observed, it was discovered that the housekeeping staff used a hose to spray a water-disinfectant mixture into the operating room when they were cleaning the room. This mixture was sprayed very close to the pressure-monitoring equipment. Contamination of the equipment by the spray was thought to be responsible for the bacteremias because the outbreak was terminated when cleaning practices were changed and pressure-monitoring equipment was set up immediately before each open-heart procedure.[48]

Investigators should consider using the opportunity of an outbreak investigation to identify other practices that may contribute to a future outbreak. These practices can than be reviewed, analyzed, and corrected after the outbreak investigation is completed.

Determining the Need for Additional Cultures or Other Diagnostic Tests

The investigative team must determine the need for collecting microbiologic cultures or conducting other diagnostic tests, such as serologic studies or skin tests. Additional testing will depend on the circumstances of the outbreak.

Microbiologic cultures. If microbiologic culturing of personnel, patients, residents, or the environment is to be done, arrangements should be made with the laboratory, with personnel in areas where testing will occur, and with the facility's administrator, who must determine how to cover the expenses involved. The required specimens and culture methods should then be identified and the specimens should be collected and processed. The appropriate typing methods for the organism being studied must also be identified and arrangements must be made to have these tests done on any isolates of epidemiologic importance.

The decision whether or not to culture personnel, equipment, devices, or environmental surfaces should be based on evidence that a person or an environmental reservoir is epidemiologically linked to the outbreak.[2] It is important to remember that a person, item, or surface is not necessarily the source of the outbreak just because it is culture-positive; any of these may have become contaminated by the true source or by an infected or colonized person. Extensive microbiologic culturing of personnel or the environment is generally not warranted and should not be done unless a full-scale epidemiologic study is conducted and the study implicates a personnel carrier or an environmental source and the significant isolates are typed for evidence of strain relatedness.

If culturing is done, the isolates should be typed to determine strain relatedness. There are many methods for typing microbial isolates.[49] Phenotypic techniques, which detect characteristics that are expressed by an organism, include biotyping, serotyping, antimicrobial susceptibility, bacteriophage and bacteriocin typing, polyacrylamide gel electrophoresis (PAGE), multi-locus enzyme electrophoresis (MLEE), and immuno-blotting. Genotypic (or molecular) techniques, which examine an organism's genetic content, include plasmid profiles, restriction endonuclease analysis (REA), ribotyping, pulsed-field gel electrophoresis (PFGE), and polymerize chain reaction (PCR). Typing systems have been shown to be a powerful tool for investigating outbreaks of nosocomial infection when they are used as an adjunct to an epidemiologic investigation.[50] They must be used and interpreted with caution, however, to avoid erroneous conclusions.[49] For instance, the finding that there is only one strain circulating in a facility does not necessarily mean that all of the infections are related—there may be only a single strain circulating in the community even though there may be many reservoirs or sources. Conversely, if multiple strains are found, there may still be an outbreak, as multiple strains have been found to cause an outbreak (based on epidemiologic evidence). The use, advantages, and disadvantages of the various typing methods are discussed in Chapter 11.

If culturing of personnel is done, specimens should be labeled with a code, rather than with a health care worker's name, to protect the identity of anyone who is culture-positive for the organism being studied. Only one person should hold the key connecting the codes and names. Culturing creates substantial anxiety among personnel because they will be concerned that they may be involved in causing the outbreak. Therefore, the decision to culture personnel must be made carefully, based on epidemiologic evidence, and personnel need to be assured that the results of testing will remain confidential—to allay concerns that they will be blamed for the outbreak if they are culture-positive.

If an infectious agent has a carrier state or can cause colonization, it may sometimes be desirable to culture patients or residents to determine the extent of the spread in the population at risk. Culture surveys should not be done unless the significant organisms that are isolated are typed or otherwise characterized to determine if they are related strains.

Other diagnostic tests. For those diseases in which infection may occur without signs or symptoms, other tests may be needed to determine if persons were infected as a result of exposure during the outbreak. For instance, skin testing with purified protein derivative (PPD) would be needed to identify persons who become infected following exposure to *M tuberculosis* because most infections with this organism are asymptomatic. Those who are identified as newly infected could then be given prophylaxis to prevent the development of disease. When investigating an outbreak of measles, serologic testing is frequently done to identify susceptible persons so they can be immunized to prevent infection and further transmission of the disease.

Formulating a Tentative Hypothesis

One of the objectives of an outbreak investigation is to determine why certain individuals in a population develop disease. This is done by collecting information on possible risk factors (exposures) and generating hypotheses. Based upon an evaluation of the information collected up to this point, a tentative hypothesis should be formulated regarding the likely causative factors of the outbreak (e.g., reservoir, source, and mode of transmission of the agent if the outbreak is of infectious etiology).

For example, a multidrug-resistant *Pseudomonas aeruginosa* has been isolated from the respiratory tract of three patients in the intensive care unit (ICU) during a three-week period. The ICU, laboratory, and infection control personnel recognize that this represents more cases of this organism than expected. An initial review of the cases shows that one patient has pneumonia and two are colonized. All three patients are on ventilators. Since mechanical ventilation has been shown to be a risk factor for infection and colonization with *P aeruginosa*, a tentative hypothesis could be that exposure to mechanical ventilation is associated with the nosocomial acquisition of a multidrug-resistant strain of *P aeruginosa*.

Control Measures

Control measures should be implemented as soon as possible during the investigative process. For an infectious disease outbreak of known etiology, preventive interventions should be based on the characteristics of the causative agent, including possible reservoirs and sources and the most likely mode of transmission. Measures that have been shown to be effective in interrupting the transmission of a variety of organisms have been discussed in Chapters 3–7. The identified control measures could be as simple as stressing good hand washing and adherence to contact precautions to help control an outbreak or cluster of MRSA. To interrupt outbreaks of noninfectious etiology, control measures should be based on the nature of the disease or event. For example, in one published report, an excess number of needlestick injuries in hospital personnel was traced to needles piercing the walls of infectious waste containers.[6] The outbreak was terminated when a different type of container was used.

Evaluating Control Measure Efficacy

Surveillance activities should be continued to determine if any new cases are occurring. If new cases continue to occur, control measures may need to be reevaluated and a more extensive epidemiologic investigation may be needed.

Statistical Hypothesis Testing

In a full-scale investigation, statistical tests are done to test the hypotheses that explain the likely cause(s) of the outbreak. Many investigations do not reach this stage. The investigation may end prior to this point if the control measures are working and if the situation does not require further study. The following outbreak situations should be pursued further: those associated with considerable morbidity or mortality, those that continue to occur despite the implementation of control measures, those that are suspected to be facility-wide, and those adverse events that are associated with a medical device or a commercial product.

This phase poses one of the greatest challenges when conducting an outbreak investigation. The investigators must carefully review the clinical, laboratory, and epidemiologic findings and hypothesize which risk factors or exposures could plausibly lead to disease. The hypotheses are then tested by comparing the population with the disease (cases) with a population without the disease (controls) in regards to exposures to postulated risk factors. These comparisons are usually done by conducting a case-control or cohort study, as discussed in Chapter 10. To ensure that the appropriate study design and statistical tests are used, health care facility personnel should consult a trained statistician before beginning a case-control or cohort study. For a discussion of the use of case-control studies in outbreak investigations, the reader is referred to a review article by Dwyer et al.[51]

When testing a hypothesis, investigators need to keep in mind the criteria that should be used to judge if an association is causal: strength of association, dose-response relationship, consistency of association, chronological relationship, specificity of association, and biological plausibility, as discussed in Chapter 1. Data should also be evaluated to determine if (1) there are any persons who were not exposed to a particular risk factor who are affected or (2) if there are persons who were exposed to a particular risk factor who are not affected.

For example, over a nine-day period, five personnel and 15 residents in a long-term care facility develop a febrile illness with diarrhea or vomiting. *Salmonella enteritidis* is isolated from several cases and is determined to be the etiologic agent of the outbreak. Because an investigation shows that no other cases have recently been reported in the community, the investigators hypothesize that exposure to the source of the organism occurred in the long-term care facility. Because *S enteritidis* outbreaks are most frequently associated with a foodborne source, a further hypothesis could be that consumption of some food or beverage in the facility was the exposure necessary to develop disease. Therefore, the likely period of exposure, based on the usual incubation period of the disease (6 to 48 hours), would be identified and the cases would be interviewed to determine what they had to eat or drink at the facility during that period. To determine if exposure to certain foods eaten by the ill persons (cases) was associated with disease, these exposures would be compared with exposures of persons who were not ill (controls) by conducting statistical tests of association and significance, as explained in Chapter 10.

Without a computer, it would take much time (and patience) to perform the calculations needed to test the hypotheses. Epi Info, a software program developed by the CDC to manage and analyze data collected during an epidemiologic investigation, can be downloaded from the CDC's Web site at http://www.cdc.gov.[52] Epi Info can be used to organize epidemiologic data and to calculate odds ratios, relative risk, 95 percent confidence intervals, Chi-squares, *P* values, etc. The *Epi Info User's Manual* and the Epi Info Tutorial can also be ordered or accessed through the CDC's Web site.

Further Analysis and Investigation

Investigators should continue to seek additional cases by searching both retrospectively and concurrently. Concurrent (ongoing) surveillance should be used to assess the effectiveness of the implemented control measures. The investigative team should meet to review findings up to this point and to formulate and test additional hypotheses, as needed.

If other testing is warranted, such as microbiologic culturing or serologic tests for hepatitis A or measles, these tests should be completed. The results of all laboratory tests should be carefully recorded and analyzed by the investigative team.

Preparing and Distributing Written Reports

Investigators should carefully document their actions and organize their findings at each step in the investigation. Interim reports should be prepared and distributed, as needed, to the facility's administrative staff, to those who are affected by the outbreak, to the infection control committee, and to relevant government or public health agencies. When the investigation is completed, a final report should be prepared and submitted to the departments, areas, or units involved in the outbreak, to the facility's administrative staff, to the infection control committee, and to the health department and other authorities, as appropriate.

The final report should follow the usual scientific format: introduction/background, methods, results, discussion, and summary/recommendations and should include the names and titles of those who prepared it and those to whom it was provided. Guidelines for preparing a report of an outbreak investigation are shown in Table 8–3. A good example of a detailed report of an outbreak is the article by White et al. who described an epidemic of giardiasis in a nursing home.[53]

PUBLISHING AN ARTICLE ON AN OUTBREAK INVESTIGATION

A literature search is one of the crucial steps in conducting an outbreak investigation because it helps the investigator to identify potential risk factors associated with a disease and control measures that have been shown to be effective in preventing that disease in similar situations. Preparing a written report of an outbreak investigation using the outline provided in Table 8–3, provides the investigator the basis for writing an article and submitting it for publication. Infection control, infectious disease, and quality management personnel who conduct outbreak investigations in health care facilities should consider publishing their findings—especially if the outbreak involves an unusual organism or a previously unrecognized risk factor, source, reser-

Table 8–3 Guideline for Preparing a Report of an Outbreak Investigation

Section	Describes or Explains, When Appropriate
1. Introduction/background	Similar outbreaks that were previously reported; how the outbreak was detected; who conducted the investigation; the type of facility and area(s) where the outbreak occurred.
2. Methods	
a. Laboratory methods	Types of culture media used; method for collecting specimens; identification and typing systems used for microorganisms isolated; serologic or other tests used.
b. Epidemiologic methods	Type of study used (e.g., case-control or cohort); case definition (possible, probable, definite; asymptomatic vs. symptomatic); how the cases and controls were selected; sources of the data collected (e.g., patient or resident medical records, infection control surveillance data, quality management data, laboratory records, reports from health care workers, health department records, phone or written surveys, interviews with patients, personnel, or visitors).
c. Statistical methods	Statistical tests used.
3. Results	Findings of the study (facts only, with no discussion); may also include tables of cases and risk factors, an epidemic curve, and spot maps, as appropriate.
4. Discussion	The interpretation and discussion of the results.
5. Summary/recommendations	The summary of the findings and recommendations.
6. Distribution of report	Notes the names and titles of those to whom the report was given.
7. Author(s)	Notes the names and titles of those who prepared the report.

voir, or mode of transmission of an infectious agent. Since outbreak investigations frequently advance knowledge of the epidemiology of infections and other adverse outcomes in health care institutions, health care professionals who investigate clusters and outbreaks of health care-related events should publish their findings to assist others who are investigating similar conditions.

RISK MANAGEMENT ISSUES

Outbreaks can result in claims and lawsuits being filed against a health care facility. In rare cases, members of the infection control department have been named in these suits. Facility personnel, including the infection control staff, may be subpoenaed to give a deposition or testify in court. In addition, during the discovery process of a lawsuit, the defendant(s) will be required to produce documents relating to the case. During an outbreak investigation, the investigators should be careful to record facts, and not speculations or personal comments, because documents produced during the investigation may be subpoenaed. The facility's risk management and legal departments should be consulted to answer questions about risk and legal issues surrounding an outbreak investigation.

OUTBREAK INVESTIGATION SKILLS

According to Goodman et al., "The concepts and techniques used in field investigations derive from clinical medicine, epidemiology, laboratory science, decision analysis, skilled communications, and common sense."[54(p10)] In order to successfully apply epidemiologic methods to recognizing, investigating, and controlling an outbreak, the investigator must be skilled in a unique set of tasks:[55]

- surveillance—the ongoing, systematic collection of data
- investigation—careful observation and gathering of data for a detailed descriptive study
- analysis—observation followed by comparison of groups
- evaluation—the assessment of the effectiveness of the actions and control measures taken to resolve a problem

In addition, the investigator should possess skills in communication, management, consultation, presenting epidemiologic findings, and human relations.[55]

PUBLIC HEALTH ISSUES

Recognizing and Reporting Clusters and Suspected Outbreaks

Health care facilities are well suited to assisting health departments in the recognition and follow-up of community outbreaks of disease because persons who are ill frequently present to a hospital emergency department or to a health care provider for treatment. Community outbreaks of salmonellosis and staphylococcal food poisoning have been first recognized by hospital personnel, especially those in emergency departments, when several patients presented during a short time period with gastrointestinal illnesses.[56,57] In 1994 the staff of a community hospital reported a cluster of community acquired cases of Legionnaires' disease (LD) and this led to the detection of an outbreak of LD among passengers of a cruise ship.[58]

Health care facilities should have a mechanism for reporting suspected community outbreaks of infectious and noninfectious conditions to the local health department as soon as possible. All 50 states have reportable disease requirements and health care providers have the responsibility for reporting cases of communicable diseases and other conditions to the health department. Even though one case may not seem important, that one individual may be involved in a larger outbreak that may not be recognized unless many cases are reported.

Community Outbreaks and Health Care Facilities

Widespread community outbreaks of infectious diseases such as salmonellosis and influenza may cause community-acquired infections in health care personnel and their families and may result in increased admissions of persons with communicable diseases and in nosocomial spread to other patients, residents, or personnel.[59] In addition, health care facilities may be asked to assist health departments provide prophylaxis, immunization, or other follow-up for persons potentially exposed to a communicable disease. Sinai Hospital of Baltimore has assisted the local and state health departments provide prophylaxis for family members of patients with meningococcal meningitis and immunization for contacts of a patient with measles. If outbreaks affect many persons, it may be necessary to set up special clinics and telephone hotlines.[60] Guidelines for developing a written plan to address infectious disease emergencies have been published and these can be used to develop a facility-specific plan.[60]

When widespread outbreaks are associated with commercial products, such as food or medication, health care facility personnel must determine if the facility has received that product and has used it. Foodborne outbreaks associated with intrinsically contaminated commercial products put patients, residents, personnel, visitors, and guests at risk—especially if the facility is involved in catering meetings attended by members of the community.[61]

Biological Weapons and Terrorist Attacks

There is increasing concern that the use of biological agents during a war or for a terrorist attack could cause widespread outbreaks and paralyze the health care system. A religious cult intentionally contaminated salad bars at 10 restaurants in Oregon and this resulted in at least 751 cases of *Salmonella typhimurium* in a county that typically reports fewer than five cases per year.[62] Health care personnel should be familiar with the biological agents most likely to be used—especially with their disease manifestations and modes of transmission and with the measures that can be used to control their spread.[63] A Bioterrorism Readiness Plan for Healthcare Facilities is available from the Association for Professionals in Infection Control and Epidemiology and can be downloaded from the association's Web site at http://www.apic.org. A discussion of this topic is beyond the scope of this text; however, information can be found via the Internet through the CDC's Web site (http://www.cdc.gov), the on-line journal *Emerging Infectious Diseases* (http://www.cdc.gov/nciod/EID), and the Johns Hopkins Center for Civilian Biodefense Studies (http://www.hopkins-biodefense.org).

USING TECHNOLOGY TO AID IN OUTBREAK INVESTIGATION

Computers have greatly aided in the management and analysis of data collected during routine surveillance activities and during outbreak investigations. Other technologies can also assist in the investigation of an outbreak. Following a report that several attendees of a conference developed salmonellosis, the CDC initiated an epidemiologic investigation by sending a questionnaire to conference attendees via the e-mail system of the organization that sponsored the conference.[64] The attendees were instructed to complete the survey and return it to the CDC via fax. Since the attendees had come from all 50 states, this electronic communication facilitated the search for cases and aided in the identification and investigation of a foodborne outbreak in a widely dispersed population. Using information supplied by the attendees, the source of the organism was eventually traced to an infected foodhandler at a restaurant near the convention site.

Many health care professionals subscribe to electronic listserves that allow instant communication locally, nationally, and internationally. These systems can be used to inquire about the experiences of others during an outbreak and to alert health care institutions about outbreaks associated with medical procedures or with commercial products and devices. Technologies such as listserves, electronic mail, and fax machines will undoubtedly continue to be useful tools for the practitioner who uses them to obtain and to disseminate information.

ADDITIONAL INFORMATION

For additional information on investigating outbreaks in the health care setting, refer to the chapter on outbreak investigation in one of the infection control texts (Bennett and Brachman, Mayhall, Olmsted, or Wenzel) on the Suggested Reading list.

REFERENCES

1. Haley RW, Tenney JH, Lindsey JO, Garnet JS, Bennett JV. How frequent are outbreaks of nosocomial infection in community hospitals? *Infect Control*. 1985;6:233–236.

2. Beck-Sague C, Jarvis WR, Martone WJ. Outbreak investigations. *Infect Control Hosp Epidemiol*. 1997;18:138–145.

3. Smith PW, Rusnak PG. Infection prevention and control in the long-term care facility. *Am J Infect Control*. 1997;25:488–512.

4. Martone WJ, Williams WW, Mortensen ML, et al. Illness with fatalities in premature infants: association with intravenous vitamin E preparation, E-Ferol. *Pediatr*. 1986;78:591–600.

5. Shay DK, Fann LM, Jarvis WR. Respiratory distress and sudden death associated with receipt of a peripheral parenteral nutrition admixture. *Infect Control Hosp Epidemiol*. 1997;18:814–817.

6. Anglim AM, Collmer JE, Loving J, et al. An outbreak of needlestick injuries in hospital employees due to needles piercing infectious waste containers. *Infect Control Hosp Epidemiol*. 1995;16:570–576.

7. Sacks JJ, Stroup DF, Will ML, Harris EL, Israel E. A nurse-associated epidemic of cardiac arrests in an intensive care unit. *JAMA*. 1988;295:689–695

8. Franks A, Sacks JJ, Smith JD, Sikes RK. A cluster of unexplained cardiac arrests in a surgical intensive care unit. *Crit Care Med*. 1987;15:1075–1076.

9. Kafrissen ME, Grimes DA, Hogue CJ, Sacks JJ. Cluster of abortion deaths at a single facility. *Obstet Gynecol*. 1986;68:387–389.

10. Centers for Disease Control and Prevention. National Nosocomial Infections Surveillance (NNIS) System Report, Data Summary from October 1986—April 1998, Issued June 1998. *Am J Infect Control*. 1998;26:522–533.

11. Centers for Disease Control and Prevention. Nosocomial group A streptococcal infections associated with asymptomatic health-care workers—Maryland and California, 1997.

12. Centers for Disease Control and Prevention. Recommendation of the Immunization Practices Advisory Committee: measles prevention. *MMWR*. 1987;36:409–425.

13. Benenson AS. Staphylococcal disease in hospital nurseries. In: *Control of Communicable Diseases Manual*. 16th ed. Washington, DC: American Public Health Association; 1995:432–435.

14. Wenzel RP, Reagan DR, Bertina JS, Baron EJ, Arias K. Methicillin-resistant *Staphylococcus aureus* outbreak: a consensus panel's definition and management guidelines. *Am J Infect Control*. 1998;26:102–110.

15. Centers for Disease Control and Prevention. Sustained transmission of nosocomial Legionnaires' disease—Arizona and Ohio. *MMWR*. 1997;46:416–421.

16. Centers for Disease Control and Prevention. Prevention and control of tuberculosis in facilities providing long-term care to the elderly. Recommendations of the Advisory Committee for Elimination of Tuberculosis. *MMWR*. 1990;39(RR-10):7–20.

17. Centers for Disease Control and Prevention. Renal insufficiency and failure associated with immune globulin intravenous therapy—United States, 1985–1998. *MMWR*. 1999;48:518–521.

18. Centers for Disease Control and Prevention. Endotoxin-like reactions associated with intravenous gentamicin—California, 1998. *MMWR*. 1998;47:877–880.

19. Geiss HK, Schmitt J, Frank SC. Bleeding after cardiovascular surgery caused by detergent residues in laparotomy sponges. *Infect Control Hosp Epidemiol*. 1997;18:579–581.

20. Beck-Sague CM, Jarvis WR, Bland LA, Arduino MJ, Aguero SM, Verosic G. Outbreak of gram-negative bacteremia and pyrogenic reactions in a hemodialysis center. *Am J Nephrol*. 1990;10:397–403.

21. Dixon RE. Investigation of endemic and epidemic nosocomial infections. In: Bennett JV, Brachman PS. *Hospital Infections*. 3rd ed. Boston: Little, Brown and Company; 1992:109–133.

22. Centers for Disease Control. Guidelines for investigating clusters of health events. *MMWR*. 1990;39(RR-11):1

23. Birnbaum D. Analysis of hospital infection surveillance data. *Infect Control*. 1984;5:332–338.

24. McGuckin MB, Abrutyn E. A surveillance method for early detection of nosocomial outbreaks. *Am J Infect Control*. 1979;7:18–21.

25. Childress JA, Childress JD. Statistical test for possible infection outbreaks. *Infect Control*. 1981;2:247–249.

26. Mylotte JM. The hospital epidemiologist in long-term care: practical considerations. *Infect Control Hosp Epidemiol*. 1991;12:439–442.

27. Birnbaum D. Nosocomial infection surveillance programs. *Infect Control*. 1987;8:474–479.

28. Jacquez GM, Waller LA, Grimson R, Wartenberg D. The analysis of disease clusters, Part I: state of the art. *Infect Control Hosp Epidemiol*. 1996;17:319–327.

29. Jacquez GM, Waller LA, Grimson R, Wartenberg D. The analysis of disease clusters, Part II: introduction to techniques. *Infect Control Hosp Epidemiol*. 1996;17:385–397.

30. Selleck JA. Statistical process control charts in hospital epidemiology. *Infect Control Hosp Epidemiol*. 1993;14:649–656.

31. Brewer JH, Gasser CS. The affinity between continuous quality improvement and epidemic surveillance. *Infect Control Hosp Epidemiol*. 1993;14:95–98.

32. Benneyan JC. Statistical quality control methods in infection control and hospital epidemiology, Part I: introduction and basic theory. *Infect Control Hosp Epidemiol*. 1998;19:194–214.

33. Benneyan JC. Statistical quality control methods in infection control and hospital epidemiology, Part II: chart use, statistical properties, and research issues. *Infect Control Hosp Epidemiol*. 1998;19:265–283.

34. Birnbaum D. CQI tools: sentinel events, warning, and action limits. *Infect Control Hosp Epidemiol*. 1993;14:537–539.

35. Verweij PE, Bilj D, Melchers W, et al. Pseudo-outbreak of multiresistant *Pseudomonas aeruginosa* in a hematology unit. *Infect Control Hosp Epidemiol*. 1997;18:128–131.

36. Kline MW. *Citrobacter* meningitis and brain abscess in infancy: epidemiology, pathogenesis, and treatment. *J Pediatr*. 1988;113:430–434.

37. Graham DR, Anderson RL, Ariel FE, et al. Epidemic nosocomial meningitis due to *Citrobacter diversus* in neonates. *J Infect Dis*. 1981;144:203–209.

38. Centers for Disease Control and Prevention. Outbreak of cryptosporidiosis associated with a water sprinkler fountain—Minnesota, 1997. *MMWR*. 1998;47:856–860.

39. Standaert SM, Hutcheson RH, Schaffner W. Nosocomial transmission of *Salmonella* gastroenteritis to laundry workers in a nursing home. *Infect Control Hosp Epidemiol*. 1994;15:22–26.

40. Centers for Disease Control and Prevention. Transmission of measles among a highly vaccinated school population—Anchorage, Alaska, 1998. *MMWR*. 1999;47:1109–1111.

41. Sheretz RJ, Reagan DR, Hampton KD, et al. A cloud adult: the *Staphylococcus aureus*-virus interaction revisited. *Ann Intern Med*. 1996;124:539–547.

42. Boyce JM. Methicillin-resistant *Staphylococcus aureus* in hospitals and long-term care facilities: microbiology, epidemiology, and preventive measures. *Infect Control Hosp Epidemiol*. 1992;13:725–737.

43. Ridgeway EJ, Allen KD. Clustering of group A streptococcal infections on a burns unit: important lessons in outbreak management. *J Hosp Infect*. 1993;25:173–182.

44. Viglionese A, Nottebart V, Bodman HA, Platt R. Recurrent group A streptococcal carriage in a health care worker associated with widely separated nosocomial outbreaks. *Am J Med*. 1991;91(Suppl 3B):329S–333S.

45. Paul SM, Genese C, Spitalny K. Postoperative group A beta-hemolytic *Streptococcus* outbreak with the pathogen traced to a member of a health care worker's household. *Infect Control Hosp Epidemiol*. 1990;11:643–646.

46. Decker MD, Lavely GB, Hutcheson RHU, Schaffner W. Food-borne streptococcal pharyngitis in a hospital pediatrics clinic. *JAMA*. 1986;353:679–681.

47. Reboli AC, Koshinski R, Arias K, Marks-Austin K, Stieritz D, Stull TL. An outbreak of *Burkholderia cepacia* lower respiratory tract infection associated with contaminated albuterol nebulization solution. *Infect Control Hosp Epidemiol*. 1996;17:741–743.

48. Redneck JR, Beck-Sague CM, Anderson RL, Schable B, Miller JM, Jarvis WR. Gram-negative bacteremia in open-heart-surgery patients traced to probable tap-water contamination of pressure-monitoring equipment. *Infect Control Hosp Epidemiol*. 1996;17:281–285.

49. Maslow J, Mulligan ME. Epidemiologic typing systems. *Infect Control Hosp Epidemiol*. 1996;17:595–604.

50. Jarvis WR. Usefulness of molecular epidemiology for outbreak investigations. *Infect Control Hosp Epidemiol*. 1994;15:500–503.

51. Dwyer DM, Strickler H, Goodman RA, Armenian HK. Use of case-control studies in outbreak investigations. *Epidemiol Rev*. 1994;16:109–123.

52. Epi Info [computer program]. Version 6. Atlanta: Centers for Disease Control and Prevention; 1994.

53. White KE, Hedberg CW, Edmonson LM, Jones DBW, Osterholm MT, MacDonald KL. An outbreak of giardiasis in a nursing home with evidence for multiple modes of transmission. *J Infect Dis*. 1989;160:298–304.

54. Goodman RA, Buehler JW, Kaplan JP. The epidemiologic field investigation: science and judgment in public health practice. *Am J E Epidemiol*. 1990;132:9–16.

55. Last JM, Tyler CW. Epidemiology. In: Last JM, Wallace RB, eds. *Maxcy-Rosenau-Last Public Health and Preventive Medicine*. 13th ed. Norwalk, CT: Appleton & Lange; 1992:11–39.

56. Goodman LJ, Lisowski JM, Harris AA, et al. Evaluation of an outbreak of foodborne illness initiated in the emergency department. *Ann Emerg Med*. 1993;22:62–65.

57. Centers for Disease Control and Prevention. Outbreak of staphylococcal food poisoning associated with precooked ham—Florida, 1997. *MMWR*. 1997;46:1189–1191.

58. Guerrero IC, Filippone C. A cluster of Legionnaires' disease in a community hospital—a clue to a larger epidemic. *Infect Control Hosp Epidemiol*. 1996;17:177–178.

59. Jarosch MJ, Sinwell G, Galviz CJ, et al. Activities of infection control practitioners during an outbreak of *Salmonella typhimurium*. *Am J Infect Control*. 1989;17:159–161.

60. Frace RM, Jahre JA. Policy for managing a community infectious disease outbreak. *Infect Control Hosp Epidemiol*. 1991;12:364–367.

61. Gellert GA, Tormay M, Rodriguez G, Brougher G, Dessey D, Pate C. Food-borne disease in hospitals: prevention in a changing food environment. *Am J Infect Control*. 1989;17:136–140.

62. McDade JE, Franz D. Bioterrorism as a public health threat. *Emerg Infect Dis*. 1998;4:493–494.

63. Franz DR, Jahrling PB, Friedlander AM, et al. Clinical recognition and management of patients exposed to biological warfare agents. *JAMA*. 1997;278:399–411.

64. Mahon BE, Rohn DD, Pack SR, Tauxe RV. Electronic communication facilitates investigation of a highly dispersed foodborne outbreak: Salmonella on the superhighway. *Emerg Infect Dis*. 1995;1:94–95.

SUGGESTED READING

American Academy of Pediatrics. *1997 Red Book: Report of the Committee on Infectious Diseases*. Elk Grove Village, IL: American Academy of Pediatrics; 1997.

Beck-Sague C, Jarvis WR, Martone WJ. Outbreak investigations. *Infect Control Hosp Epidemiol*. 1997;18:138–145.

Benenson AS, ed. *Control of Communicable Diseases Manual*. 16th ed. Washington, DC: American Public Health Association; 1995.

Bennett JV, Brachman PS, ed. *Hospital Infections*. 4th ed. Baltimore, MD: Williams & Wilkins; 1998.

Centers for Disease Control and Prevention. *Principles of Epidemiology: An Introduction to Applied Epidemiology and Biostatistics*. 2nd ed. Atlanta, GA: US Department of Health and Human Services, Public Health Service, Centers for Disease Control and Prevention, Epidemiology Program Office; 1992. (This is the textbook used in the CDC Principles of Epidemiolgy course noted below.)

Dwyer DM, Strickler H, Goodman RA, Armenian HK. Use of case-control studies in outbreak investigations. *Epidemiol Rev*. 1994;16:109–123.

Last JM, Wallace RB, eds. *Maxcy-Rosenau-Last Public Health and Preventive Medicine*. 13th ed. Norwalk, CT: Appleton & Lange; 1992.

Mayhall GC, ed. *Hospital Epidemiology and Infection Control*. 2nd ed. Baltimore, MD: Williams & Wilkins; 1999.

Olmsted R, ed. *APIC Infection Control and Applied Epidemiology: Principles and Practice*. St. Louis: Mosby; 1996.

Reingold AL. Outbreak investigations—a perspective. *Emerg Infect Dis*. 1998;4:21–27.

Roueche B. *The Medical Detectives*. New York: Washington Square Press; 1986.

Roueche B. *The Medical Detectives*, Vol. II. New York: Washington Square Press; 1986.

Roueche B. *The Medical Detectives*. Reprint edition. New York: Plume; 1991.

Wenzel RP, ed. *Prevention and Control of Nosocomial Infections*. 3rd ed. Baltimore, MD: Williams & Wilkins; 1997.

OTHER RESOURCES

The Centers for Disease Control and Prevention's Web site (http://www.cdc.gov) can be used to access the *Morbidity and Mortality Weekly Report*, the on-line journal *Emerging Infectious Diseases*, the Hospital Infections Program, and other information on outbreaks, infection control, and infectious diseases.

Two training courses are available from the Centers for Disease Control and Prevention:

- Principles of Epidemiology, 3030-G. This is a print-based self-study course covering basic epidemiology principles, concepts, and procedures generally used in the surveillance and investigation of health-related events. The key features and applications of descriptive and analytic epidemiology, an in-depth study of public health surveillance, and a step-by-step description of outbreak investigations are presented in this course. The course also addresses how to calculate and interpret frequency measures (ratios, proportions, and rates) and measures of central tendency, and how to use tables, graphs, and charts to organize, summarize, and display data. This course may be ordered by calling 1-800-41-TRAIN. Press 1,4,1 and choose PHF, Public Health Foundation, the distributor of this course.

- Investigating an Outbreak: Pharyngitis in Louisiana, 3050-G. This case study simulates an outbreak investigation in which the student is lead investigator and conducts epidemiologic detective work, leading to the source of the outbreak. Undertaking a variety of investigative activities, the student uncovers important information that leads to the source of the outbreak. Investigating an Outbreak: Pharyngitis in Louisiana is a CBT (computer-based training) program that runs on a computer in DOS or Windows without the need of an Internet connection. This CBT is available to download from the CDC Web site at http://www.cdc.gov. There is also a packaged version of the CBT. The content of the downloadable version is identical to the packaged version. To order the packaged version call 1-800-41-TRAIN. (Note: A prerequisite for taking this course is completion of an introductory epidemiology course such as the CDC's Principles of Epidemiology self-study course 3030-G noted above.)

Additional information on these courses can be obtained from the CDC Web site at http://www.cdc.gov.

CHAPTER 9

Conducting a Literature Search

Georgia Phelps Dash

When an outbreak occurs, whether it is suspected to have an infectious or a noninfectious etiology, a critical component of the investigation is searching the literature, as well as other sources, for pertinent information. There are a number of reasons to conduct such a search, among them the following:

- identification of other outbreaks with the same etiologic agent
- formulation of a case definition
- determination of the incidence and prevalence of disease in the population at risk
- generation of a hypothesis regarding risk factors, mechanisms of exposure, and transmission
- development of prevention and control measures

During an outbreak investigation, the need for rapid and reliable information that aids in the investigation is critical. Literally thousands of potential sources of information exist. The objective of this chapter is to discuss high-yield strategies for searching not only published literature, but also other information sources that may be helpful in investigating disease outbreaks.

SEARCHING MEDICAL LITERATURE— SEARCH SERVICES

A logical starting point for identifying published information regarding an outbreak is to conduct a literature search of one or more of the databases/data banks (Table 9–1) maintained by the National Library of Medicine's (NLM) Medical Literature Analysis and Retrieval System (MEDLARS). MEDLARS comprises two computer subsystems, ELHILL and TOXNET, on which reside 40 on-line databases containing about 18 million references.

For those who do not have a personal computer and access to the Internet, the majority of medical libraries and public libraries will permit use of their computer facilities to access the databases either on CD/ROM (produced by commercial vendors and subscribed to by the library) or via the World Wide Web (WWW). If the library does not permit its patrons to perform electronic searches, one may ask to see *Current Contents*, which is a weekly index of biomedical literature, or *Index Medicus*, published yearly since 1966, which is a compendium of the biomedical literature published during the year.

The most efficient way to search the databases/data banks in Table 9–1 is to utilize an electronic search service accessible through the WWW. The WWW is one of the easiest resources to use, and a number of services provide free searching (e.g., PubMed, Internet Grateful Med, and Medscape). These electronic search services can be accessed by keying in the appropriate Universal Resource Locator (URL). A URL functions as an address that directs a computer to the site where the information being sought is stored so that the searcher can view it, download it to a computer file, print it out, or order a copy. The WWW browser will have a prompt or a space where the URL can be entered.

Medical Matrix, an Internet provider of clinical medicine resources, has recently rated 18 of the leading electronic search services on variables such as cost to user, accessibility, concept matching, search interface, query features, access to full-text articles and associ-

Table 9–1 National Library of Medicine Electronic Databases/Data Banks Useful for Outbreak Investigation

Database/ Data Bank	Description
MEDLINE	Database covers fields of medicine, nursing, dentistry, veterinary medicine, health care systems, and preclinical sciences. Includes 3,900 current biomedical journals published in the United States and 70 foreign countries. Dates back to 1966.
PREMEDLINE	Introduced in 1996, database provides basic citations, information, and abstracts before the full records are prepared for addition to the MEDLINE database.
CINHAL	Nursing and allied health database covers all aspects of nursing, health education, and related disciplines from 1983 to the present.
RTECS	Registry of Toxic Effects of Chemical Substances database, built and maintained by the National Institute for Occupational Health and Safety (NIOSH); focuses on acute and chronic effects of toxic and potentially toxic chemicals.
TOXLINE	Database contains 2 million records covering the toxicological, pharmacological, biochemical, and physiological effects of drugs and other chemicals. Data from 1981 to the present.

ated costs, field searches, and results display. It may be beneficial to look at this report before selecting a search service to use. The URL for Medical Matrix is http://www.medmatrix.org. One of the nice features of the report is that it allows a searcher to click on the name of a rated service and be connected to its home page, where all of the details of its service provision can be found. The number one–rated service is Ovid, which charges a fee to users, as does the number two–rated service, Silver Platter. Among Medical Matrix's top-rated electronic search services—numbers three and four, respectively—are PubMed and Internet Grateful Med, both of which are available for free through the National Library of Medicine. The URL for PubMed is http://www.ncbi.nlm.nih.gov/PubMed. The URL for Internet Grateful Med is http://igm.nlm.nih.gov. Table 9–2 lists

other free services that allow MEDLINE searches and provides their URLs.

PubMed

PubMed is an electronic search tool, developed by the National Center for Biotechnical Information (NCBI) at the National Library of Medicine, for accessing the medical/scientific literature. It is a user-friendly tool with many useful features, including

- capability to search all of the databases/data banks in Table 9–1, plus 40 other NLM databases
- automatic mapping of search terms to the appropriate medical subject headings by which biomedical journal literature is indexed
- Cubby Service, where users can sign up for a "cubby," a place to store individual information and preferences, which permits the development and storage of search strategies for future reference and also allows the storage of tailored print commands
- Clinical Alert Service, which provides on-line information regarding findings from National Institutes of Health (NIH) clinical trials
- Clinical Query Services, which permits a search of a subject by specifying one or more of the four focus areas: (1) therapy; (2) diagnosis; (3) etiology; or (4) prognosis, and by indicating whether the emphasis should be on sensitivity or specificity (Note: This is a rapid search that focuses on the four listed parameters and does not allow a searcher to specify the parameters or to restrict the focus of the search, as is possible when performing a search of one of the databases such as MEDLINE.)

Table 9–2 Services with Free MEDLINE Search Access

Service	Universal Resource Locator (URL)
Avicenna	http://www.avicenna.com
HealthCare	http://www.healthgate.com
Helix	http://www.helix.com
Internet Grateful Med	http://igm.nlm.nih.gov
Medscape	http:///www.medscape.com
PubMed	http://www.ncbi.nlm.nih.gov/PubMed

- Loansome Doc Service, which allows a searcher to order from participating health science libraries the articles revealed by the search (A searcher may inquire at a nearby health science library to see if it participates in this service.)

Information on participating libraries is available from the National Network of Libraries of Medicine at (800)-338-RMLS (7657). Calls are automatically routed to the Regional Medical Library serving each caller's area code. Business hours for the Regional Medical Libraries are 9 AM to 5 PM; at other times there is a prompt to leave a message.

It is not necessary to be a physician to use Loansome Doc. There is a simple on-line registration to fill out. After a searcher completes the registration, Loansome Doc supplies a user identification (ID), a password, and a service agreement. A participating health sciences library in the user's area can provide the Ordering Library ID to use when requesting an article. Loansome Doc then sends the requested articles to the local health sciences library. There is usually a nominal fee charged by the local health sciences library for this service. Loansome Doc allows users to request document delivery through mail, fax, pickup, or the Internet. Before initiating a search, it is important first to find out which delivery options the participating library offers.

Internet Grateful Med

Internet Grateful Med has most of the features listed above, including Loansome Doc. It has some additional databases such as TOXLINE and RTECS (see Table 9–1), available by clicking on the "Search Other Files" button. In addition, it has features such as a new user's survival guide (this title makes it sound harder to use than it really is), a list of recommended Web browsers; and the extremely useful "Find MeSH Meta Terms " that helps with finding medical subject headings (MeSH) essential for performing a search.

WHAT IS "MeSH" AND WHY IS IT IMPORTANT?

The National Library of Medicine uses a system of medical subject headings for indexing articles, for cataloging books and other holdings, and for searching MeSH-indexed databases. A subject heading is assigned to every article in each database. These head-

ings are organized in a hierarchical structure so that searches of a broad concept may include articles indexed to narrower concepts. There are 18,000 MeSH headings. It is not necessary to know the headings because the software automatically maps a search topic to the correct medical subject heading. When a subject is entered, the search system displays a list of MeSH headings from which the searcher may choose the most appropriate. Some systems, such as PubMed and Internet Grateful Med, will automatically match the search subject to MeSH headings. A MeSH fact sheet is available from the National Library of Medicine Web site at http://www.nlm.nih.gov/mesh/meshhome.html.

MEDLINE DATABASE

The most commonly searched database is MEDLINE, and as such it is a logical starting point for searching the literature on disease outbreaks. MEDLINE is one of the MEDLARS databases offered by the National Library of Medicine. It contains data from 3,900 biomedical journals published in the United States and 70 medical journals published in other countries. Citations and abstracts for articles from 1966 to the present are given when available.

It is important to know several points to ensure a successful MEDLINE search.

- The MEDLINE database system searches only subject headings unless a text word, author, or journal search is specified.
- The journal articles are indexed to the most specific MeSH available, so selecting a heading that accurately reflects the search topic is important.
- Sometimes a searcher wants to retrieve articles on all facets of the subject. Some search systems, such as Internet Grateful Med, automatically "explode the heading." This option uses the broad heading and all narrower and more specific terms as well. Many search systems do not do this automatically and some do not even provide the option.
- After "exploding the headings," a searcher may wish to restrict the focus, an option that MEDLINE permits. For example, a searcher may wish to restrict the focus of the search to those terms that are the most important. This restriction is indicated by an asterisk preceding the terms. Restricting the focus will limit the number of articles received.

- After restriction of the focus of a search on MEDLINE, a further restriction can also be performed. The system displays a listing of subheadings that describe aspects of the subject, such as diagnosis, complications, etiology, therapy, prevention, and control. Proper selection from the menu of subheadings will eliminate retrieval of articles that do not pertain to the specific area of interest of the search. Retrieval of articles can be further reduced by selection of articles limited to, for example, humans, specific journals, publications in English, year of publication, or articles with abstracts displayed.
- Additionally, a search can be performed by text word, rather than by subject. This type of search is useful when a subject is new and a MeSH heading has not yet been assigned or when a MeSH heading may not be specific enough to limit retrieval to a certain topic. Searches can also be done by author and by journal title.

If a search yields zero articles, the following possibilities should be considered and a new search initiated:

- Check the search terms for typos and misspellings.
- Avoid use of acronyms; spell out the full term (e.g., Magnetic Resonance Imaging , not MRI).
- Spell out the first few letters of the name of a particular journal (do not abbreviate, as some systems require the full name).
- Simplify the number of terms used in the search.
- Avoid overuse of subheadings or the "limit set" options.
- Attempt a search under text words as well as MeSH headings.
- Use the "explode" command, if the search service doesn't do it automatically. Failure to do this results in retrieval only of articles indexed to the main MeSH term used in the search, and articles indexed to the more specific terms within the search subject are overlooked. An excellent resource on MEDLINE searching, including search strategies and exercises, can be found in Chapter 2 of Greenhalgh's text *How to Read a Paper*, BMJ Publishing Group, 1997.

Performing a MEDLINE search, followed by a search of other relevant databases, such as CINHAL or TOXLINE, should be the first strategy employed in a quest for relevant published literature because it is most likely to yield rapid results. However, there are many other information resources that, depending on the type of outbreak, are important to query. A brief description of some of the most useful resources that individual health care professionals or any member of the public can query follows below. This is not meant to be an exhaustive list, nor does it contain those databases such as the National Electronic Telecommunications System for Surveillance (NETSS), access to which is restricted to state/city public health officials. Rather, it is a listing of resources that may be useful to a health care professional investigating an outbreak of infection in an acute, intermediate, long-term, or ambulatory health care facility. While these databases/data banks are publicly available for searching, the Centers for Disease Control and Prevention (CDC) recommends first contacting an epidemiologist in the state's health department or the Investigation and Prevention Branch of the Hospital Infections Program at CDC (telephone: 404-639-6139) for assistance in investigation of nosocomial infection outbreaks.

U.S. GOVERNMENTAL AGENCY RESOURCES

Centers for Disease Control and Prevention and Agency for Toxic Substances and Disease Registry Information Resources

The Centers for Disease Control and Prevention and the Agency for Toxic Substances and Disease Registry (ATSDR) are resources for public health information and for information retrieval tools. Information is available via computer and automated telephone systems, as discussed below.

CDC Voice Information System

The CDC's Voice Information System (VIS) provides telephone access to prerecorded messages on many communicable diseases. As the messages are often written at the level of the lay person, they may be useful for patient education purposes. This service also provides information on late-breaking news and outbreaks. VIS may be called at 404-332-4555, or a request for information may be faxed to 404-332-4565. There is no charge for documents faxed or mailed to users.

CDC Home Page

The CDC home page (http://www.cdc.gov) is the jumping-off point for information on a variety of CDC resources (e.g., press summaries regarding infectious and noninfectious diseases of public health interest, health information brochures for the general public, training opportunities, information on CDC software and publications, and links to related sites). An excellent option available on the CDC home page is a link to data and statistics on various communicable diseases. It is possible to obtain, for example, the number of cases of tuberculosis, salmonellosis, hepatitis B, etc., in the United States. This site can be accessed directly at http://www.cdc.gov/nchswww/fastats/infectis.htm.

Rates of various nosocomial infections, updated semiannually, from the National Nosocomial Infections Surveillance system can be found at the CDC Hospital Infections Program (HIP) home page at http://www.cdc.gov/ncidod/hip/default.htm. Information on outbreak management and CDC guidelines on topics such as vancomycin-intermediate-resistant *Staphylococcus aureus*, Infection Control in Health Care Personnel, and Prevention of Surgical Site Infections are available at the HIP home page. It is also possible to link to a section entitled Epidemiologic Studies and Outbreaks, where information regarding other links to publications on outbreaks of hepatitis A, B, and C, as well as to the investigation of bacterial contamination of blood- and transfusion-associated reactions, can be found.

Guidelines for prevention and control of infection, access to the *Morbidity and Mortality Weekly Report* (MMWR), and links to many other public health resources are also available from the CDC home page.

Morbidity and Mortality Weekly Report *Journal*

The MMWR contains reports on outbreaks of infectious and noninfectious diseases and statistics on notifiable diseases and conditions reported by state health departments to CDC. The MMWR can be accessed in a variety of ways: through the CDC home page, via CDC Wonder (see below), via Medscape, or by subscribing to a CDC e-mail list. The MMWR is searchable by subject and date. Two additional MMWR publications, "Surveillance Summaries" and "Reports and Recommendations," are available electronically through the CDC home page or CDC Wonder. All of these reports can be downloaded as Acrobat (pdf) files, which can be read using a software program called Adobe Acrobat Reader that is available (for free) on the CDC home page. A full-text version of these reports is also available (for free) on Medscape (http://www.medscape.com) and can be read using a Web browser.

An e-mail subscription to the MMWR list can be obtained by sending an e-mail to lists@list.cdc.gov and typing in the body of the message the following: subscribe mmwr-toc. A weekly notification of the contents of MMWR and instructions on how to access the contents is then sent via e-mail to the subscriber.

Emerging Infectious Diseases *Journal*

Emerging Infectious Diseases (EID) is a peer-reviewed Internet journal that is published quarterly by the National Center for Infectious Diseases. The purpose of the journal is to improve the understanding of new and reemerging infectious diseases and to delineate prevention and control strategies. The journal includes a section entitled Perspectives that discusses social and biological factors that influence disease emergence. The Synopses section summarizes current knowledge regarding specific infectious diseases. The Dispatch section contains epidemiologic reports of outbreaks throughout the world. EID also contains a letters section, book reviews, guidelines published by national and international agencies, and information about national and international conferences. EID can be accessed from the CDC home page or directly at http://www.cdc.gov/ncidod/eid/eid.htm. Contents of past and upcoming issues can be viewed easily by clicking on the hypertext (boldfaced text) at the top of the electronic page. Articles can be viewed on screen by selecting the hypertext. Options given for downloading are Adobe PDF, ASCII Text, or Postscript. The journal can be searched by subject and issue.

CDC Wonder

CDC Wonder was developed for the public health professional to provide access to morbidity and mortality data for infectious and noninfectious diseases and for occupational injuries. Features of CDC Wonder that may be helpful in the investigation of an outbreak are:

- A listing of objectives and related data for the Healthy People 2000 initiative. One of the objectives of the Healthy People 2000 initiative is to lower the rate of surgical site infection in the United States by 20 percent. If a facility is experiencing an increased incidence of surgical site infection, infection control personnel may wish to obtain national rates for surgical site infection for comparison purposes. A request may be submitted for data on surgical site infections that give rates per 100 operations. This may be useful for obtaining a rough estimate of the rate; however, it should be noted that to obtain risk-adjusted rates for specific types of operations, the CDC Hospital Infections Program, National Nosocomial Infection Surveillance (NNIS) system, data should be queried at http://www.cdc.gov.

- Full text of the MMWR from February 12, 1982, forward is available for downloading, including associated tables and figures.
- Mortality counts and rates by age, race, gender, year, state and county of residence, and underlying causes of death can be found here.
- Surveillance statistics and national trends for tuberculosis and sexually transmitted diseases are available from this site.

CDC Wonder can be obtained in two ways. The easiest way is via the CDC home page (http://www.cdc.gov). If Internet access is unavailable, the CDC Wonder databases can also be accessed via computer (DOS-based) and modem (the information from the databases is downloaded to your computer via the modem). Special software and an account are required. The software, instruction manual, and account cost can be obtained from USD, 2075 A West Park Place, Stone Mountain, GA 30087. The phone number for USD is 770-469-4098; the fax number is 770-469-0681. The cost of the account is $23 and there are no usage fees. Since the software and manual are in the public domain, it is permissible to obtain them from a colleague and duplicate them.

National Center for Infectious Diseases

The National Center for Infectious Diseases (NCID) mission is to prevent illness, disability, and death from infectious diseases in the United States and around the world. The NCID home page can be reached either via a link from the CDC home page or directly at http://www.cdc.gov/ncidod/diseases/diseases.htm.

The NCID home page provides links to EID and to Pulse Net, a national network of public health laboratories that perform DNA fingerprinting on bacteria associated with foodborne outbreaks. The NCID data bank can be searched; however, the search parameters cannot be limited in the same way that some search ser-

vices allow (e.g., by English language, humans, year of publication, etc.).

National Institute for Occupational Safety and Health Information System

The National Institute for Occupational Safety and Health (NIOSH) home page can be found at http://www.cdc.gov/niosh/home page.html. Statistics on occupational injury as well as information on prevention and control are found on NIOSH's home page. Information on how to request a NIOSH investigation of a hazard in the workplace is also given. Information on requesting a NIOSH investigation can also be obtained by calling 800-356-4674.

Agency for Toxic Substances and Disease Registry

The Hazardous Substance Release/Health Effects Database (HazDat) contains substance-specific information on hazardous substances in the Agency for Toxic Substances and Disease Registry. Included are health effects of toxic substances by route and duration of exposure. HazDat is accessible through the Internet at http://atsdrl.atsdr.cdc.gov:8080/hazdat.html. The database can be searched by single words.

WORLD HEALTH ORGANIZATION

The World Health Organization (WHO) can be accessed at http://www.who.ch. *The Weekly Epidemiological Record* published by WHO provides information on infectious disease incidence and outbreaks worldwide. Adobe Acrobat Reader, available for free from the CDC home page, is needed to read these reports.

In May 1998, the Canadian government, in cooperation with WHO, launched a system called the Global Public Health Intelligence Network (GPHIN) that continuously scans the Internet, news wires, public health e-mail systems, and local on-line newspapers worldwide looking for information about disease outbreaks. The system extracts meaningful and properly validated information, which is transmitted to public health experts at Health Canada and at the World Health Organization, making possible timely reporting, investigation, and control of outbreaks.

OTHER NONGOVERNMENTAL ELECTRONIC RESOURCES FOR OUTBREAK INVESTIGATION

Program for Monitoring Emerging Diseases

The Program for Monitoring Emerging Diseases (ProMed) is a resource for monitoring disease outbreaks around the world. Reports describing outbreaks of disease in humans, domestic and wild animals, and plants, made by scientists and public health workers from all over the globe, are posted daily to the ProMed mailing list. The mailing list is monitored and the subjects are indexed. Questions can be posted to this list. It is probably the premier mailing list devoted to communicating information on outbreaks of infectious disease.

This resource can be accessed in one of two ways. A subscription to the ProMed mailing list can be obtained by sending an e-mail message to majordomo@usa. healthnet.org and in the body of the message typing the following: subscribe ProMed-digest. Subscribers receive a daily e-mail of the discussions taking place via this mailing list, as well as instructions on posting queries and reviewing the indexes of past discussions. The other way to view ProMed without actually subscribing is to visit the Medscape home page (http://www. medscape.com) and look at the Infectious Diseases section.

Association for Professionals in Infection Control and Epidemiology

The Association for Professionals in Infection Control and Epidemiology (APIC) provides several resources for health care professionals with queries regarding outbreak investigation. APIC maintains a mailing list using e-mail-based technology to host queries and discussion from infection control professionals regarding investigation, prevention, and control of infection in health care facilities. The list is open to anyone with an interest in the practice of infection control and applied epidemiology. Membership in APIC is not a prerequisite to participation in the list. A subscription to the list can be obtained by sending an e-mail to listserv@peach.ease.com and in the body of the message typing: subscribe APIC. An e-mail response will request confirmation of the sender's e-mail address, after which the subscriber will receive confirma-

tion of the subscription and further instructions on list usage.

APIC also maintains a discussion forum section on its Web site (http://www.apic.org) to promote communication and exchange of information regarding infection control issues. The Web site features the ability to search published abstracts in the area of clinical epidemiology and infection control, presented at the APIC Annual Educational and International Conference. CDC and APIC guidelines that address various topics for prevention and control of infection are available through APIC by calling 202-789-1890 to request a hard copy.

Another service provided by APIC that may be helpful in searching the literature when investigating an outbreak is the APIC Resource Line. The Resource Line was started to provide informative responses to infection control professionals who have exhausted their available searching resources on their topic of interest. The Resource Line is provided as a membership service for current APIC members; however, the service is available to nonmembers at a cost of $50 per inquiry. The APIC Resource Line does not provide specific answers to clinical questions; rather, it identifies resources and information for individuals to use in making informed decisions. Resource Line requests can be made by calling 202-789-1890 or by sending an e-mail to resource@apic.org. APIC members must include their membership number with their request. Responses to Resource Line requests typically take 10 business days.

WEB DIRECTORIES AND SEARCH ENGINES

The discussion of medical literature search strategies for outbreak investigation began with the strategy that should yield the most rapid and sensitive search for information, i.e., MEDLINE searching or searching of the other databases and data banks listed in Table 9–1. The logical second-line strategy is to search government agency resources such as those provided by CDC and ATSDR. The resource chosen for search should be determined by the nature of the outbreak under investigation. It is equally important to use nongovernment resources such as ProMed and APIC. While ProMed provides an excellent resource for discussion of worldwide community-based outbreaks, APIC is a premier

Table 9–3 World Wide Web Search Directories

Directory	Description	URL
Achoo	Directory to health care-related information.	http://www.achoo.com
EINet Galaxy	Directory of Web pages, gopher, and telnet sites.	http://galaxy.einet.net
LookSmart	Directory that provides a road map to the Web.	http://www.looksmart.com
Magellan	Evaluated sites, including newsgroups, listservs, and mailing lists.	http://www.magellan.com
Yahoo	Weekly updates on new Web sites and daily headlines.	http://www.yahoo.com

resource for discussion and information on a wide variety of health care facility-based outbreaks, as well as guidelines for prevention and control. Once all of these resources have been exhausted, it is advisable to search the World Wide Web, utilizing one of the Web directories or search engines.

Web directories provide a hierarchically organized subject access to the World Wide Web and other Internet functions. Most provide a function for searching within sections of their directories. Some popular directories are listed in Table 9–3.

Search engines are programs or services that allow you to enter specific words or phrases. The program looks for Web pages that contain those search strings in titles or content. Each search engine has different ways of entering search strings, and indexes different, but overlapping, selections of Web sites and other Internet services. Table 9–4 contains a list of popular search

Table 9–4 Popular Search Engines

Search Engine	Description	URL
AltaVista	Index of over 22 million Web pages. Full-text index of more than 13,000 newsgroups. Offers simple word, phrase, and advanced queries. Searches text words of page. Very comprehensive database.	http://www.altavista.digital.com
Excite	Includes database of 50,000 reviewed Web pages. Can do simple as well as advanced searches.	http://www.excite.com
InfoSeek	Indexes Web pages, usenet newsgroups, FTP and gopher sites, e-mail addresses, and frequently asked questions. Does not use Boolean operators—AND, OR—in searching. Search results cannot be bookmarked, i.e., stored for future reference.	http://guide.infoseek.com
Lycos	Indexes URLs and links to pages. Searches on title, headings, links, keywords, and first 20 lines of Web pages.	http://www.lycos.com
Health A to Z	Medical search engine that ranks results based on a reliable site review and categorizes them according to audience, i.e., patient or professional or both. Information provided is oriented more to the lay person but would be useful for health education.	http://www.healthatoz.com
Medis Search	Uses the Lycos search engine to find URLs of more than 70 journals with established reputations that have content on-line, either as abstracts or, in some instances, full-text articles. The reader should recall that a MEDLINE search indexes 3,900 U.S. journals alone!	http://www.docnet.org.uk/medisn/searchs.html
Medical World Search	Produced by Brooklyn Polytechnic University. Indexes information from reputable educational facilities, agencies, and organizations.	http://www.mwsearch.com/

engines with their features and includes two medical search engines.

Is it better to use a search directory or a search engine? The answer depends on what the searcher is looking for. If a searcher is seeking general information on a topic (e.g., urinary tract infection), a directory will be the best choice. But if a searcher is looking for something very specific (e.g., urinary tract infection and indwelling catheters), the outcome will probably be more successful using a search engine. A good discussion of when to use a search engine and when to explore with a directory can be found in the help pages for LookSmart at http://www.looksmart.com/h/info/exploreorsearch.html.

Caution should be exercised when evaluating information found as a result of searching the WWW. Individuals, organizations, medical centers, companies, and governmental agencies produce Web documents. Very little of the information published on the WWW is peer reviewed, with the exception of the specific governmental and nongovernmental sites listed above.

Therefore, a searcher must use the utmost of care in assessing the value of what is found on the Web. To judge a document's validity, a searcher should consider the sponsoring body. Generally government organizations, known national organizations, and academic institutions are reliable sources of factual information. Information about the author and the publication date is usually available at the end of a document, along with an e-mail address for directing comments or questions. Some sites have editorial boards and include details about their members. In attempting to judge the validity of information, a searcher should see if it can be confirmed by other sources as well. These are all caveats to keep in mind when searching the World Wide Web. A generalized Web search should be undertaken only after exhausting the other strategies listed above. Caution should be the byword! A carefully conducted search of the medical literature, utilizing the resources listed in this chapter, is a critical step in outbreak investigation and management.

CHAPTER 10

Statistical Methods Used in Outbreak Investigation

Deborah Y. Phillips and Kathleen Meehan Arias

The source(s) and route(s) of exposure must be determined to understand why an outbreak occurred, how to prevent similar outbreaks in the future, and, if the outbreak is ongoing, how to prevent others from being exposed to the source(s) of infection.

Arthur L. Reingold[1]

INTRODUCTION

It can be frustrating to have a sense that there is an outbreak occurring and yet have no data to substantiate this belief. Basic statistical methods can be used to organize, summarize, and analyze data to determine if there are trends or associations in observations. Statistical methods allow the researcher to find the answers to epidemiologic questions such as the following:

- Are there more cases of a disease than usual or expected? (Note: The term "disease" is used in this chapter to describe an adverse health-related event such as an infection, illness, or injury.)
- Is there a cause-and-effect relationship between an exposure and a disease?
- Could the event be random occurrence?

This chapter includes a basic description of the statistical measures used to describe and analyze an outbreak and is intended to be an introduction to the statistical methods commonly used in health care epidemiology, such as frequency measures and measures of central tendency, association, and dispersion. It includes a brief discussion on the use of analytic studies (cohort and case-control studies) and on statistical inference theory (including the concepts of hypothesis testing, probability, and statistical significance). Since a thorough discussion of each of these concepts cannot be accomplished in one chapter, the reader who wishes to obtain more information on these topics is referred to the references noted or to one of the textbooks listed in the Suggested Reading list at the end of this chapter. For those seeking an explanation of the statistical methods commonly used to analyze data presented in the medical literature, the series of six articles by Gaddis and Gaddis is recommended.[2–7]

Numerous computer database and statistical programs are available and these have virtually eliminated the need to calculate complicated statistical formulas by hand or by using a handheld calculator. Nevertheless, those responsible for implementing infection control and quality management programs still need to be familiar with the statistical measures discussed in this chapter and when these measures are used.

When investigating an outbreak, the investigator begins by using descriptive statistics to describe the person, place, and time characteristics of the outbreak, as described in Chapter 8. If the most likely risk factors responsible for the outbreak cannot be identified during the descriptive phase, then an analytic study is designed and conducted. An analytic study attempts to associate potential risk factors or exposures with the development of disease and to determine the strength of that association. Case-control or cohort studies are the analytic study methods that are most frequently used in outbreak investigations to compare rates of disease in various populations in order to determine which exposures or risk factors are most likely responsible for the disease. Although the investigator must be familiar with the use and limitations of these studies, the authors recommend that a statistician be consulted if advanced statistical analysis is necessary when conducting an outbreak investigation.

DESCRIPTIVE STATISTICS

Frequency Measures

Frequency measures are used to characterize the occurrence and risk of disease in a given population during a specified time period. The frequency measures commonly used in health care epidemiology are ratios, proportions, and rates. These three measures are based on the same formula:

$$\frac{x}{y} \times 10^n$$

in which x (the numerator) and y (the denominator) are the two groups that are being compared and 10^n is a constant that is used to transform the result to a convenient number (usually a number that has at least one digit to the left of the decimal place).

Ratios and Proportions

A ratio is a fraction in which the values in the numerator are not necessarily included in the denominator. This means that a ratio can be used to express the relationship between a numerator (x) and a denominator (y) when the two have independent values. One may use a ratio to indicate a relationship between two groups. The odds ratio and the risk ratio (or relative risk), which are discussed later in the chapter, are commonly used to measure associations between two groups.

A proportion is a type of ratio in which the values in the numerator are included in the denominator. A proportion is often expressed as a percentage. For example, in a sample of 69 case patients who developed a nosocomial urinary tract infection (UTI) over a 1-year period, 46 cases are females and 23 cases are males.

To calculate the ratio of female cases to male cases, the following formula is used:

$$x/y \times 10^0$$

in which x is 46 female cases, y is 23 male cases, and 10^0 is 1.

The ratio of females to males would be $46/23 \times 1 = 2/1$. Thus there are two females for each male who developed a nosocomial urinary tract infection. Note that the values in the numerator (the female patients) are not included in the denominator (the male patients).

To calculate the proportion of cases who are males, the following formula is used:

$$x/y \times 10^0$$

in which x is equal to 23 male cases, y is equal to 69 total cases who have a nosocomial UTI, and 10^0 is equal to 1.

The proportion of cases who are males would be $23/69 \times 1 = 1/3$. This means that one in every three cases is a male. If 10^n is 10^2 (100), then the proportion can be expressed as a percentage: $23/69 \times 100 = 33\%$. In this calculation, the values in the numerator (the male cases) are included in the denominator (the total number of cases).

Rates

As Last explains, "rates describe the frequency with which events occur."[8(p.28)] In other words, a rate measures the occurrence of an event in a defined population over time. Rates are used to track trends, such as the occurrence of nosocomial infections, over time. The rates most frequently used in health care epidemiology are incidence, prevalence, and attack rates. When an increase in a disease or other health-related event is suspected, rates can be calculated and used to determine if there is a change in the occurrence of disease from one period of time to the next.

Incidence rates. Incidence rates are used to measure and compare the frequency of new cases or events in a population. The formula is as follows:

$$\text{Incidence rate} = \frac{\text{the number of new cases that occur in a defined period}}{\text{the population at risk during the same period}} \times 10^n$$

One type of incidence rate is incidence density, which incorporates time (such as person-years, person-days, or device-days) in the denominator. This gives a more accurate reflection of the population at risk when the likelihood of developing a disease increases as the time of exposure increases. In health care epidemiology, incidence density is commonly used to calculate the incidence of nosocomial infections because the risk of developing a nosocomial infection increases as the length of time of exposure to the health care environment increases, as discussed in Chapter 2. Nosocomial infection rates are generally expressed as the number of infections per 1,000 person-days (such as patient-days or resident-days, depending on the type of facility). Incidence density is used to express the incidence of nosocomial infections that are associated with medical devices, such as mechanical ventilators or intravascular catheters, because the risk of developing an infection increases with the length of time the device is used. These rates are commonly expressed as the number of infections per 1,000 device-days (such as 3.2 bloodstream infections per 1,000 central line-days). The formula is as follows:

$$\text{Incidence density} = \frac{\text{the number of new cases that occur in a defined period}}{\text{the time each person in population at risk is observed, totaled for all persons}} \times 10^n$$

in which 10^n is usually 1,000 (to provide uniformity of results and to have the final value displayed with at least one digit to the left of the decimal point).

Another type of incidence rate, attack rate, is an incidence rate that is expressed as cases per 100 population (or as a percentage). It is used to describe the new cases of disease that have been observed in a particular group during a limited time period in special circumstances, such as during an epidemic. The formula is as follows:

$$\text{Attack rate} = \frac{\text{the number of new cases that occur in a population in a specified time period}}{\text{the population at risk at the beginning of time period}} \times 100$$

For example, a newborn nursery reports 17 infants with loose stools in 1 month. During this month, there were 120 patients and 480 patient-days in the newborn nursery. Using the formula above, the incidence rate would be calculated as follows:

$$\frac{\text{17 cases of loose stools in 1 month}}{\text{120 patients in newborn nursery during the month}} \times 100 = .142 \times 100 = \frac{\text{14.2 cases}}{\text{per 100 patients}}$$

In this example, the incidence rate is expressed as an attack rate (i.e., 14.2 percent of patients were affected)

because $10^n = 10^2$ or 100. Using the formula above, the incidence density would be calculated as follows:

$$\frac{\text{17 cases of loose stools in 1 month}}{\text{480 patient-days in the same month}} \times 1,000 = 0.0354 \times 1,000 = \frac{\text{35.4 cases}}{\text{per 1,000 patient-days}}$$

To determine if this incidence is higher than expected, this rate can be compared to the rates for the prior months. Sometimes it may not even be necessary to calculate a rate to determine if an event is unusual; it may be apparent if the disease is rare (such as a nosocomial infection with group A streptococcus). For example, during a 2-month period there were 175 patients admitted to the medical/surgical intensive care unit. Forty of the patients subsequently developed an infection with vancomycin-resistant *Enterococcus* (VRE). Eighty of the patients were medical patients and the remainder were surgical patients. Of the 40 patients with VRE infection, 30 were medical patients. The patient-days for this period were 450 for medical patients and 110 for surgical patients.

The overall attack rate for VRE infection in the unit would be calculated as follows:

$$40/175 \times 100 = 22.8\%$$

The VRE attack rate for medical patients would be calculated as follows:

$$30/80 \times 100 = 37.5\%$$

The VRE attack rate for surgical patients would be calculated as follows:

$$10/95 \times 100 = 10.5\%$$

The incidence density of VRE infection for medical patients would be calculated as follows:

$$30/450 \times 1,000 \text{ patient-days} = 66.7 \text{ infections per 1,000 patient-days}$$

The incidence density of VRE infection for surgical patients would be calculated as follows:

$$10/110 \times 1,000 \text{ patient-days} = 90.9 \text{ infections per 1,000 patient-days}$$

When analyzing the incidence of infections over time among patients on a hospital unit, an investigator should calculate the incidence density using patient-days as the denominator, because incidence density more accurately reflects the population at risk than the incidence rate.

Finally, in determining incidence rates, numerators and denominators must be chosen with care. As soon as an outbreak is suspected, cases should be identified using a case definition. When calculating incidence rates, the cases are included in the numerator data. Those in the population at risk are placed in the denominator data. It is important that those who are identified as the population at risk (i.e., the denominator) are free of the disease at the beginning of the study period. The selection of an appropriate denominator is one of the most important aspects of measuring disease frequency, as discussed in Chapter 2.

Prevalence rate. Prevalence is a measure of the number of active (new and old) cases in a specified population either during a given period of time (period prevalence) or at a given point in time (point prevalence). The formula for calculating the prevalence rate is as follows:

$$\text{Prevalence rate} = \frac{\begin{array}{c}\text{all new and existing cases} \\ \text{during a given period} \\ \text{or a given point in time}\end{array}}{\begin{array}{c}\text{population at risk} \\ \text{during same time period}\end{array}} \times 10^n$$

A prevalence rate is used to describe the current status of active disease at a particular time in a particular population. It is sometimes helpful to review the incidence and prevalence simultaneously. A low incidence (new cases) may be due to a high prevalence (new and existing cases) in a given population. For instance, if the incidence of infection or colonization with methicillin-resistant *Staphylococcus aureus* (MRSA) is relatively low on a patient care unit, but colonized patients remain in this unit for prolonged periods, an explanation for the low incidence (number of new cases) may be the high prevalence. This is because there are very few patients who are at risk, or free of MRSA, to become a new case.

Under stable conditions, that is, when incidence is not changing, the following formula can be used to show the relationship between incidence and prevalence[9]:

$$P = I \times D$$

where P is prevalence, I is incidence, and D is the average duration of disease. A high prevalence of disease in a population can occur if the incidence is high or if the duration of disease is long (such as occurs with chronic diseases or long-term colonization or infection with an infectious agent).

Adjusting rates. The rates of two dissimilar populations should not be compared unless the rates are adjusted for appropriate risk factors, such as age, gender, or other factors that affect the risk of disease. For instance, rates of infection in a population exposed to a medical device are frequently risk adjusted by incorporating into the denominator the number of days the medical device is in use (e.g., rates of central line–associated bloodstream infections are calculated using central line-days as the denominator). Similarly, rates of ventilator-associated pneumonia are calculated using ventilator-days as the denominator. The Centers for Disease Control and Prevention's (CDC) National Nosocomial Infection Surveillance (NNIS) system is an example of a system in which rates are risk adjusted to allow for interhospital comparison.[10]

Measures of Central Tendency

Measures of central tendency describe the values around the middle of a set of data. The mean, median, and mode are the principal measures of central tendency.

Mean

The mean, $\bar{x}$, is the mathematical average of the values in a set of data. The formula is as follows:

$$\bar{x} = \sum \frac{x_i}{n}$$

in which $\sum x_i$ is the sum of the individual values in a set and n is the number of values in the set. For example, if the ages among cases in an outbreak are 11, 7, 5, 3, and 4 years, then the mean is:

$$\frac{11 + 7 + 5 + 3 + 4}{5} = 30/5 = 6 \text{ years}$$

The value of the mean is affected by extreme values in the data set. For example, if a 65-year-old patient is added to the cases in the above data set, the mean, or average, would be $(11 + 7 + 5 + 3 + 4 + 65)/6 = 15.8$ years. When extreme values are in a data set, the data become skewed and the mean does not give a representative picture of the data, as shown in Figure 10–1. When there are extreme values in a data set, the median should be calculated.

Median

The median is the middle point—the value at which half the measurements lie below the value and half the measurements lie above the value.[8(p.80)] The median is useful when there are extreme values in a data set (i.e., the data are skewed).

The median in a data set is calculated as follows:

1. Rank order the values in either ascending or descending order.
2. Identify the midpoint of the sequence.
   a. If there are an odd number of values, the median is the middle value. For example, in the data set 11, 7, 5, 4, 3, the median is the middle value of 5.
   b. If there are an even number of values, then the midpoint between the two middle values is calculated. For example, if the ages in the data set are 11, 7, 6, 5, 4, 3 years, then the median is the midpoint between 6 and 5, or (6 + 5)/2 = 5.5 years.

Mode

The mode is the most frequently occurring value in a set of observations. For example, if the ages in a group of controls are 5, 6, 7, 7, 7, 8, 12, then the mode would be 7.

Some data sets are characterized as bimodal, or having two modes. For example, a sample of ages of cases consisting of the values 3, 4, 4, 5, 5, 5, 5, 5, 5, 6, 7, 8, 9, 9, 9, 9, 9, 13 would be bimodal, the two modes being 5 and 9 years of age. Some authors have described such a distribution by identifying the major and the minor modes (in this case, the value 5 would be the major mode because it occurs six times, and the value 9 would be the minor mode because it occurs five times). The mode is less affected by skewness (outliers) than is the mean or the median. Mode is not often used as a measure of central tendency, particularly in small data sets.[8(p.82)]

Skewness

In a normal (symmetric) distribution, the mean, median, and mode have the same value. A curve or histogram that is not symmetrical is referred to as skewed or asymmetrical, as shown in Figure 10–1. A curve that is said to be negatively skewed, as shown in this figure, has a tail off to the left and most of the values lie above the mean. The mean is less than the median, which is less than the mode. In contrast, a positively skewed curve would depict a mirror image of this and the mean will be greater than the median, which will be greater than the mode.

Measures of Dispersion

The measures of dispersion describe the distribution of values in a data set around its mean. The most commonly used measures of dispersion are range, deviation, variance, and standard deviation.

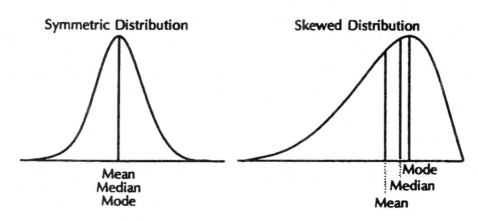

Figure 10–1 Effect of Skewness on the Mean, Median, and Mode. *Source:* Reprinted from *Principles of Epidemiology: An Introduction to Applied Epidemiology and Biostatistics,* 2nd ed., p. 187, 1992, Centers for Disease Control and Prevention, Department of Health and Human Services.

Range

The difference between the highest and lowest values in a data set is termed the "range."[8(p.110)] For example, if the length of antibiotic use among cases is 7, 8, 9, 10, and 14 days; the range is $14 - 7 = 7$ days.

Deviation

The deviation is the difference between an individual measurement in a data set and the mean value for the set. It is expressed as follows:

$$\text{deviation} = x_i - \bar{x}$$

in which x_i is the i-th observation and $\bar{x}$ is the mean.

A measurement may have no deviation (it is equal to the mean), a negative deviation (it is less than the mean), or a positive deviation (it is greater than the mean).

Variance

The variance measures the deviation around the mean of a distribution. It is also called the mean sum of squares or mean square because it is the sum of the squares of deviations from the mean divided by the number of degrees of freedom in the sample set. The variance (s^2) for a sample is expressed as follows:

$$s^2 = \frac{\sum \left(x_i - \bar{x}\right)^2}{n - 1}$$

in which Σ is the sum of, i is the i-th observation ($x_1 =$ first observation, $x_2 =$ second observation, etc.), $\bar{x}$ is the mean, and n is the number of observations.

Standard Deviation

The standard deviation, which may be represented as s or SD, is a measure of dispersion that reflects the distribution of values around the mean. When calculating the standard deviation for a sample, the following formula is used:

$$SD = \sqrt{\frac{\sum \left(x_i - \bar{x}\right)^2}{n - 1}}$$

in which Σ is the sum of, x_i is the i-th observation, $\bar{x}$ is the mean, and n is the number of observations.

As can be seen by comparing the two formulas, the standard deviation is the square root of the variance. The standard deviation is always a non-negative quantity. If the values in a data set are close to the mean, the standard deviation is small (i.e., the values are distributed closely around the mean). If the values in a data set are not close to the mean, the standard deviation is large. For example, the incubation periods for six cases of hepatitis A related to a foodborne outbreak range from 24 to 31 days. Calculate the variance and standard deviation to describe this distribution. Use the data shown in Table 10–1, and the formulas above to calculate the variance and standard deviation.

1. Calculate the mean using the data in the first column (x_i).

$$\bar{x} = \Sigma x_i / n = 168/6 = 28.0$$

2. Subtract the mean from each observation to find the deviations from the mean (shown in the second column). (Note: the sum of the deviations from the mean will always equal zero because the mean is the arithmetic center of the distribution.)
3. Square the deviations from the mean (shown in the third column).
4. Sum the squared deviations (see the third column):

$$\Sigma (x_i - \bar{x})^2 = 40$$

5. Divide the sum of the squared deviations by $n - 1$ to find the variance:

$$\Sigma (x_i - \bar{x})^2 / n - 1 = 40/5 = 8$$

Table 10–1 Calculating the Variance and Standard Deviation

x_i (Observations)	$x_i - \bar{x}$ (Deviations from the Mean)		$(x_i - \bar{x})^2$ (Square of the Deviations)
24	$24 - 28.0 = -4.0$		16
25	$25 - 28.0 = -3.0$		9
29	$29 - 28.0 =$	$+1.0$	1
29	$29 - 28.0 =$	$+1.0$	1
30	$30 - 28.0 =$	$+2.0$	4
31	$31 - 28.0 =$	$+3.0$	9
168	$-7.0 + 7.0 = 0$		40

Note: x_i = i-th observation; $\bar{x}$ = mean.

Source: Reprinted from *Principles of Epidemiology: An Introduction to Applied Epidemiology and Biostatistics,* 2nd ed., pp. 174–175, 1992, Centers for Disease Control and Prevention, Department of Health and Human Services.

6. Take the square root of the variance to calculate the standard deviation:

$$SD = \sqrt{s^2} = \sqrt{8} = 2.8$$

Normal Distribution

A normal distribution represents the natural distribution of values around the mean with progressively fewer observations toward the extremes of the range of values. A normal distribution plotted on a graph shows a bell-shaped curve, in which 68.3 percent of the values will fall within one standard deviation of the mean, 95.5 percent of the values will fall within two standard deviations of the mean, and 99.7 percent of the values will fall within three standard deviations of the mean as shown in Figure 10–2. Statistical inferences about a sample, such as the cases of disease in a population, are frequently based on a normal distribution.

Measures of Association

Measures of association are used during outbreak investigations to evaluate the relationship between exposed and unexposed populations. These statistical measures can express the strength of association between a risk factor (exposure) and an outcome (disease). The measures of association used for outbreak investigations are the risk ratio (or relative risk) and the odds ratio. A two-by-two table (shown in Table 10–2) is used to show comparisons between exposures and outcomes and to calculate risk ratios and odds ratios.

The Risk Ratio (Relative Risk)

The risk ratio is the ratio of the attack rate (or risk of disease) in the exposed population to the attack rate (or risk of disease) in the unexposed population. Using Table 10–2, the attack rate for the exposed population would be a/a + b and the attack rate for the unexposed population would be c/c + d. The risk ratio is therefore calculated as follows:

$$\text{Risk ratio (relative risk)} = \frac{a/a + b}{c/c + d}$$

If the value of the risk ratio (relative risk) is equal to 1, the risk is the same in the two groups and there is no evidence of association between the exposure and outcome.

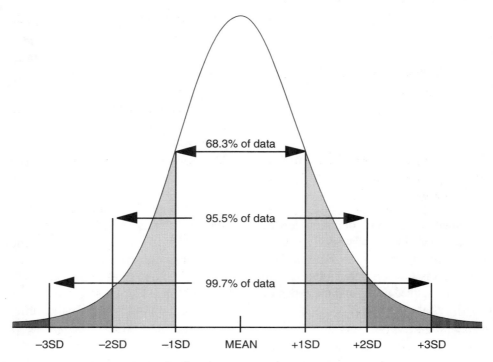

Figure 10–2 Areas under the Normal Curve That Lie between 1, 2, and 3 Standard Deviations on Each Side of the Mean. *Source:* Reprinted from *Principles of Epidemiology: An Introduction to Applied Epidemiology and Biostatistics,* 2nd ed., p. 177, 1992, Centers for Disease Control and Prevention, Department of Health and Human Services.

Table 10–2 The Two-by-Two Table

	Disease	No Disease	Total
Exposed	a	b	a + b
Unexposed	c	d	c + d
Total	a + c	b + d	N

Note: a, those with exposure and disease; b, those with exposure and no disease; c, those with no exposure and disease; d, those with no exposure and no disease; a + c, total of those with disease; b + d, total of those with no disease; a + b, total of those with exposure; c + d, total of those with no exposure; N = a + b + c + d, total population in the study.

If the risk ratio is greater than 1, the risk is higher for the exposed group and the exposure may be associated with the outcome. If the risk ratio is less than 1, the risk is lower for the exposed group and the exposure may possibly protect against the outcome. An investigator can calculate a risk ratio, or relative risk, from the data collected in a cohort study, which is discussed later.

The Odds Ratio

The odds ratio is similar to the risk ratio except that the odds, instead of the risk (attack rates), are used in the calculation. An odds ratio can be used to approximate the strength of association between an exposure and a disease (outcome). The odds ratio is the ratio of the probability of having a risk factor if the disease is present to the probability of having the risk factor if the disease is absent. Using the two-by-two table, it is calculated as follows:

$$\frac{a/b}{c/d} = \frac{a \times d}{b \times c} \text{ or}$$

$$\text{Odds ratio} = \frac{\dfrac{\text{exposed cases}}{\text{exposed controls}}}{\dfrac{\text{unexposed cases}}{\text{unexposed controls}}} = \frac{\text{exposed cases} \times \text{unexposed controls}}{\dfrac{\text{unexposed cases}}{\text{exposed controls}}}$$

If the odds ratio is equal to 1, the odds of disease are the same if the exposure is present and if it is absent (i.e., there is no evidence of association between the exposure and disease). If the odds ratio is greater than 1, the odds of disease are higher for the exposed group and the exposure is probably associated with the disease.

Confidence Intervals

In an outbreak investigation, if the exposure rates of the cases differ from those of the controls, statistical tests of significance can be done to determine if the difference was likely to have occurred by chance alone or if there may indeed be a causal relationship between the exposure and disease. Probability, or *P*, values traditionally have been used to describe the significance of the findings; however, many authors have recommended that confidence intervals be used, either in place of or in addition to the *P* value to explain the findings.[11–16] A *P* value (discussed below) provides information on statistical significance but does not provide information on the magnitude or precision of the findings. By computing an odds ratio or a risk ratio (which are termed "point estimates") and a confidence interval, the investigator can provide information on the strength of an association, the precision of the estimate, and the statistical significance.

The confidence interval (CI), sometimes referred to as the margin of error of a study, has been defined as "the computed interval with a stated probability (usually 95%) that the true value of a variable, such as the mean, proportion, or rate, falls within the interval."[17(p.26)] In other words, a person using a 95 percent CI can be confident that if a study were repeated many times, the observed value would fall within the confidence interval in 95 out of 100 studies. Unlike the *P* value, which provides information on statistical significance only, the confidence interval expresses the statistical precision of a point estimate (an observed effect, such as a risk ratio or odds ratio) and the strength of an association. The statistical precision is measured by the size (range) of the confidence interval: the narrower the computed interval, the more precise the estimate. The strength of the association is measured by the magnitude of the difference in the measured outcomes between the two groups (e.g., the higher the numerical value of the risk ratio, the more likely the exposure is related to the outcome).

Confidence intervals provide an alternative to hypothesis testing when ratios of risk or rates are being compared. A 95 percent CI provides information on whether or not an observation is statistically significant with a *P* value less than or equal to 0.05. As noted previously, an odds (or risk) ratio of 1.0 means that the odds (or risk) of disease are the same between the comparison groups whether or not the exposure occurs. If the value of an odds ratio is greater than one, the probability of having a risk factor if the disease is present is greater than the probability of having the risk factor if the disease is absent. If the value of a risk ratio is greater than one, the risk of disease in the exposed population is greater than the risk of disease in the unexposed population. If a ratio's 95 percent CI does not include 1.0, then statistical significance is implied ($P \leq 0.05$). If the CI for an odds or risk ratio includes 1.0, then the findings are not statistically significant.

For example, if the odds ratio (the point estimate) for an exposure is said to be 8.2 with a 95 percent confidence interval of 6.2–10.6, this means: (1) persons with the disease were 8.2 times more likely to have been exposed to the risk factor than those without the disease and (2) one can be 95 percent confident (probability of 0.95) that the odds ratio in the population is between the confidence limits of 6.2 and 10.6 (i.e., it may be as low as 6.2 or as high as 10.6). In addition, since the lower limit of this observed confidence interval is well above 1.0 (which equals no association), it is implied that the results are statistically significant at the 0.05 level.

As another example, if an odds ratio is 1.6 with a 95 percent CI of 0.8–2.4, then the findings are not statistically significant because unity (one) is included in the confidence interval.

Although *P* values alone traditionally have been used to show the statistical significance between disease and risk factors in outbreaks, odds ratios/risk ratios and 95 percent confidence intervals are now frequently reported. For example, in a report of a 1998 outbreak of *Shigella sonnei* infection associated with eating fresh parsley, the Centers for Disease Control and Prevention presented the following data:

> In a case-control study of 172 ill and 95 well restaurant patrons, five items were associated with illness: water (odds ratio {OR} = 1.9; 95% confidence interval {CI} = 1.0–3.8); ice (OR = 3.7; 95% CI = 1.6–8.6); potatoes (OR = 2.6; 95% CI = 1.5–4.6); uncooked parsley (OR = 4.3; 95% CI = 2.4–8.0); and raw tomato (OR = 1.9; 95% CI = 1.0–3.9). In a multivariate analysis, only uncooked parsley (OR = 4.3; p less than 0.01) and ice (OR = 6.9; p less than 0.01) remained significantly associated with illness.[18]

As illustrated by this report, when a point estimate and confidence interval are given, the reader has more information with which to interpret the results than if a *P* value alone is reported because the magnitude of the odds ratio provides an estimate of the strength of association between a disease and a risk factor and the con-

fidence interval provides an estimate of the statistical significance and the precision of this finding. For instance, in this report the odds ratio for uncooked parsley was 4.3, which means that those who were ill were 4.3 times more likely to have eaten uncooked parsley than those who were not ill. The CI of 2.4–8.0 infers that these findings are statistically significant because the lower confidence limit of 2.4 is well above 1.0.

Confidence intervals can be computed using computer programs, formulas, tables, or graphs—the method varies according to the type of data. Because the methods used to calculate them are complex, a discussion of the computation of confidence intervals is beyond the scope of this chapter. For more information, the reader should refer to the references given[11–16] or to one of the statistics texts listed in the Suggested Reading list at the end of this chapter. In practice, an investigator should consult a statistician to ensure that the correct method will be used to compute any confidence intervals used to describe the findings of an outbreak investigation.

ANALYTIC STUDIES

Analytic studies are used to compare rates of disease between two groups. This comparison allows an investigator to (1) quantify relationships between risk factors and disease and (2) to determine the strength of association in these causal relationships. Analytic studies are used to test the hypotheses proposed to explain the occurrence of an outbreak.

There are two major categories of epidemiologic studies used to examine cause and effect: experimental and observational. In experimental studies, the investigator controls the exposures to specific factors and then follows the subjects to determine the effect of the exposure (e.g., a clinical trial of a new drug). In observational studies, the investigator observes the natural course of events. Observational studies are used to analyze outbreaks because the investigator is observing the outcomes to prior exposures over which the investigator has no control. The two types of observational studies most commonly used in outbreak investigations are the retrospective cohort study and the case-control study.

Cohort Studies and the Risk Ratio (Relative Risk)

In a cohort study, subjects are categorized based on their *exposure* to a specific factor and then they are observed to see if they develop a disease. A cohort study may be conducted prospectively or retrospectively. In a prospective cohort study, subjects may be observed over a prolonged period of time in order to examine the natural history or incidence (risk) of a disease. The Framingham Study is an example of a well-known, long-term prospective cohort study that has produced many reports on cardiovascular disease.[19] Using a retrospective cohort study, an event that has already occurred (such as an outbreak) can be analyzed by reconstructing records of exposures and studying their outcomes. A retrospective cohort study can be used only when studying a well-defined population, such as the attendees of a luncheon or the patients of a surgeon. It cannot be used if the true population at risk cannot be identified (such as an outbreak associated with a widely distributed commercial product because it would not be possible to identify all the users of the product).

When conducting a cohort study, it is helpful to develop a spreadsheet listing potential risk factors and attack rates, as shown in the example in Table 10–3. The investigator can then scan the data to look for three characteristics[20(p.375)]:

1. a high attack rate in those exposed to the factor
2. a low attack rate in those not exposed to the factor
3. a factor to which most of the cases were exposed (so that exposure could possibly be implicated as a risk factor responsible for the outbreak)

For example, residents, personnel, and visitors developed acute gastroenteritis after attending a Sunday luncheon at a long-term care facility that provides assisted living and nursing care. Of the 90 persons who attended the luncheon, 86 were available for interview and 41 met the case definition for acute gastroenteritis. Attack rates for those who did and those who did not eat particular food items are shown in Table 10–3.

According to the data in Table 10–3: (1) the ice cream is the item that has the highest attack rate (88%), (2) the attack rate is low among those who did not eat ice cream (9.1%), and (3) most of those who met the case definition for gastroenteritis ate ice cream (37/41). Therefore, it is likely that the ice cream was the vehicle.

The risk ratio (relative risk) can be calculated to show the association between eating ice cream and developing gastroenteritis. The relative risk is the ratio of the attack rate in the exposed population to the attack rate in the unexposed population. A two-by-two table (Table 10–4) can be used to demonstrate the comparison of attack rates between the exposed (ate ice cream) and unexposed (did not eat ice cream) groups. Using the data in Table 10–4, the risk ratio would be the attack rate for those who ate ice cream (88) divided by the attack rate for those who did not eat ice cream (9.1), or 88/9.1 = 9.7.

Once a measure of association, such as a risk ratio, has been computed to quantify a relationship between exposure and outcome, the investigator can use a statistical test of significance, such as a chi-square test, to determine the likelihood of this relationship occurring by chance alone. In practice, a combination of cohort and case-control studies are frequently used when investigating clusters and outbreaks. Exhibit 10–1 demonstrates the use of rates and the risk ratio to identify an apparent risk factor for developing an MRSA infection. A case-control study could then be designed to further delineate risk factors associated with developing disease (in this example, a case-control study could be designed to identify risk factors that may exist on a trauma service but not on a surgical service).

Table 10–3 Attack Rates by Items Served at a Luncheon at a Long-term Care Facility, Anywhere, USA, 1999

	Number of Persons Who Ate Item				Number of Persons Who Did Not Eat Item			
	Ill	Well	Total	Attack Rate (%)	Ill	Well	Total	Attack Rate (%)
Egg salad	20	17	37	54	18	27	45	40
Ham sandwich	23	18	41	56	19	36	55	35
Turkey sandwich	22	18	40	55	8	40	48	17
Ice cream	37	5	42	88	4	40	44	9.1
Water	27	17	44	61	22	20	42	52
Milk	18	25	43	42	17	26	43	40
Coffee	17	32	49	35	21	16	37	57

Table 10–4 Attack Rate by Consumption of Ice Cream, Anywhere, USA, 1999

	Ill	Well	Total	Attack Rate (%)
Ate ice cream	37	5	42	88
Did not eat ice cream	4	40	44	9.1
Total	41	45	86	48

As discussed in the previous section, confidence intervals of the risk ratio are frequently determined and presented in the final report of an outbreak investigation. This is illustrated in a 1998 report of an outbreak of gram-negative bacterial bloodstream infections (BSIs) associated with contamination of the waste drain port in hemodialysis machines[21(p.56)]:

> Results of a cohort study of all patients receiving dialysis at the center during the 2-month epidemic period indicated that the risk for gram-negative BSI was associated with exposure to any of three particular dialysis machines (seven BSIs in 20 patients who were exposed to one or more of the three machines versus three BSIs in 64 patients who were exposed to the other machines; relative risk = 7.5; 95% confidence interval = 2.1–26.2).

The interpretation of this report is that persons who were exposed to the particular dialysis machines were 7.5 times more likely to develop a gram-negative bloodstream infection than those who were not exposed to the machines. This finding is statistically significant at $P \leq 0.05$ because the confidence interval does not include 1.0.

The Case-Control Study and the Odds Ratio

The case-control study is used to demonstrate whether or not an association exists between a disease (outcome) and a risk factor (exposure) in an outbreak investigation. A case-control study begins with the identification of persons with the *disease* being studied (the cases). A suitable comparison group of persons without the disease (the controls) is then chosen and the two groups are compared in relation to their exposures. As in the cohort study, associations and quantitative

Exhibit 10–1 Using Rates and Ratios (Measures of Association) To Identify Risk Factors

The following information was collected during an investigation of an outbreak of infections caused by methicillin-resistant *Staphylococcus aureus* (MRSA) in a surgical intensive care unit (SICU):

During a 3-month period, 180 patients were admitted to the SICU and 15 patients developed an MRSA infection. Twenty-five patients were on the Trauma Service and the other patients were on the Surgical Service. Of the 15 patients who developed MRSA infection, 10 were on the Trauma Service. From the information presented, it appears that being on the Trauma Service may be a risk factor for developing an MRSA infection. An investigator can use a two-by-two table to display this data and to calculate attack rates (incidence or risk of disease) and a risk ratio:

Number of Cases of MRSA and Attack Rates, by Service, in the SICU During a 3-Month Period

	MRSA Infection Present	MRSA Infection Absent	Total	Attack Rate (%)
Trauma service	a = 10	b = 15	a + b = 25	40
Surgical service	c = 5	d = 150	c + d = 155	3.2
Total	a + c = 15	b + d = 165	a + b + c + d = 180	8.3

Calculate the following rates:
1. Overall attack rate of MRSA infection in the SICU: a + c/ a + b + c + d × 100 = 15/180 × 100 = 8.3%
2. Attack rate for patients on the Trauma Service: a/a + b × 100 = 10/25 × 100 = 40%
3. Attack rate for patients on the Surgical Service: c/c + d × 100 = 5/155 × 100 = 3.2%

Calculate the risk ratio (RR) between patients on the Trauma Service and those on the Surgical Service:
RR = attack rate (risk of disease) for Trauma Service/attack rate (risk of disease) for Surgical Service
RR = (a/a + b)/ (c/c + d) = 40/3.2 = 12.5

Interpretation: The risk for MRSA infection for patients on the Trauma Service (40%) appears to be 12.5 times higher than the risk for patients on the Surgical Service (3.2%). Therefore, being a patient on the Trauma Service appears to be a risk factor for developing an MRSA infection.

comparisons of risk are made through the use of two-by-two tables, as shown in Table 10–2. A cohort study allows the computation of a risk ratio; however, a case-control study yields an odds ratio. This is because attack rates (needed to compute the risk ratio) cannot always be calculated in a case-control study because the entire population at risk may not be defined. Once the strength of association is measured (i.e., the odds ratio is calculated), the investigator can use statistical tests of significance and confidence intervals to evaluate the likelihood of the association occurring by chance.

The case-control study is the method most commonly used to investigate outbreaks because it is relatively inexpensive to conduct, is usually of short duration, can be used for rare diseases, requires relatively few study subjects, and allows for testing of multiple hypotheses.[17,22] A case-control study can be used when the population at risk (the cohort) cannot be adequately defined or cannot be fully identified (such as may occur in a multistate outbreak of salmonellosis associated with a contaminated food).

(Note: A case-control study differs from a cohort study in that the subjects are enrolled into a case-control study based on whether or not they have a *disease*. In a cohort study subjects are included in the study based on their *exposure* and are then followed for the development of disease.)

In an outbreak investigation, the magnitude of an odds ratio is indicative of the strength of an association between an exposure and a disease. As in a cohort study, it has become common practice to compute the confidence intervals of the odds ratio as shown in this report of an outbreak of gastrointestinal illness associated with eating burritos[23]:

> In a case-control study at one school, eight (57%) of 14 case-patients and five (13%) of 38 well children ate burritos (odds ratio {OR} = 8.8; 95% CI = 1.8–47.6). In the other school, 11 (85%) of 13 case-patients and 11 (33%) of 33 well children ate burritos (OR = 11.0; 95% CI = 1.8–87.6).

An odds ratio of 8.8 implies that those who were ill were 8.8 times more likely to have eaten a burrito than those who were not ill. A 95 percent confidence interval (CI) of 1.8–47.6 means that these odds could be as low as 1.8 or as high as 47.6. Since the CI does not include 1.0, the findings are statistically significant at a *P* value less than or equal to 0.05.

Designing and Conducting a Case-Control Study

Case-control studies must be carefully designed and conducted in order to ensure valid results. Although a detailed explanation of the design of a case-control study is beyond the scope of this chapter, the reader should be aware of several methodological problems that can affect the study results: improper or biased selection of cases or controls, information bias, confounding, and too small a sample size.

The reader who wishes detailed information on designing and conducting a case-control study may refer to the text by Schlesselman in the Suggested Reading section of this chapter or to one of the references listed.[24–26] In practice, a statistician should be consulted before conducting a case-control study to ensure that the study is appropriately designed.

Bias

Bias is "the deviation of results or inferences from the truth, or processes leading to such deviation."[8] Bias can lead to conclusions that are distorted (different from the truth). Some types of bias may occur in either a case-control or cohort study. Selection bias can occur when the cases selected for study do not represent the entire population at risk. This can occur if a nonrandom method is used to select study subjects (e.g., the selection is unconsciously or consciously influenced in some way) or if some of the study subjects are unavailable (e.g., they refuse to participate, their records are missing, their disease is mild and they do not seek medical care and are therefore not detected, or they seek medical care and their disease is undiagnosed or misdiagnosed). Information bias can occur if the information collected is incorrect because of inaccurate recall (e.g., a participant at a luncheon does not correctly remember what he ate) or because it is inconsistently collected (observer bias). Observer bias occurs when collection or interpretation of data about exposures is systematically different for persons who have the disease than those who do not or data about outcomes is systematically different for persons who are exposed than for persons who are not exposed.

Selecting Cases

Cases are selected based on a case definition, as discussed in Chapter 8. A case-control study conducted as part of an outbreak investigation differs from other case-control studies in that the case definition in an outbreak investigation frequently changes during the course of the investigation. In the initial stages, a case definition may be broad in order to identify all potential cases (e.g., all persons who developed gastroenteritis from April 10 through 17). The case definition may be refined as the investigation progresses and potential risk factors are identified (e.g., all persons who developed gastroenteritis from April 11 through April 15 and who ate food prepared by the hospital kitchen).

In many outbreaks in health care facilities, the number of cases is small and it is possible to include all of them in a case-control study. All of the cases should be included whenever possible to avoid the need to select a sample and introduce biases. In a large outbreak, however, it may not be practical, or possible, to identify or include all of the cases. In this instance, cases may be selected (sampled) from those who are ill. Care must be taken to ensure that the cases sampled are representative of the entire population with disease so that the study findings can be validly extrapolated to the whole population. To help eliminate some sampling biases, additional cases should be sought out during an outbreak to determine the magnitude of the problem.

Selecting Controls

Controls must come from the same environment where the cases' exposures occurred (i.e., they must be from the same population at risk for exposure and must be at the same risk of acquiring the disease).[24] Controls should be similar to the cases in many respects except for the presence of the disease being studied. For instance, if a case-control study is being designed to investigate an outbreak of group A streptococcal infections in postpartum patients, then the controls should be selected from postpartum patients who were hospitalized at the same time as the cases but who did not develop a streptococcal infection. Ideally, controls should be randomly selected from the population at risk to avoid selection bias.

Confounding Variables

"Comparisons may differ from the truth and therefore be biased when the association between exposure and the health problem varies because a third factor confounds the association."[17(p.24)] This difference can happen when a third factor is associated with both the exposure and the disease. Confounding factors that can bias results include age, sex, length of stay in a health care facility, or underlying disease. For example, confounding could occur if there were a community outbreak of foodborne disease and the investigators selected only those cases who were seen in a hospital. If most of the cases seen at a hospital were elderly, it could be inferred that the illness had struck the elderly

population when in fact this population may be more likely to become clinically ill and then go a hospital for treatment. One method of reducing confounding errors is to choose controls that are the same age and sex as each case.

Sample Size

A case-control study must contain a sufficiently large number of study subjects in order to be able to detect an association, if one exists, between an exposure and a disease. Multiple mathematical formulas are available to determine an appropriate sample size and these can be found in many statistics textbooks and articles.[27–30] However, it is advisable to consult a trained statistician to assist with this task. As the number of study subjects increases, the power to detect a statistically significant association increases. In an outbreak of 50 or more cases, one control for each case will usually suffice.[20(p.380)] Since outbreaks in health care facilities generally involve fewer than 50 cases, two controls are frequently selected for each case whenever possible.

For example, if investigating an outbreak of six cases of aspergillosis that occurred among patients on a bone marrow transplant unit, the investigator would want to select at least two controls for each case, and the controls would be chosen from the population of patients who were on the bone marrow transplant unit at the same time as the cases but who did not develop aspergillosis.

HYPOTHESIS TESTING (INFERENTIAL STATISTICS)

(NOTE: The following is a simplified explanation of statistical significance testing as it is used for investigating an outbreak. The reader is referred to one of many statistics textbooks for a detailed discussion of the concepts noted here.)

During an outbreak investigation, descriptive studies are used to describe those who are ill, when they became ill, and where they were when they became ill. From this information, the population at risk can generally be identified. Although this information may be enough to allow the investigator to identify potential risk factors and implement control measures that will interrupt the outbreak, it may sometimes be necessary, or desirable, to more specifically pinpoint the exposure that resulted in the disease. This is done by conducting an analytic epidemiologic study (usually a case-control or retrospective cohort study). Before conducting an analytic study, the investigator must first formulate a hypothesis (a statement that says a specific exposure results in disease) and then design the analytic study to test this hypothesis (i.e., use tests of statistical significance to assess the relationship between the specific exposure and the disease being studied). Statistical significance testing helps the investigator evaluate the role of chance by determining the probability that an association between an exposure and a disease actually exists.

There are six steps in the statistical significance testing process[31(p.22)]:

1. State the hypothesis.
2. Formulate the null hypothesis.
3. Choose a statistical significance cutoff level.
4. Conduct an analytic study.
5. Apply statistical significance test.
6. Reject, or fail to reject, the null hypothesis.

State the Hypothesis

To generate a hypothesis about the likely causative risk factor(s) or exposure(s) responsible for disease in an outbreak situation, the investigator should carefully review the existing epidemiologic and laboratory data and conduct a literature search, as discussed in Chapter 8. The hypothesis states that a difference exists between the study group and the control group. Care must be taken when generating the hypothesis. Although the source of an outbreak may appear to be obvious, it is prudent to hold an open mind and look for answers that may not have been considered. For example, an investigation of an outbreak of nosocomial legionellosis at a hospital in Rhode Island revealed that *Legionella pneumophila* was in the hospital potable water supply and this was the likely source for the outbreak. When a sudden increase in new cases occurred, it was believed to be related to the potable water, however, an extensive epidemiologic investigation demonstrated that a new cooling tower at the hospital was the source of the second outbreak.[32]

Formulate the Null Hypothesis

A null hypothesis is generated before testing for statistical significance. The null hypothesis states that no difference exists between the study group and the control group (i.e., the results observed in a study are no different from what might have occurred by chance alone). In other words, the null hypothesis states that the proportion of disease in the exposed group is the same as the proportion of disease in the nonexposed group (i.e., the exposure has no effect on the development of disease). It should be noted that an investigator can never "prove" an association between a factor (exposure) and an outcome (disease); however, inferences can be made based on statistical testing.

For example, if investigating an outbreak of group A streptococcal surgical site infections, an investigator could state that a likely risk factor for developing disease would be exposure to a colonized or infected health care worker. A possible study hypothesis would be, patients exposed to surgeon N are more likely to develop a group A streptococcal surgical site infection than patients not exposed to surgeon N. This hypothesis is based on published reports of investigations of outbreaks of group A streptococcal surgical site infections in which a colonized or infected member of the surgical team was found to be the most likely source of the organism. The null hypothesis for this study hypothesis could be, there is no difference in group A streptococcal surgical site infection rates between patients who were exposed to surgeon N and patients who were not exposed to surgeon N.

Choose a Statistical Significance Cutoff Level

In outbreak investigations, a 5 percent chance of occurrence is traditionally used as the statistical cutoff level. This means that the investigator will accept the fact that an association that is found between an exposure and the disease being studied may occur by chance alone 5 percent of the time. This also means that the *P* value must be less than 0.05 in order for the investigator to be able to reject the null hypothesis.

Conduct an Analytic Study

When conducting an outbreak investigation in a health care facility, a case-control or retrospective cohort study is usually used to allow the investigator to collect data on a study group (the cases or the cohort) and a control group so the two groups can be compared in relationship to their exposures and the presence or absence of disease.

Apply Statistical Significance Test

Tests of statistical significance are then used to determine the probability that the results of comparison testing could have occurred by chance alone if the exposure is not related to the disease. If differences are found between the study group and the control group, the investigator must choose which test of statistical significance to use to determine the probability that these differences would occur if no true difference exists (i.e., if the null hypothesis were true). In outbreak investigations in health care facilities, the most commonly used tests of significance are the chi-square and Fisher exact tests, which will be discussed later.

Reject, or Fail to Reject, the Null Hypothesis

If 5 percent is used as the statistical cutoff level, the investigator can reject the null hypothesis (and thus can accept the study hypothesis) if the statistical test shows that the association is likely to occur less than 5 percent of the time by chance alone (i.e., the P value is less than 0.05).

Type I and Type II Errors

An investigator's inference about an association can be wrong if the findings are due to bias or confounding in the study or to chance alone. A Type I error occurs when an investigator states that there is an association when in fact there is no association (i.e., the investigator rejects a null hypothesis that is actually true). A Type II error occurs when the investigator states that there is no association when in fact there is an association (i.e., the investigator fails to reject a null hypothesis that is actually false). Table 10–5 uses a two-by-two table to illustrate the four possible outcomes of statistical significance testing.

Although these errors are not always avoidable, the likelihood of making a Type II error can be minimized by using a larger sample size. By choosing the statistical cutoff level, the investigator decides before beginning the study what probability of committing a Type I error can be accepted (usually 5 percent).

TESTS OF STATISTICAL SIGNIFICANCE

The Chi-Square Test

The chi-square test is commonly used in outbreak investigations to evaluate the probability that observed differences between two populations, such as cases and controls, could have occurred by chance alone if an exposure is not truly associated with disease. There are several variations of the chi-square test.[6] Since a detailed explanation of this test is beyond the scope of this chapter, the reader is referred to the article by Gaddis and Gaddis[6] or to one of the statistics textbooks noted in the Suggested Reading section at the end of the chapter.

Using the two-by-two table shown in Table 10–2, a frequently used formula for calculating chi-square is as follows[20(p.377)]:

$$\text{chi-square} = \frac{N[|ad - bc| - N/2]^2}{(a+b)(c+d)(a+c)(b+d)}$$

Once the value for chi-square has been calculated, the investigator then uses a table of chi-squares (found in a textbook of statistical tables) to look up the associated P value. An example of a table of chi-squares is shown in Table 10–6.

To use a table of chi-squares, the degrees of freedom, defined as the number of independent comparisons that can be made between the members of a sample, must be known. A two-by-two table has one degree of freedom. Using Table 10–6 and a statistical cutoff point of 0.05, if the computed chi-square value is greater than 3.841, then the probability, or P value, would be less than 0.05 and the null hypothesis can be rejected.

Because it takes a lot of patience to calculate chi-square by hand, most investigators opt to use a computer with a statistical software package.

The chi-square test can be used if the number of subjects in a study is approximately 30 or more.[20(p.378)] For

---

Table 10–5 The Four Possible Outcomes of Statistical Significance Testing

	Association between Factor and Outcome Exists (Null Hypothesis Is Not True)	No Association between Factor and Outcome Exists (Null Hypothesis Is True)
Reject null hypothesis	Correct	Type I error
Fail to reject null hypothesis	Type II error	Correct

Table 10–6 Table of Chi-Squares

Degree of Freedom	Probability						
	0.50	0.20	0.10	0.05	0.02	0.01	0.001
1	.455	1.642	2.706	3.841	5.412	6.635	10.827
2	1.386	3.219	4.605	5.991	7.824	9.210	13.815
3	2.366	4.642	6.251	7.815	9.837	11.345	16.268
4	3.357	5.989	7.779	9.488	11.668	13.277	18.465
5	4.351	7.289	9.236	11.070	13.388	15.086	20.517
10	9.342	13.442	15.987	18.307	21.161	23.209	29.588
15	14.339	19.311	22.307	24.996	28.259	30.578	37.697
20	19.337	25.038	28.412	31.410	35.020	37.566	43.315
25	24.337	30.675	34.382	37.652	41.566	44.314	52.620
30	29.336	36.250	40.256	43.773	47.962	50.892	59.703

Source: Reprinted from *Principles of Epidemiology: An Introduction to Applied Epidemiology and Biostatistics,* 2nd ed., p. 378, 1992, Centers for Disease Control and Prevention, Department of Health and Human Services.

smaller populations, or if the value of any of the cells in a two-by-two table is less than 5, the Fisher exact test should be used.[6]

Fisher Exact Test

The Fisher exact test, which is used for evaluating two-by-two contingency tables, is a variant of the chi-square test. The Fisher exact test is the preferred test for studies with few subjects. The formula for the Fisher exact test calculates the P value directly, so a table of chi-squares is not needed. Using the two-by-two table shown in Table 10–2, the formula for the Fisher exact test is as follows[33]:

$$p = \frac{(a+c)! \times (b+d)! \times (c+d)! \times (a+b)!}{N! \times a! \times b! \times c! \times d!}$$

where ! = factorial (for example, $4! = 4 \times 3 \times 2 \times 1 = 24$).

However, in order to calculate the P value for the study, one must calculate the P value for the observations in the study and then add this P value to the P values of all possible combinations that have lower P values. This calculation should be done with the aid of a computer!

USING COMPUTERS TO MAKE LIFE EASIER

Computers have greatly enhanced accuracy and reduced the time it takes to calculate complex mathematical formulas; however, the investigator still needs to understand which statistical methods to use and when to use them. There are two basic types of software programs that can be used to manage epidemiologic data: database managers, which store and organize data, and statistical packages, which can analyze it. There are several computer software programs that can be used to store, manage, and analyze epidemiologic data. Examples are SPSS® (*Statistical Package for the Social Sciences,* Inc., Chicago, IL), SAS (SAS Institute, Cary, NC), AICE® (*Automated Infection Control Expert,* Infection Control and Prevention Analysts, Inc., Austin, TX) and *Epi Info. Epi Info* is a software program that was developed by the Centers for Disease Control and Prevention (CDC) to manage and analyze data collected during an epidemiologic investigation. *Epi Info,* which can be used to calculate odds ratios, relative risk, 95 percent confidence intervals, chi-squares, P values, etc., can be downloaded from the CDC Web site (www.cdc.gov).[34] The *Epi Info User's Manual*[35] and the *Epi Info Tutorial* can also be ordered or accessed through the CDC Web site.

INTERPRETING RESULTS: THE MEANING OF STATISTICAL SIGNIFICANCE

A result is said to be statistically significant if the computed P value is lower than the significance level chosen for the study because this means that it is highly unlikely that the observed association occurred by chance alone. If an investigator is using a significance level of $P = 0.05$, and the computed P value is lower than 0.05, this result is said to be statistically significant because the probability that the findings occurred by chance alone are less than 1 in 20. As discussed earlier in the chapter, many researchers recommend using the *P* value in addition to a measurement of association, such as an odds ratio, when analyzing the findings of an epidemiologic study.

The results of statistical significance tests and other statistical measurements, such as rates, ratios, and proportions, must be interpreted with caution. As discussed in Chapter 1, two important concepts in analytic epidemiology are cause and association. A cause is a factor that directly influences the occurrence of a disease. An association is a statistical relationship between two or more variables, such as an exposure and a disease. While an investigator cannot use statistics to prove that a particular factor caused a disease, if statistical testing shows that a group of people with exposure to a specified factor are more likely to have a disease than a group of people who are not exposed to that factor, then the factor is said to be associated with the disease. It is important to keep in mind that findings may be statistically significant but clinically irrelevant. This is because a statistically significant finding may be artifactual or spurious (i.e., a Type I error, which is a false association due to chance or some bias in the study) or may be the result of confounding (e.g., a third factor may account for an apparent association). The following criteria can be used to judge whether or not an association is causal (i.e. the suspected factor is the likely cause of the event)[17(p.27)]:

1. Strength of association: The prevalence of disease is higher in the exposed group than in the nonexposed group.

2. Dose-response relationship: There is a quantitative relationship between the amount of exposure to the factor and the frequency of disease.
3. Consistency of association: The findings have been confirmed by different investigators in different populations.
4. Chronological relationship: Exposure to the factor precedes the onset of disease.
5. Biologically plausible: The findings are coherent with existing information; they are acceptable in light of current knowledge.

SUMMARY

When investigating an outbreak, the investigator should conduct a literature search to gather clues about the possible risk factors associated with the disease or condition. Data should be collected to describe the characteristics of the cases so that potential risk factors can be identified and analyzed and a hypothesis explaining the occurrence of an outbreak can be generated. In many outbreak investigations, the information gathered in a descriptive epidemiologic study will be sufficient to identify likely risk factors so that effective control measures can be implemented to interrupt the outbreak. Further statistical analysis will be needed to pinpoint the associated risk factors more precisely if the problem continues or recurs, if the disease or condition involves significant morbidity or mortality, or if the outbreak is unique and the investigator wishes to publish the findings of the investigation. The authors strongly recommend that those who are investigating an outbreak consult a statistician before conducting an analytic epidemiologic study such as a case-control or cohort study.

REFERENCES

1. Reingold AL. Outbreak investigations—a perspective. *Emer Infect Dis.* 1998;4:24.
2. Gaddis ML, Gaddis GM. Introduction to biostatistics: part 1, basic concepts. *Ann Emerg Med.* 1990;19:86–89.
3. Gaddis ML, Gaddis GM. Introduction to biostatistics: part 2, descriptive statistics. *Ann Emerg Med.* 1990;19:309–315.
4. Gaddis ML, Gaddis GM. Introduction to biostatistics: part 3, sensitivity, specificity, predictive value, and hypothesis testing. *Ann Emerg Med.* 1990;19:591–596.
5. Gaddis ML, Gaddis GM. Introduction to biostatistics: part 4, statistical inference techniques in hypothesis testing. *Ann Emerg Med.* 1990;19:820–825.
6. Gaddis ML, Gaddis GM. Introduction to biostatistics: part 5, statistical inference techniques for hypothesis testing with nonparametric data. *Ann Emerg Med.* 1990;19:1054–1059.
7. Gaddis ML, Gaddis GM. Introduction to biostatistics: part 6, correlation and regression. *Ann Emerg Med.* 1990;19:1462–1468.
8. Last JM. *A Dictionary of Epidemiology.* New York: Oxford University Press; 1988.
9. Freeman J, Hitchison GB. Prevalence, incidence and duration. *Am J Epidemiol.* 1980;112:707–723.
10. Centers for Disease Control and Prevention. National nosocomial infections surveillance system (NNIS) report. *Am J Infect Control.* 1996;24:380–388.

11. Young KD, Lewis RJ. What is confidence? Part 1: the use and interpretation of confidence intervals. *Ann Emerg Med.* 1997;30:307–310.

12. Young KD, Lewis RJ. What is confidence? Part 2: detailed definition and determination of confidence intervals. *Ann Emerg Med.* 1997;30:311–318.

13. Gardner MJ, Altman DG. Confidence intervals rather than *P* values: estimation rather than hypothesis testing. *Br Med J.* 1986;292:746–750.

14. Morris JA, Gardner MJ. Calculating confidence intervals for relative risks (odds ratios) and standardized ratios and rates. *Br Med J.* 1988;296:1313–1316.

15. Birnbaum D, Sheps SB. The merits of confidence intervals relative to hypothesis testing. *Infect Control Hosp Epidemiol.* 1992;13:553–555.

16. Woolson RF, Kleinman JC. Perspectives on statistical significance testing. *Ann Rev Public Health.* 1989;10:423–440.

17. Last JM, Tyler CW. Epidemiology. In: Wallace RB, ed. *Maxcy-Rosenau-Last Public Health and Preventive Medicine.* 14th ed. Stamford, CT: Appleton & Lange; 1998:5–33.

18. Centers for Disease Control and Prevention. Outbreaks of *Shigella sonnei* infection associated with eating fresh parsley—United States and Canada, July–August 1998. *MMWR.* 1999;48:285–289.

19. Kennel WB, Wolf PA, Garrison RJ, eds. *The Framingham Study: An Epidemiologic Investigation of Cardiovascular Disease.* Washington DC: National Technical Information Service; 1988. DHHS Publication No. (NIH) 88–2969.

20. Centers for Disease Control and Prevention. *Principles of Epidemiology: An Introduction to Applied Epidemiology and Biostatistics.* Atlanta, GA: US Dept of Health and Human Services; 1992.

21. Centers for Disease Control and Prevention. Outbreaks of gram-negative bacterial bloodstream infections traced to probable contamination of hemodialysis machines—Canada, 1995, United States, 1997, and Israel, 1997. *MMWR.* 1998;47:55–58.

22. Dwyer DM, Strickler H, Goodman RA, Armenian HK. Use of case-control studies in outbreak investigations. *Epidemiol Rev.* 1994;16:109–123.

23. Centers for Disease Control and Prevention. Outbreaks of gastrointestinal illness of unknown etiology associated with eating burritos—United States, October 1997–October 1998. *MMWR.* 1999;48:210–213.

24. Wacholder S, McLaughlin JK, Silverman DT, Mandel JS. Selection of controls in case-control studies. I. Principles. *Am J Epidemiol.* 1992;135:1019–1028.

25. Wacholder S, McLaughlin JK, Silverman DT, Mandel JS. Selection of controls in case-control studies. II. Types of controls. *Am J Epidemiol.* 1992;135:1029–1041.

26. Wacholder S, McLaughlin JK, Silverman DT, Mandel JS. Selection of controls in case-control studies. III. Design options. *Am J Epidemiol.* 1992;135:1042–1050.

27. Kelsey JL, Thompson WD, Evans AS. *Methods in Observational Epidemiology.* New York: Oxford University Press; 1986.

28. Kleinbaum D, Rosner B. *Fundamentals of Biostatistics.* Boston: Duxbury Press; 1982.

29. Hennekens CH, Buring J. *Epidemiology in Medicine.* Boston: Little, Brown and Company; 1987:260.

30. Edmiston CE, Josephson A, Pottinger J, Ciasco-Tsivitis M, Palenik C. The numbers game: sample-size determination. *Am J Infect Control.* 1993;21:151–154.

31. Riegelman RK, Hirsch RP. Analysis. In: *Studying a Study and Testing a Test: How to Read the Health Science Literature.* 3rd ed. Philadelphia: Lippincott-Raven Publishers; 1996:22–39.

32. Garbe PL, Davis BJ, Weisfeld JS. Nosocomial Legionnaires' disease: Epidemiologic demonstration of cooling towers as a source. *JAMA.* 1985;254:521–524.

33. Checko PJ. Use of statistics for epidemiology. In: Olmsted R, ed. *APIC Infection Control and Applied Epidemiology: Principles and Practice.* St. Louis, MO: Mosby; 1996:2-1–2-24.

34. *Epi Info* [computer program]. Version 6. Atlanta, GA: Centers for Disease Control and Prevention; 1994.

35. Dean AG, Dean SA, Columbier D, et al. *Epi Info, Version 6: A Word Processing, Database, and Statistics Program for Microcomputers.* Stone Mountain, GA: USD, Inc; 1994.

SUGGESTED READING

Campbell MJ, Machin D. *Medical Statistics: A Common Sense Approach.* Chichester: John Wiley & Sons; 1990.

Centers for Disease Control and Prevention. *Principles of Epidemiology: An Introduction to Applied Epidemiology and Biostatistics.* 2nd ed. Atlanta, GA: US Dept of Health and Human Services, Public Health Service; 1992.

Checko PJ. Use of statistics for epidemiology. In: Olmsted R, ed. *APIC Infection Control and Applied Epidemiology: Principles and Practice.* St. Louis, MO: Mosby; 1996:2-1–2-24.

Dwyer DM, Strickler H, Goodman RA, Armenian HK. Use of case-control studies in outbreak investigations. *Epidemiol Rev.* 1994;16:109–123.

Fletcher RH, Fletcher SW, Wagner EH. *Clinical Epidemiology: The Essentials.* Baltimore: Williams & Wilkins; 1996.

Hennekens CH, Buring J. *Epidemiology in Medicine.* Boston/Toronto: Little, Brown and Company; 1987.

Hulley SB, Cummings SR. *Designing Clinical Research: An Epidemiologic Approach.* Baltimore: Williams & Wilkins; 1988.

Kleinbaum D, Kupper L, Morgenstern H. *Epidemiologic Research: Principles and Quantitative Methods.* Belmont, CA: Lifetime Learning Publications; 1982.

Last JM, Tyler CW. Epidemiology. In: Wallace RB, ed. *Maxcy-Rosenau-Last Public Health and Preventive Medicine.* 14th ed. Stamford, CT: Appleton & Lange; 1998:5–33.

Muñoz A, Townsend T. Design and analytical issues in studies of infectious diseases. In: Wenzel RP. *Prevention and Control of Nosocomial Infections.* Baltimore: Williams & Wilkins; 1997:215–230.

Ning L. Statistics in infection control studies. In: Wenzel RP. *Prevention and Control of Nosocomial Infections.* Baltimore: Williams & Wilkins; 1997:231–240.

Reingold AL. Outbreak investigations—a perspective. *Emerg Infect Dis.* 1998;4:21–27.

Riegelman RK, Hirsch RP. *Studying a Study and Testing a Test: How to Read the Health Science Literature.* 3rd ed. Philadelphia: Lippincott-Raven; 1996.

Schlesselman JJ. *Case-Control Studies: Design, Conduct, Analysis.* New York: Oxford University Press, 1982.

Selvin S. Estimating and comparing means and proportions: the t-test and the chi-square test. In: Olmsted R, ed. *APIC Infection Control and Applied Epidemiology: Principles and Practice.* St. Louis, MO: Mosby; 1996:3-1–3-22.

Zar JH. *Biostatistical Analysis.* Englewood Cliffs, NJ: Prentice-Hall, Inc.; 1981.

OTHER RESOURCES

Principles of Epidemiology, 3030-G is a training course that is available from the Centers for Disease Control and Prevention. It is a print-based self-study course covering basic epidemiology principles, concepts, and procedures generally used in the surveillance and investigation of health-related events. It includes information on the applications of descriptive and analytic epidemiology and addresses how to calculate and interpret frequency measures (ratios, proportions, and rates) and measures of central tendency. This course may be ordered by calling 1-800-41-TRAIN. Press 1, 4, 1 and choose PHF, Public Health Foundation, the distributor of this course.

CHAPTER 11

The Role of the Laboratory in Outbreak Investigation

Robert L. Sautter

The practice of clinical microbiology in the United States is a relatively young science, dating back fewer than 100 years.[1] The study of epidemiology is much older but has only recently been widely applied to the health care setting.[2] Early physicians and microbiologists were unable to associate a causative agent for disease.

As early as 1717, Giovanni Lancisi postulated that malaria was a poison that could possibly be transmitted by mosquitoes. However, as of the mid-1800s, the causative agent of the disease had not been elucidated.[3] The following quote is taken from the 1863 medical school notebook of William Brooks Bigler, a Pennsylvania physician who practiced during the Civil War:

> Malaria: what is it? Malaria has a real existence but cannot be detected. There is (or may be) a latent period which the poison does not exhibit itself. One room in a house may be malarious, the others not. Intermittent may leave a locality for a number of years and then return. With us, moisture, heat and low grounds favor the existence of malaria. Hence malaria must have weight. As our winds are mostly from south and west, in summer, hence eastern and northern sides of streams and swamps are most subject to malaria. Drinking the water of malarious districts to be avoided, as it may have absorbed the poisons.[3(p.427)]

Although the disease was described by Hippocrates, the causative agent of malaria (*Plasmodium malariae*) was not identified until the late 1800s.

Since 1970, many outbreaks of diseases caused by previously unrecognized agents have been documented. Examples include Legionnaire's disease (*Legionella pneumophila*) in the mid-1970s; Lyme disease (*Borrelia burgdorferi*), acquired immune deficiency syndrome (human immunodeficiency virus), and diarrhea caused by *Cyclospora* species in the 1980s; and Navaho fever (Hanta virus) and hemolytic uremic syndrome caused by *Escherichia coli* O157:H7 in the 1990s.[4,5] Table 11–1 lists examples of pathogenic microbes and infectious diseases recognized since 1973.[5] Clearly, the role of health care professionals, including those in the clinical microbiology laboratory, has become challenging.

Clinical microbiology laboratories are vital in identifying the agents of newly recognized diseases and in tracking diseases caused by well-characterized nosocomial and community-acquired pathogens.[4] The microbiology laboratory plays an integral role in a health care facility's infection control program by providing a coordinated approach to the diagnosis of disease, offering the most updated and clinically reliable tests, supplying useable surveillance data, tracking antimicrobial resistance, assisting in outbreak investigations, and serving as a resource for consultation.[6–9] This chapter discusses the role of the laboratory in the surveillance,

Table 11–1 Examples of Pathogenic Microbes and Infectious Diseases Recognized Since 1973

Year	Microbe	Type	Disease
1973	Rotavirus	Virus	Major cause of infantile diarrhea worldwide
1975	Parvovirus B19	Virus	Aplastic crisis in chronic hemolytic anemia
1976	*Cryptosporidium parvum*	Parasite	Acute and chronic diarrhea
1977	Ebola virus	Virus	Ebola hemorrhagic fever
1977	*Legionella pneumophila*	Bacteria	Legionnaire's disease
1977	Hantaan virus	Virus	Hemorrhagic fever with renal syndrome
1977	*Campylobacter jejuni*	Bacteria	Enteric pathogens distributed globally
1980	Human T-lymphotropic virus I (HTLV-I)	Virus	T-cell lymphoma-leukemia
1981	Toxic-producing strains of *Staphylococcus aureus*	Bacteria	Toxic shock syndrome (tampon use)
1982	*Escherichia coli* O157:H7	Bacteria	Hemorrhagic colitis; hemolytic uremic syndrome
1982	HTLV-II	Virus	Hairy cell leukemia
1982	*Borrelia burgdorferi*	Bacteria	Lyme disease
1983	Human immunodeficiency virus	Virus	Acquired immune deficiency syndrome (AIDS)
1983	*Helicobacter pylori*	Bacteria	Peptic ulcer disease
1985	*Enterocytozoon bieneusi*	Parasite	Persistent diarrhea
1986	*Cyclospora cayetanensis*	Parasite	Persistent diarrhea
1988	Human herpesvirus 6 (HHV-6)	Virus	Roseola subitum
1988	Hepatitis E	Virus	Enterically transmitted non-A, non-B hepatitis
1989	*Ehrlichia chafeensis*	Bacteria	Human ehrlichiosis
1989	Hepatitis C	Virus	Parenterally transmitted non-A, non-B hepatitis
1991	Guanarito virus	Virus	Venezuelan hemorrhagic fever
1991	*Encephalitozoan hellem*	Parasite	Conjunctivitis, disseminated disease
1991	New species of *Babesia*	Parasite	Atypical babesiosis
1992	*Vibrio cholerae* O139	Bacteria	New strain associated with epidemic cholera
1992	*Bartonella heneselae*	Bacteria	Cat-scratch disease; bacillary angiomatosis
1993	Sin Nombre virus	Virus	Adult respiratory distress syndrome
1993	*Encephalitozoan cuniculi*	Parasite	Disseminated disease
1994	Sabia virus	Virus	Brazilian hemorrhagic fever
1995	HHV-8	Virus	Associated with Kaposi's sarcoma in patients with AIDS

Source: Reprinted from J. Lederberg, Infectious Disease as an Evolutionary Paradigm, *Emerging Infectious Diseases,* Vol. 3, p. 419, 1997, Centers for Disease Control and Prevention.

recognition, and investigation of outbreaks using examples drawn from actual hospital situations as well as from the literature.

THE ROLE OF THE LABORATORY IN THE SURVEILLANCE AND RECOGNITION OF OUTBREAKS

Communication and Collaboration

An effective surveillance program requires good communication and collaboration among the laboratory, the other departments in a health care facility, and outside agencies such as the health department. The infection control department relies on the microbiology laboratory to serve as an early detection or warning mechanism.[8]

An infection surveillance system should monitor the results of cultures, antimicrobial susceptibility tests, direct examination of samples using appropriate stains (e.g., gram stain for bacteria, acid-fast stains for *Mycobacterium* species), toxin assays (*Clostridium difficile*), serologic tests (hepatitis viruses), and rapid methods for the identification of epidemiologically important viruses and bacteria (such as rotavirus and *Neisseria meningitidis*). Rapid methods, such as enzyme-linked immunoassay, polymerase chain reaction, and ligase chain reaction, allow the detection of some organisms that may have previously gone undetected (e.g., *Bordetella pertussis*).[10]

Infection control and laboratory personnel should review test results for unusual organisms (such as *Sphingomonas paucimobilus* from patients on mechanical ventilation),[11] organisms of public health significance, or organisms that are either potential causes of an outbreak or have caused an outbreak at the institution in the past.

Each laboratory should have a list of organisms or occurrences that are immediately reported to the infection control department. This list should be developed with input from the infection control committee. Examples of organisms or occurrences that may require immediate notification include *N meningitidis*, methicillin-resistant *Staphylococcus aureus* (MRSA), vancomycin-resistant *Enterococcus* species (VRE), *Mycobacterium tuberculosis* (MTB), enteric bacilli exhibiting unusual resistant mechanisms (extended spectrum beta-lactamase), *Salmonella* or *Shigella* species, sputum smears positive for acid-fast bacilli, and clusters of organisms isolated from anywhere in the institution.

Each state has disease regulations that require health care providers and laboratories to report specific diseases and conditions, as discussed in Chapter 2. The laboratory plays a key role in identifying organisms of public health significance and reporting them to the infection control department and the health department.

A well-educated and informed microbiology staff can be of utmost importance in recognizing clusters of nosocomial and community-acquired infections. One summer in the author's laboratory, technologists noticed an unusual number of *Salmonella* isolates and they notified the state department of health. This call prompted an investigation that uncovered a community outbreak of *Salmonella* food poisoning associated with contaminated meat products. Observations of this type serve the public health community as well as the medical community by enabling the health department to recognize community outbreaks of disease and by alerting the infection control department to the possibility that contaminated products may be used in a health care facility.

The laboratory must collaborate with the primary caregiver as well as with the infection control department. In the author's laboratory, a cluster of nontuberculous mycobacteria isolates was detected in respiratory cultures from one of the laboratory's outpatient clients. The isolates were identified as *Mycobacterium gordonae*. Because none of the patients had evidence of mycobacterial infection, the cluster was thought to be a pseudo-outbreak (a cluster of false infections). Epidemiologic investigation of the cases revealed the source of the organism to be the water supply at the outpatient facility. False-positive specimens complicate the diagnosis of infections caused by nontuberculous mycobacteria as well as other microorganisms. The laboratory can aid in detecting clusters of false-positive cultures and alerting the clinician.

Infection control personnel must be informed about which routine procedures are used in the laboratory, which organisms are identified in routine cultures, and which organisms are included in the catch-all term of "normal flora." Walsh et al[12] showed that the respiratory tract often is the first positive culture site for the isolation of MRSA. After isolation from the respiratory tract, other sites became colonized with the organism. Infection control personnel should be aware that most laboratories identify isolates of *S aureus* from the lower respiratory tract only when it is found in predominant numbers and do not identify isolates from the upper respiratory tract. Therefore, the infection control practitioner should not rely on routine cultures to identify colonized patients or residents but must request that a special surveillance culture be collected from those patients or residents who are suspected of carrying MRSA. The usual susceptibility patterns of organisms isolated in the facility should be shared with the infection control personnel, and changes noted by the technologists should be brought to the attention of the infection control department.

In the hospital, the clinical microbiologist or the microbiology supervisor should be an active member of the infection control committee.[9] This participation allows the microbiologist to explain the methods that are used in the laboratory to detect and identify microorganisms and to assess antimicrobial susceptibility. It also provides the opportunity for the microbiologist to become aware of the nosocomial pathogens that are endemic to the facility and to discuss problems and issues confronting the infection control department.

Computerization of Laboratory Data: Provision of Test Results

The increase in the number of computer programs and systems to enhance data management has revolutionized the practice of microbiology and infection control.[13] Many laboratories are computerized and capable of offering data to aid their users.[14,15] Some of the advantages of computerization include accurate and consistent information retrieval for the infection control and other departments, tracking of abnormal results, automatic notification of results to physicians by e-mail, evaluation of the quality and reliability of laboratory tests offered, automatic downloading of data to personal computers in different areas of the hospital, and storage and management of voluminous quantities of data.

The infection control department should identify test results that it needs to conduct routine surveillance and should meet with laboratory and computer systems personnel to set up a mechanism for having these results provided daily. Examples of test results useful for surveillance include all positive culture results from any site, all wound cultures (whether positive or negative), positive toxin assays for *C difficile*, positive respiratory syncytial virus and rotavirus tests, positive results of antigen testing on cerebral spinal fluid, and any tests (such as syphilis tests and hepatitis serology) that are needed for reporting diseases to the health department.

Most laboratory computer database systems and automated or semiautomated microbial identification and susceptibility systems have the capability of generating special reports that are useful to the infection control department (e.g., antibiograms, epidemiology reports, incidence and trending analysis, and significant finding reports). The automated systems contain epidemiologic database packages that allow searches to be performed to track microorganisms by ward, service, or patient population. Many of these systems allow an additional terminal to be placed in the infection control department or the pharmacy, thus supplying immediate information to these areas. Unfortunately, most of these systems require much manual intervention to be able to provide accurate information.

Relational databases, such as Microsoft Access and Oracle RDBMS (Relational Database Management System), provide cross-referencing of data from different sources,[14] allowing almost any combination of data to be analyzed. For instance, a search including all organisms can be sorted by patient, unit, antimicrobial susceptibility, biotype, and other factors. An automatic download of information from databases such as the laboratory information system or the hospital information system to personal computers can also be achieved.[15] Key to achieving the goal of combining data from different sources is using a language that is interpretable by all systems. Many of the insurance providers have accomplished this by using Health Level 7, a standard format for electronic data interchange.[14]

One innovative laboratory developed a computer system that compares isolation rates of all organisms from the current week's culture results to data archived from previous weeks and reports microorganisms that exceed a chosen limit.[16] This system uses a time series analysis with the capability of detecting potential nosocomial infections and clusters. Another microbiology laboratory has been tracking nosocomial infections for many years by downloading data each day to a database in the laboratory director's personal computer. The director can manipulate this information to trend nosocomial infections and antibiotic susceptibility results.[15] For more information, the reader is referred to two excellent articles detailing the possibilities that microbiology laboratory information systems can offer.[14,15]

More and more hospital laboratories have been marketing to physician offices, nursing homes, and other facilities to become more cost-effective by increasing the volume of testing. This trend becomes an advantage for the hospital-based infection control department that is responsible for managing the infection control programs at off-site or ambulatory care locations. When the hospital laboratory services the physician's offices, nursing homes, and other institutions that admit patients or are part of the hospital's health system and the microbiological history of a patient is in the laboratory's database, then the infection control personnel can be alerted to potential nosocomial problems.

Care must be taken in offering infection control services "free of charge" to outside clients. This practice may be viewed as violating Medicare "kickback" laws if the laboratory and infection control share the same site as a client. The institution's compliance officer should be consulted prior to the laboratory or infection control department performing these duties.

Laboratory Methods Affecting Surveillance

Accurate and consistent identification of microorganisms is crucial for an effective infection surveillance and control program. Many different methods are available to identify microorganisms. To identify isolates of *S aureus,* most laboratories use classical methods such as the coagulase slide or tube test, the thermonuclease test, or the mannitol fermentation test. Other laboratories use commercial systems such as Microscan® (Dade Behring, Inc., West Sacramento, CA) or BBL Crystal™ ID (Becton Dickinson and Company, Cockeysville, MD) to identify staphylococcal isolates.[17] Although these systems compare well in published studies, laboratories may misclassify individual isolates if they do not use consistent methodologies. For instance, an organism may be identified as *S aureus* by the coagulase test, but subsequent cultures from the same patient may be identified as another species of *Staphylococcus* if a different test method is used. Commercial latex agglutination tests can misidentify an MRSA as a methicillin-resistant coagulase-negative *Staphylococcus*.[18–21] This misidentification could be a potentially serious error if therapy is withheld. In addition, the infection control and patient care personnel would be unaware that MRSA is present and would not institute control measures such as contact isolation. The microbiology laboratory must limit the number of different methods used to provide consistent information.

It has become more difficult to identify gram-negative bacilli over the past two decades. Extrachromosomal elements have been able to transfer not only resistance factors between organisms but also the ability of a microbe to produce a biochemical reaction.[22] For example, *E coli* can gain the ability to use urea or citrate from a *Proteus* or *Salmonella* species,[22] and this can make the *E coli* more difficult to identify. However, unique strains such as these may allow them to be monitored using phenotype typing methods discussed later in this chapter.

There are many excellent commercially available systems for the identification of gram-negative bacilli; however, not all of these systems use the same biochemical tests for identification.[23] It is not possible to use biotyping (epidemiologic typing using biochemical reactions) to determine strain relatedness if a laboratory does not consistently use the same method for identification of isolates.[24]

Some laboratory methods, such as direct antigen testing of clinical specimens, can aid in rapidly evaluating clusters or potential outbreaks. Examples of rapid methods include direct detection of *Streptococcus pneumoniae* or *S aureus* in positive blood cultures[25,26] and antigen tests used to identify group B streptococcus or *N meningitidis* in cerebral spinal fluid. Identification of *S aureus* may be obtained within 4 hours of detection of a positive blood culture.[26] Laboratories that this author has been associated with have been using a direct coagulase test on positive blood culture bottles containing gram-positive cocci for approximately 20 years. During that time, only one false-positive result has been noted, misidentifying an isolate as *S aureus*.

Test Reliability

Statistical information concerning the reliability of laboratory tests should be shared with the infection control staff. The sensitivity (probability of a positive test result in a person with the disease), specificity (probability of a negative test result in a person without the disease), and positive and negative predictive values (measure of the likelihood that a positive or negative test represents a true positive or negative result) of particular tests influence the ability of the infection control department to analyze data from the laboratory.[27] For instance, the results of direct fluorescent antibody tests (DFA) for different agents (e.g., *L pneumophila*, *B pertussis*, and influenza virus) should not be interpreted in the same manner. Kits using monoclonal antibody for detection of an agent will be more specific than those using polyclonal antibody; however, when changes in the target organism occur (such as antigenic drift), the sensitivity of tests using monoclonal antibodies is decreased. Because different methodologies are available to detect almost every organism imaginable[23] and these methodologies do not always perform the same, the laboratory must choose appropriate tests for the circumstances and share the reliability of each with its clients.

Each test result is interpreted based on the statistical information peculiar to the individual test kit and the prevalence of the disease in the patient populations evaluated. For example, DFA tests for *L pneumophila*[28] and enzyme-linked immunosorbent assay tests for *Cryptosporidium* species[29] are known to generate false-positive and -negative results. The sensitivity and specificity of tests depends mostly on the test methodology, whereas the positive and negative predictive values vary with sensitivity, specificity, and the disease prevalence. The DFA tests for influenza virus have sensitivity <70 percent, with a specificity of 98 percent.[30] These figures mean that a positive test and not a negative test may be relied on. Prevalence of the disease also affects the reliability of results. As the incidence of disease decreases, the reliability of a positive result also decreases. With the decline in incidence of tuberculosis in the early 1970s, positive smears for acid-fast bacilli became less reliable.[31] However, in areas that have an increased incidence of typical and atypical acid-fast infections, the smear remains a reliable test method. Laboratory test results must always be interpreted in relationship to clinical findings.

An epidemiologist looks at test results from a different angle than a clinician. The epidemiologist is interested not only in the presence of disease but also in accurately tracking the number of cases, pinpointing the likely source of the agent, and determining the need for isolation precautions. The use of an inaccurate single test, such as DFA for *B pertussis,* can be misleading. This particular test has a very low sensitivity and specificity; therefore, a negative DFA test means little for this organism. However, a positive test should direct the infection control department to take action. For this reason, the pertussis DFA test should be coupled with a culture, if it is to be used at all.[32]

When investigating an outbreak, tests that display high sensitivity should be chosen. Otherwise, cases will be inappropriately excluded from the investigation. Specificity is less important when screening cases in the early stages of an outbreak investigation and becomes more critical when confirming cases for inclusion in an outbreak and treating the affected individuals. For instance, during flu season, outbreaks occur in the community as well as in health care institutions.[33] Screening kits are popular for the detection of influenza A and have been marketed extensively. These kits provide rapid results, are easy to perform, and are cost-effective.[34] However, their use may be drastically misleading for identifying cases of the disease during outbreaks. The sensitivity of these screening tests ranges between 42 and 84.7 percent.[30,34] For accurate identification of patients with influenza, a combination of direct antigen testing and culture will increase the sensitivity of the test results to close to 100 percent.[34]

THE ROLE OF THE LABORATORY IN THE INVESTIGATION OF AN OUTBREAK

Saving Isolates of Potential Epidemiologic Significance

The laboratory plays a key role in identifying clusters of infections and sporadic infections caused by uncommon pathogens. The laboratory should have a mechanism for routinely saving potentially significant isolates in case epidemiologic typing is later desired.

In the 1970s, methods became available to enable the microbiology department to precisely identify many microorganisms to the species level with minimal cost.[35] One of the biggest advances in that decade was the use of computer-assisted databases to assess the probability or likelihood that an organism was identified correctly. A series of biochemical reactions could be used to generate a code number that corresponded to the identity of microorganisms. This biochemical phenotyping enabled infection control practitioners to compare isolates from different sources and make a determination whether they may be related and an outbreak may have occurred.[24] During the 1980s and

1990s, decreased reimbursement and cost-containment incentives have forced many laboratories to use abbreviated screening methods to identify commonly isolated microorganisms.[36,37] For these methods, immediate epidemiologic surveillance using biochemical phenotypic characteristics to determine relatedness is no longer possible. However, retrospective analysis of the organisms can occur if the laboratory routinely saves microorganisms of potential epidemiologic significance. The infection control professional, the hospital epidemiologist, and the laboratory personnel should decide which organisms to save and how long to archive them. This decision is often dictated by the available space and staffing in the laboratory. Many hospitals archive all isolates from normally sterile body fluids (e.g., blood and cerebrospinal fluid). Each laboratory should develop a policy for saving microorganisms and make the policy available to clinical departments.[8]

Infection control personnel should immediately notify the laboratory in the event of an suspected cluster or outbreak and request that all relevant isolates be saved for possible future testing. In the words of Weber et al, "Organisms cannot be tested unless they are available. It is easy to throw out saved isolates, but impossible to recover them from the trash."[38(p.275)]

Performing Special Cultures or Other Tests

The laboratory can assist in investigating an epidemic by performing special cultures or other tests:

- patient or resident cultures for resistant microorganisms such as MRSA, VRE, or resistant gram-negative bacilli
- stool cultures for investigating a foodborne outbreak
- staff cultures for *S aureus* or group A beta-hemolytic streptococci to detect personnel carriers
- microbiologic evaluation of the environment (e.g., analysis of hemodialysis water)
- serology for measles
- microbiologic evaluation of medical devices (e.g., bronchoscopes) or pharmaceutical products that are epidemiologically implicated in an outbreak

Focused cultures for many of these studies require specialized procedures and media; therefore, these cultures must be ordered in consultation with the infection control personnel, hospital epidemiologist, and microbiologist. Infection control programs should have policies in place that specify when these focused surveillance cultures may be initiated. Prior approval by the infection control committee, or its designee, should be required before any special surveillance cultures are collected to maximize the data from such studies and ensure that specimens are collected and processed appropriately.[2]

During the course of an outbreak investigation, culturing of personnel or the environment is frequently done to identify a common source or reservoir. The Hospital Infections Program of the Centers for Disease Control and Prevention (CDC) traditionally discourages such cultures unless a prior epidemiologic investigation provides evidence that a personnel or environmental source is linked to the outbreak.[39–41] In 1985, the CDC noted that "Microbiologic sampling is indicated during investigation of infection problems if environmental reservoirs are implicated epidemiologically in disease transmission. It is important, however, that such culturing be based on epidemiologic data and follow a written plan that specifies the objects to be sampled and the action to be taken based on culture results."[41(p.14)] There are several arguments in support of this stance.

- It may be difficult, or impossible, to interpret the presence of microorganisms from environmental surfaces such as walls, floors, or sinks because there are no standards for the numbers or types of organisms on most environmental surfaces.[40]
- Laboratory-based investigations (i.e., extensive culture surveys) are expensive, consume valuable laboratory resources, and can be misdirected in the absence of a carefully conducted epidemiologic study.[39]
- The fact that a health care worker is culture-positive for the organism being studied does not necessarily mean that the health care worker was the source of the outbreak. The worker could have become colonized or infected as a result of the outbreak or could have been colonized or infected before the outbreak and may not have transmitted the organism to another person.

An outbreak investigation should include a careful epidemiologic study and the generation of hypotheses about the potential sources or reservoirs. Culture surveys of these potential sources or reservoirs should be considered if the outbreak involves an unusual pathogen or results in considerable morbidity or mortality, if control measures fail to stop the outbreak, or if the investigators wish to publish their findings. If culture surveys are conducted, the isolates should be typed to determine whether the strains are related.

The scope of the laboratory's expertise should be considered when conducting an outbreak investigation or performing surveillance cultures. For example, media and procedures for the culture of food are not routinely available in most clinical microbiology laboratories,[8,42] and the clinical microbiologist, unless trained in food microbiology, may not be familiar with the common microorganisms found in food. To complicate the situation further, many of the organisms present in the environment and in food are not in the databases supplied by the commercial identification systems commonly used in clinical microbiology laboratories.[43]

Specimen Selection and Collection

Once the decision to culture patients, residents, or the environment has been made, the laboratory should assist the investigators in choosing the proper types of specimens, culture sites, and appropriate collection and transportation methods. It is important when performing specialized cultures during an outbreak to maximize the recovery of the organism. The specimen collection sites vary for the types of organisms targeted; however, some examples are listed below:

- *S aureus* (including MRSA): cultures from the anterior nares, surgical wounds, decubiti, and hands[44–47]
- *Enterococcus* species (including VRE): rectal swab or stool sample[48]
- *Streptococcus pyogenes* (group A streptococci): oropharynx or rectal cultures[49]
- *Streptococcus agalactiae* (group B streptococci): vaginal or rectal cultures[50]
- Enteric bacilli (i.e., *Salmonella* species): stool sample (preferred) or rectal culture[49,51]
- *C difficile:* stool sample or rectal swab[52,53] (Note: Toxin assays, rather than cultures, should be used when conducting surveillance for *C difficile* infection because asymptomatic rectal carriage of *C difficile* can occur.[52,53] In addition, care should be taken when interpreting the results of positive toxin assays because these may occur in the absence of clinical symptoms.)
- Enteric viruses: stool sample[51,54]

The following methods are recommended for collection of common samples taken during an outbreak investigation:

- Anterior nares culture: Use swab premoistened with sterile saline. Insert approximately 2 cm into nares. Rotate the swab against the nasal mucosa.[49]
- Rectal culture: Carefully insert swab approximately 1 inch (2.54 cm) beyond the anal sphincter. Gently rotate the swab to sample the anal crypts.[49]
- Hand culture: "Pour 50 mL of hand wash broth . . . over the dominant hand of the subject. Massage the hand in the broth" for 1 minute.[55(p.11.17.1)]

Sampling guidelines for the collection of specimens have been published by the American Society for Microbiology,[56] the CDC,[51,54] and by many state health departments. Guidelines for collecting specimens when investigating outbreaks of acute respiratory diseases, scabies, or gastroenteritis in long-term care facilities can be found in Appendixes H, I, and J.

The methods used to collect cultures of environmental and medical device surfaces depend on the surface being cultured. Guidelines for culturing inanimate surfaces have been published by the American Society for Microbiology.[57]

Procedures for the Selective Isolation of Microorganisms from Animate and Inanimate Surfaces

In consultation with the investigators, the laboratory must select the appropriate culture method and medium that will selectively isolate the organism from health care workers, patients or residents, or an inanimate surface. The culture techniques used for these purposes are different than those used for routine microbiologic cultures. Antibiotic drugs are often incorporated into culture media to selectively inhibit normal flora at the site and thus allow the target organism to be isolated. A prime example would be the incorporation of 6 μg of oxacillin into mannitol salt agar or blood agar plates to isolate MRSA.[44,45] Salt broth may also be used for this reason; however, care must be taken to ensure that the strain of the target organism is not susceptible to the concentrations of salt used.[58]

Table 11–2 provides some examples of procedures that can be used to selectively isolate microorganisms from animate or inanimate surfaces.[55,57,59–64] Culture of medical devices, some inanimate surfaces, equipment, soaps, lotions, intravenous fluids, and medications may be beyond the scope and expertise of routine laboratory procedures. Filtration techniques and media that includes neutralizers should be used for many of these cultures.[57] The routine clinical laboratory does not have these items and would have difficulty getting them delivered in time to act on the sample. These cultures may be sent out to reference laboratories. Personnel from state health departments or the CDC Hospital Infections Program can usually arrange for these studies to be done.

Analysis of potentially contaminated intravenous or hemodialysis fluids should include tests for pyrogens, including gram-negative endotoxin (limulus lysate).[65] This endotoxin is a lipopolysaccharide that can be found in intravenous fluid and can cause a severe endotoxic shock. The organisms need not be living for the syndrome to occur.[65]

If intravenous or other medications are believed to be intrinsically contaminated, the Food and Drug Administration should be notified immediately (http://www.fda.gov/medwatch). All lots of the product that is suspected to be contaminated should be pulled from the facility's shelves and quarantined.

Epidemiologic Typing Methods for Outbreak Investigation

Once an organism is isolated, the next step is to determine whether the isolates are the same strain (i.e., can be from the same source). The methods that are used to determine whether isolates are related can be divided into two groups: phenotypic and genotypic methods. A phenotypic method uses expressed traits that a microorganism displays, and a genotypic method examines the genetic structure of an organism (its chromosomal or plasmid DNA). An example of a phenotypic method is the classification of an organism based on pigment production, such as the distinct red pigment of *Serratia marcesans*. An example of a genotypic method is pulsed-field gel electrophoresis, which can be used to type many nosocomial pathogens.

Examples of phenotypic and genotypic methods that are used to discriminate whether a bacterial strain is similar to another strain of the same species are listed in Table 11–3. During an outbreak, the laboratory must move expediently to identify the most appropriate techniques that will supply useful information to the investigators.[66]

Table 11–2 Procedures for the Selective Isolation of Microorganisms from Animate and Inanimate Sources

Culture	Purpose	Methods Employed/Reference	Interpretation	Availability
Air	To assess the dissemination of fungal spores	Settling plates; sieve sampler, slit sampler, and other sampling devices[59]	Qualitative fungal spores for settling plates; air samplers can provide quantitative data	Settling plates widely available; air sampling equipment must be purchased or rented or services can be contracted with an environmental reference laboratory
Water for *Legionella* species	To assess the presence of *Legionella* in the environment	Selective charcoal yeast extract agar (BCYE, ACES) with acid pretreatment or filtration[60]	Controversial; organisms are present in most water delivery systems	Environmental reference laboratories and some hospital laboratories
Dialysis water	To assess level of contamination of dialysis water	Plate count agar, Mueller Hinton agar, or Trypticase soy agar; inoculation by lawn streak method or agar dilution[61]	Acceptable limits: 1. <200 colony-forming units (CFU) before dialysis 2. <2,000 CFU after dialysis	Hospital laboratories
Environmental surfaces and medical devices	To assess the presence of organisms on environmental surfaces and medical devices	Nutrient-rich nonselective agar, Trypticase soy agar, or brain heart infusion (with or without 5% sheep or rabbit blood); inactivation of disinfectants may be needed[57]; specific media used to qualitatively isolate pathogens	Isolation of organisms epidemiologically associated with outbreak	Hospital laboratories and environmental reference laboratories
Hands	To assess the presence of bacteria on hands	Hand wash broth technique[55]	Isolation of organisms epidemiologically associated with outbreak; assessment of carriers	Hospital laboratories
Animate or inanimate sources for resistant bacteria	To assess patients, residents, health care workers, or environment for resistant bacteria such as MRSA, VRE, and gram-negative bacilli	Mannitol salt agar with oxacillin or selective broth for MRSA; vancomycin agar screen or high salt broth for VRE; culture and susceptibility testing for aminoglycoside-resistant and ESBL producers[58,62–64]	Isolation of organisms epidemiologically associated with outbreak; assessment of carriers	Hospital laboratories

Phenotypic Methods

Phenotypic methods used for epidemiologic purposes include antimicrobial susceptibility patterns, biotyping (using the pattern of biochemical reactions), serotyping, phage typing, and bacteriocin production and susceptibility. Bacteriophage typing, once commonly used to type *S aureus*, and bacteriocin typing are now rarely used. Antimicrobial susceptibility testing and biotyping are the most readily available and easiest to perform phenotypic methods and therefore they are the most widely used. However, these methods have

Table 11–3 Typing Methods Commonly Used To Determine Strain Relatedness

Method	Application	Limitations	Availability
Phenotypic methods			
Antimicrobial susceptibility pattern	Aerobic gram-negative rods and staphylococci	Patterns may be inherently similar, thus inhibiting organism discrimination; slight between-technician variations may be noted when reading susceptibilities; not very discriminatory	Most hospital laboratories
Biotyping (pattern of biochemical reactions)	Gram-negative bacilli, *Neisseria, Haemophilus, Staphylococcus* epidermidis	Slight between-technician variations may be noted when reading biochemical panels; limited utility; does not discriminate well between strains of the same species	Most hospital laboratories
Serotyping (serogrouping)	*Streptococcus pneumoniae, Escherichia coli* O157:H7, *Salmonella* species, *Shigella* species, *Legionella pneumophila, Hemophilus influenzae, Neisseria meningitidis*	Antigenic drift or mutations make the test less desirable for organisms subject to mutation	Some hospital laboratories and all reference laboratories
Genotypic (molecular) methods			
Analysis of plasmid DNA	*Staphylococci,* gram-negative bacilli, *Neisseria,* some herpesviruses, *adenovirus*	Microorganisms potentially unstable as a result of loss of plasmids and other mutations	Reference laboratory or medical center/research laboratory
Pulsed-field gel electrophoresis	Many microorganisms (*Staphylococci, Enterococci, Mycobacteria, Enterobacteriaceae,* pseudomonads); excellent power to discriminate	Some microorganisms are difficult to lyse and others possess extracellular products that will render the methods unreadable (e.g., *Serratia* DNAase)	Reference laboratory or medical center/research laboratory
Restriction fragment length polymorphism	Many microorganisms; method of choice for *Mycobacterium tuberculosis*	Large numbers of bands, difficult to interpret	Reference laboratory or medical center/research laboratory
Restriction endonuclease analysis of chromosomal DNA	*Clostridium difficile*	Large numbers of bands, difficult to interpret	Reference laboratory or medical center/research laboratory
Ribotyping	Many microorganisms	Limited power to discriminate	Reference laboratory or medical center/research laboratory
Polymerase chain reaction; arbitrarily primed polymerase chain reaction	*Clostridium difficile*		Reference laboratory or medical center/research laboratory
Random amplification of polymorphic DNA	Many microorganisms	Difficult to standardize	Reference laboratory or medical center/research laboratory

Source: Data from S. Weber, M.A. Pfaller, and L.A. Herwaldt, Role of Molecular Epidemiology in Infection Control, *U.S. Disease Clinics of North America,* Vol. 11, pp. 257–278, © 1997 and J. Maslow and M.E. Mulligan, Epidemiologic Typing Systems, *Infection Control and Hospital Epidemiology,* Vol. 17, pp. 595–604, © 1996.

poor discriminatory power (i.e., they do not clearly differentiate epidemiologically unrelated isolates).[67] The ability of microorganisms to change their biotype or alter their antimicrobial susceptibility pattern by the acquisition or loss of genetic material in the form of plasmids or transposons hinders the use of biotyping and antimicrobial susceptibility patterns for determining strain relatedness.[67] Organisms of the same strain may in fact mutate because of the selective antibiotic pressure found in most health care settings. This mutation could result in the organism changing their phenotypic characteristics in a short period of time.[68]

Serologic typing techniques also have drawbacks. Many strains of organisms are not able to be typed if they fail to react with available antiserum. From 10 to 15 percent of *Mycobacterium avium* strains fail to react and are therefore not able to be typed.[69] However, serology is a useful adjunct when used to identify *Salmonella* species and *Shigella* species.

Whenever possible, genotypic methods, which have better discriminating power, should be used rather than phenotypic methods. Some molecular (genotypic) methods are inexpensive and may replace the use of phenotypic methods altogether in the future.[69]

The importance of identifying organisms to the species level can be illustrated with the following example. In the summer of 1991, in the neonatal intensive care unit (NICU) at this author's hospital, nurses noticed that stools from two infants smelled foul.[70] They collected samples and sent them to the laboratory for culture. Neither of the infants seemed to be infected; however, a neonate near them was gravely ill, so this infant's stool was also sent to the laboratory for culture. All three samples were positive for *Salmonella poona*. An epidemiologic investigation began with a phone call to the NICU from the microbiology laboratory. As part of the investigation, stool cultures were performed on a total of 60 employees and patients. All were negative for *Salmonella*. A nurse who was off work with a gastrointestinal illness was contacted and sent to her physician who collected a stool culture. The specimen was sent to a different laboratory, which isolated *Salmonella*, and she was diagnosed with *Salmonella* food poisoning. Because the laboratory that did the culture did not offer serotyping, it was assumed that she was the point source of the nosocomial outbreak. However, when an additional sample from this nurse was sent to the hospital laboratory for culture, serotyping of the isolate revealed that she was infected with *Salmonella*

enteritidis, and therefore she was not the source. The likely source of the organism was eventually determined to be a symptomatic, culture-positive maternity patient who passed *S poona* to her infant at the time of birth. Her infant had no signs of illness but had stool cultures that were positive for *S poona*. At the time of the NICU outbreak, there was a nationwide outbreak of *S poona* associated with contaminated cantaloupe, and 26 cases associated with that foodborne outbreak had been reported to the state health department in Pennsylvania, where the NICU is located.[70]

Some important lessons should be learned from this experience. When conducting an investigation, evaluate laboratory data cautiously, demand complete identification of the isolates with confirmatory tests, and send all organisms involved in the outbreak to the same laboratory for testing. The laboratory should have procedures and reagents available to provide complete information on common pathogens such as *Salmonella* and should be capable of serotyping these isolates even if the majority of clinical cases do not require it for therapy. There have been pseudo-outbreaks associated with failure of the laboratory to discriminate one *Salmonella* species from another.[71]

Genotypic (Molecular) Methods

Today, a laboratory's test arsenal contains sophisticated molecular methods that can ascertain whether the strains of isolates are related.[9,38–40,66–68,72–76] Genotypic, or molecular, methods that are used for the epidemiologic study of endemic and epidemic infections include

- DNA probe hybridization
- amplified molecular methods such as polymerase chain reaction
- restriction fragment length polymorphism
- ribotyping
- pulsed-field gel electrophoresis (PFGE)
- plasmid fingerprinting
- random amplification of polymorphic DNA (also known as arbitrarily primed PCR or AP-PCR)
- enterobacterial repetitive insertion

Molecular methods can be used to discriminate strains that cannot be separated by phenotypic methods.

The intent of this section is not to explain the scientific basis of the genotypic methods but rather to identify examples of how they might be applied. Molecular methods can be used to determine whether isolates of the same species are the same strain, to study antimicrobial resistance mechanisms of organisms, and to detect nonviable or noncultivable organisms. This section will focus on their use in strain typing during outbreak investigations.

There are many examples in the literature that document the use of molecular methods for investigating a potential outbreak.[38–40,68,77–89] For information on the principles, applications, advantages, disadvantages, interpretation, and costs of the various typing systems, the reader is referred to several published reviews.[38,66–69] Because methods for distinguishing among microbial strains are evolving rapidly, keep in mind that these publications become quickly outdated. At present, start-up costs for these technologies range between $8,000 and $130,000, and cost to the laboratory per analysis ranges between $11 and $40.[69] Charges to the infection control department may be considerably higher.

In 1997, the Society for Healthcare Epidemiology of America published a position paper on how to select and interpret molecular strain typing methods for epidemiologic studies of bacterial infections.[66] This paper identifies the following preferred typing techniques for nosocomial pathogens:

- Pulsed-field gel electrophoresis for *S aureus*, coagulase-negative staphylococci, enterococci, *S pneumoniae*, most of the *Enterobacteriaceae* (*E coli, Citrobacter, Proteus, Providenicia, Klebsiella, Enterobacter*, and *Serratia*), *Pseudomonas aeruginosa, Burkholderia, Stenotrophomonas, Acinetobacter*, and mycobacteria other than MTB
- restriction fragment length polymorphism for MTB
- AP-PCR for *C difficile*
- serotyping for *Salmonella* and *Shigella* species[66]

An article by Maslow and Mulligan[67] lists important caveats to keep in mind when using molecular typing during an investigation. For instance, some organisms, such as MRSA, have limited genetic diversity and isolates may be epidemiologically unrelated even though they appear to be the same strain. This lack of diversity can lead investigators to falsely conclude that an outbreak has occurred.

The following example illustrates the application of molecular methods in investigating an outbreak. This author was involved in the investigation of a suspected outbreak of *S marcescens* in a nursery. Because an epidemiologic investigation failed to implicate any potential sources, environmental cultures were performed. *S marcescens* was isolated from the wash sinks, the housekeeping equipment, and environmental surfaces, and these isolates were phenotypically indistinguishable from the patient's isolates. These organisms were saved and sent to a specialty laboratory for PFGE. Subsequently, the results of the PFGE showed that the environmental strains were not related to the patient isolates. In this instance, a molecular method (PFGE) was able to demonstrate that isolates that appeared phenotypically identical were actually different strains.

Molecular typing has been used in investigations of clusters and potential outbreaks to aid in the following:

- demonstrate that a health care worker was the likely source of an outbreak of *S aureus* in a surgical intensive care unit[87]
- allow distinction between endogenous and exogenous infection[68,86]
- confirm the suspicion of an outbreak by confirming that isolates from multiple patients were genetically similar[78,79]
- provide evidence of person-to-person transmission of an organism[80,83,88]
- demonstrate cross-contamination in the laboratory[77,81,90,91]
- demonstrate that contaminated medical devices, medication, disinfectants, or equipment were the likely source of organisms colonizing or infecting patients[82,84,85,92]
- demonstrate that more than one strain of an organism may be involved in an outbreak[84,89]
- show evidence that *S aureus* nasal colonization of pediatric patients may be a risk factor for sternal wound infections after open heart surgery[86]

PSEUDO-OUTBREAKS

Pseudo-outbreaks occur when there is a real cluster of false infections or a false cluster of real infections. Pseudo-outbreaks, discussed in detail in Chapter 6, have been attributed to laboratory contamination, improper collection of specimens, and contamination of pharmaceutical products, medical devices, municipal water supplies, and disinfectants.[77,90–97]

Infection control and microbiology laboratory personnel must be aware that laboratory contamination has been a common problem causing nosocomial pseudo-outbreaks.[77,81,94–97] Recently, several reports have detailed laboratory contamination as the cause of an increased incidence of MTB.[90,91] Pseudo-outbreaks of tuberculosis can be extremely costly for an institution because the patients involved may be unnecessarily started on antituberculous therapy, they may be placed in isolation rooms, and contact tracing may be done before the pseudo-outbreak is recognized.

The first and easiest department to evaluate in the event of a suspected pseudo-outbreak is the laboratory.[2] During 1998, the infection control department in the author's hospital noticed an increased incidence of MTB from patients seen in its health system.[90] Many patients had evidence that suggested active or past infection with MTB. However, the finding that five patients were identified with MTB over a 2-week period seemed more than a coincidence. Investigation in the laboratory revealed the potential for contamination during specimen processing. All of the samples were processed using the same decontaminating/mucolytic solution. Because all acid-fast organisms isolated in this laboratory are saved for at least 1 year, the infection control department requested that the MTB organisms be sent for typing. All of the isolates were found to be related by PFGE to the MTB from the first sample processed; therefore, the cultures were thought to have been cross-contaminated. Contamination during processing of MTB samples has often been reported, and the incidence of false-positive results can be as high as 12 percent of the total MTB isolates detected.[91]

Pseudo-outbreaks have occurred with other organisms, such as *Burkholderia (Pseudomonas) cepacia* (found in contaminated povidone iodine preparations),[92] *S marcescens* (contaminated disinfectants),[93] atypical mycobacteria (contaminated medical devices and water supplies),[97] and *Enterobacter cloacae* and *Enterococcus faecium* (contaminated chopped meat glucose broth culture media).[96]

More than 10 years ago, this author's laboratory noticed that coagulase-negative staphylococci were isolated from several specimens from chopped meat broth cultures only. Because molecular techniques were not available at that time, a study was conducted to determine the likelihood of contamination and to demonstrate to the technologists the importance of using sterile techniques. Three technologists aseptically entered five chopped meat broth media tubes (16 by 125-mm tubes with a small-bore opening) five times using the same inoculating loop. The loop was heated to sterilize it between each entry. The tubes were incubated for 2 days at 35 °C, and 40 percent of the tubes showed growth (i.e., were contaminated). The laboratory replaced the chopped meat glucose tubes with another type that had a wide-bore opening to decrease the possibility of contamination. The study was repeated, and no contamination was noted. This kind of a study can demonstrate the importance of the use of sterile techniques in the laboratory. Laboratory personnel must be able to objectively look at their processes without taking offense at the inference that their procedures might not be optimal.

LABORATORY PREPAREDNESS FOR INVESTIGATING ACTS OF BIOLOGICAL WARFARE AND BIOTERRORISM

World politics dictate that the infection control professional and the microbiologist be aware of the most common microorganisms found in the areas where armed forces service personnel have been stationed. Before and after the Gulf War, several articles[98,99] appeared in journals alerting the microbiology and infectious disease communities to microorganisms and diseases from the Middle East and the methods required to diagnose and treat them. Many laboratories in the United States have never isolated or identified causative agents of diseases endemic in third world countries.

Recently, the health care community has been asked to review procedures used to isolate and identify microorganisms used as biological weapons.[100,101] Table 11–4 lists organisms with potential for use as biological weapons.[101] In the United States, four states reported alleged bioterrorist threats in 1998 involving the use of *Bacillus anthracis* as a biological weapon.[102] All of these cases turned out to be hoaxes; however, the federal government and the health care community are taking these threats seriously.

It is likely that health care facilities will be among the first to recognize cases of infectious disease caused by a biological attack. A report by Dr. James Snyder details the pitfalls and recommendations for the microbiology laboratory's involvement.[98] The microbiology laboratory may become involved as a result of the following events:

1. An overt act of bioterrorism in which, under the direction of the Federal Bureau of In-

Table 11–4 Agents of Bioterrorism

Agent (Disease)	Comments	Laboratory Support
Bacillus anthracis (inhalation)	Endospores delivered in an aerosol expected to produce severe morbidity in unprotected populations	Most laboratories do not have policies to isolate or identify this organism
Yersinia pestis (plague)	Fulminant pneumonic form of plague is often fatal unless treatment with antibiotic drugs is initiated with 24 hours of onset of symptoms	Requires biosafety level 3; most laboratories not capable of isolating and identifying the organism
Francisella tularensis (tularemia)	Aerosol delivery produces typhoidal tularemia, often with a respiratory component; highly infectious (case fatality rate in untreated patients is 35%)	Requires biosafety level 3; most laboratories not capable of isolating and identifying the organism
Brucella species (brucellosis)	Highly infective via aerosol; febrile illness with nonspecific symptoms with low (<5%) mortality in untreated patients; symptoms may last for weeks to months; relapses common	Most laboratories can isolate the organism; however, dye test for speciation is not widely available
Coxiella burnetii (Q fever)	Highly infective (because of sporelike form); produces acute febrile illness with a low case fatality rate; treatment with antibiotic drugs shortens course or prevents disease when administered during incubation period	Most laboratories incapable of isolation and identification
Variola virus (small pox)	Stable virus, effectively spread via aerosol; mortality of 30% or higher in unvaccinated populations with increased susceptibility	Most laboratories cannot isolate; must be serologically identified at a reference laboratory
Venezuelan (VEE), Eastern (EEE), and Western (WEE) encephalitis virus (febrile illness, encephalitis)	Normally mosquito-borne febrile illness with possible neurologic sequelae; easy and inexpensive to produce in large amounts; infectious via aerosol; infections may vary from incapacitating to lethal	Most laboratories cannot isolate; must be serologically identified at a reference laboratory
Rift Valley fever, Congo-Crimean hemorrhagic fever, Junin, Machupo, Guanarito, Sabia, and Ebola viruses (hemorrhagic fevers)	Acute febrile illnesses, often with bleeding manifestations; normally transmitted through contact with animals or via arthropods but also infectious via aerosol; high morbidity and with some high mortality	Only available at a sophisticated reference laboratory

Source: Reprinted from *Clinical Microbiology Newsletter*, Vol. 20, K.L. Ruoff, Biological Warfare, p. 175, Copyright 1998, with permission from Elsevier Science.

vestigation who requests the assistance of the local microbiology laboratory to provide a preliminary analysis of an environmental sample suspected of containing a biological agent. 2. A covert act leading to a disease outbreak and during the early stages of the suspected outbreak, the laboratory receives samples from patients exhibiting varying disease etiologies and applies routine diagnostic procedures that are not targeted to the detection of biothreat agents. 3. Following the confirmation of an outbreak (late stage); specimens are received from patients who are suspected of having been exposed to a biological agent and the laboratory is requested to identify the specific agent.[98(p.524)]

Unfortunately, the report notes that most microbiology laboratories are ill equipped to handle outbreaks of this type. Very few laboratories have biosafety levels above level 2, and a biosafety level 3 is required to safely handle the organisms that would most likely be involved in a bioterrorist attack.

Every institution's safety and infection control department should work with the infectious disease staff and the laboratory to assess the facility's ability to respond to potential terrorist threats.[101–104] Bioterrorists in the United States have used *Salmonella typhimurium* in an attempt to influence polling numbers during an election.[104] The use of a potentially virulent microorganism such as small pox virus or *Bacillus anthracis* might be disastrous.[103,104] The pulmonary disease caused by *B anthracis* resembles a septic pneumonia, and anthrax is usually diagnosed late in the disease process. Because *B anthracis* could likely be isolated from blood cultures of patients infected with pulmonary anthrax, the laboratory should have policies in place to routinely identify spore-forming bacilli when found in sterile body sites. In reality, most laboratories would dismiss a spore-forming facultative bacilli found in one blood culture bottle as a contaminant.[100] In the author's laboratory, policy states that spore-forming aerobic bacilli that do not exhibit hemolysis should be identified and *B anthracis* should be ruled out as the infecting agent.

However, this policy is not extensive enough. Policies and procedures must be implemented to collect samples, contact the Federal Bureau of Investigation, and preliminarily screen or transport samples to a regional or federal laboratory for identification.[100]

Additional information on this topic can be found on the Web sites of the Association for Professionals in Infection Control and Epidemiology (http://www.apic.org), the CDC (http://www.cdc.gov), and the Johns Hopkins Center for Civilian Biodefense Studies (http://www.hopkins-biodefense.org).

CONCLUSION

The laboratory plays an integral role in a facility's infection surveillance, prevention, and control program by identifying organisms of epidemiologic significance, providing the results of laboratory tests, tracking antimicrobial resistance, assisting in outbreak detection and investigation, and serving as a resource for consultation.

Many microbiologists are trained in infection control. When a suspected outbreak occurs, the laboratory must be contacted immediately so that significant isolates and sera are saved. If microbiologic culturing is to be done, the laboratory should be consulted regarding the specimens to be collected, the method of transport, and the level of identification required for the organism being studied. Policies for outbreak investigation should be in place before an emergency.

REFERENCES

1. McClung LJ, Merger KF. Beginnings of bacteriology in California. *Bacteriol Rev.* 1974;38:251–271.

2. Gilcrest MJR. Laboratory support for infection control: optimization by policy and procedure. In: Isenberg H, ed. *Clinical Microbiology Procedure Manual.* Washington, DC: ASM Press; 1992:11.1.1.

3. Shultz SM. The medical education of William Brooks Bigler (1863). *Ann Intern Med.* 1998;129:426–430.

4. Centers for Disease Control. Preventing emerging infectious diseases: a strategy for the 21st century; overview of the updated CDC plan. *MMWR.* 1998;47:1–14.

5. Lederberg J. Infectious disease as an evolutionary paradigm. *Emerg Infect Dis.* 1997;3:417–423.

6. Emori TG, Gaynes RP. An overview of nosocomial infections, including the role of the microbiology laboratory. *Clin Microbiol Rev.* 1993;6:428–442.

7. Thomson RB Jr, Peterson LR. Role of the clinical microbiology laboratory in the diagnosis of infection. *Cancer Treat Res.* 1998;96:143–165.

8. McGowan JE Jr., Metchock BG. Basic microbiology support for hospital epidemiology. *Infect Control Hosp Epidemiol.*1996;17:298–303.

9. Pfaller MA, Herwaldt LA. The clinical microbiology laboratory and infection control: emerging pathogens, antimicrobial resistance, and new technology. *Clin Infect Dis.*1997;25:858–870.

10. McNicol P, Giercke SM, Gray M, et al. Evaluation and validation of a monoclonal immunofluorescent reagent for direct detection of *Bordetella pertussis. J Clin Microbiol.* 1995;33:2868–2871.

11. Lemaitre D, Elaichouni A, Hundhausen M, et al. Tracheal colonization with *Shingomonas paucimobilis* in mechanically ventilated neonates due to contaminated ventilator temperature probes. *J Hosp Infect.* 1996;32:199–206.

12. Walsh TJ, Vlahov D, Hansen SL, et al. Prospective microbiologic surveillance in control of nosocomial methicillin-resistant *Staphylococcus aureus. Infect Control.* 1987;8:7–14.

13. Reagan DR. Microcomputers in hospital epidemiology. *Infect Control Hosp Epidemiol.* 1997;18:440–448.

14. Baron EJ. Development in laboratory informatics. *Clin Microbiol Newsl.* 1996;18:65–70.

15. Campos JM. Use of the laboratory information system to improve the quality and reduce the cost of microbiology testing. *Clin Microbiol Newsl.* 1999;21:11–14.

16. Dessau RB, Steenberg P. Computerized surveillance in clinical microbiology with time series analysis. *J Clin Microbiol.* 1993;31:857–860.

17. Kloos WE, Lambe DW. Staphylococcus. In: Balows A, Hausler WJ, Herrmann KL, Isenburg, HD, Shadomy HJ, eds. *Manual of Clinical Microbiology.* 5th ed. Washington, DC: ASM Press; 1991:222–237.

18. Hsueh PR, Teng LJ, Yang PC, et al. Dissemination of two methicillin-resistant *Staphylococcus aureus* clones exhibiting negative staphylase reactions in intensive care units. *J Clin Microbiol.* 1999;37:504–509.

19. Smole SC, Aronson E, Brecher SM, Arbeit RD. Sensitivity and specificity of an improved rapid latex agglutination test for identification of methicillin-sensitive and -resistant *Staphylococcus aureus* isolates. *J Clin Microbiol.* 1998;36:1109–1112.

20. Wilkerson M, McAllister S, Miller JM, Heiter BJ, Bourbeau PP. Comparison of five agglutination tests for identification of *Staphylococcus aureus. J Clin Microbiol.* 1997;35:148–151.

21. Brown WJ. Comparison of a yellow latex reagent with other agglutination methods for the identification of *Staphylococcus aureus. J Clin Microbiol.* 1986;23:640–642.

22. Reanney DC. Extrachromosomal elements as possible agents of adaptation and development. *Bacteriol Rev.* 1976;40:552–590.

23. Farmer JJ III. Enterobacteriaceae: introduction and identification. In: Murray PR, Baron EJ, Pfaller MA, Tenover FC, Yolken RH, eds. *Manual of Clinical Microbiology.* 6th ed. Washington, DC: ASM Press; 1995:438–449.

24. Sautter RL, Mattman LH, Legaspi RC. *Serratia marcescens* meningitis associated with a contaminated benzalkonium chloride solution. *Infect Control.* 1984;5:223–225.

25. Rappaport T, Sawyer KP, Nachamkin I. Evaluation of several commercial biochemical and immunologic methods for rapid identification of gram positive cocci directly from blood cultures. *J Clin Microbiol.* 1988;26:1335–1338.

26. Speers DJ, Olma T, Gilbert GL. Evaluation of four methods for rapid identification of *Staphylococcus aureus* from blood cultures. *J Clin Microbiol.* 1999;36:1032–1034.

27. Valenstein PN. Evaluating diagnostic tests with imperfect standards. *Am J Clin Pathol.* 1990;93:252–258.

28. Roy TM, Flemming D, Anderson WH. Tularemic pneumonia mimicking Legionnaires' disease with false-positive direct fluorescent antibody stains for *Legionella. South Med J.* 1989;82:1429–1431.

29. Centers for Disease Control. False-positive laboratory tests for *Cryptosporidium* involving an enzyme-linked immunosorbent assay—United States: November 1997–March 1998. *MMWR.* 1999;48:4–8.

30. Marcante R, Chiumento F, Palu G, Cavedon G. Rapid diagnosis of influenza type A infection: comparison of shell-vial culture, directigen flu-A and enzyme-linked immunosorbent assay. *New Microbiol.* 1996;19:141–147.

31. Pollock HM, Wieman EJ. Smear results in the diagnosis of *Mycobacterioses* using blue light fluorescence microscopy. *J Clin Microbiol.* 1977;5:329–331.

32. Muller FM, Hoppe JE, Wirsing von Konig CH. Laboratory diagnosis of pertussis: state of the art in 1997. *J Clin Microbiol.* 1997;35:2435–2443.

33. Centers for Disease Control. Prevention and control of influenza: recommendations of the Advisory Committee on Immunization Practices (ACIP). *MMWR.* 1999;48(Suppl):1–28.

34. Reina J, Munar M, Blanco I. Evaluation of a direct immunofluorescence assay, dot-blot enzyme immunoassay, and shell vial culture in the diagnosis of lower respiratory tract infections caused by influenza virus. *Diag Microbiol Infect Dis.* 1996;25:143–145.

35. Smith PB, Tomfohrde KM, Rhoden DL, Balows A. API system: a multitube micromethod for identification of Enterobacteriaceae. *Appl Microbiol.* 1972;24:449–452.

36. Daly JA. Rapid diagnostic tests in microbiology in the 1990s. *Am J Clin Pathol.* 1994;101(4 suppl 1):S22–S26.

37. McLaughlin J. Standards for abbreviated bacterial identification. *Clin Microbiol Newsl.* 1993;15:123–125.

38. Weber S, Pfaller MA, Herwaldt LA. Role of molecular epidemiology in infection control. *Infect Dis Clin N Am.* 1997;11:257–278.

39. Jarvis WR. Usefulness of molecular epidemiology for outbreak investigations. *Infect Control Hosp Epidemiol.* 1994;15:500–503.

40. Maloney SA, Jarvis WR. Epidemic nosocomial pneumonia in the intensive care unit. *Clin Chest Med.* 1995;16:209–223.

41. Centers for Disease Control. Microbiologic sampling. In: *Guideline for Handwashing and Hospital Environmental Control, 1985.* Atlanta, GA: U.S. Department of Health and Human Services, Hospital Infections Program, Center for Infectious Diseases, Centers for Disease Control; 1985.

42. Brooks L. Policy for infection control cultures. In: Isenberg H, ed. *Clinical Microbiology Procedure Manual.* Washington, DC: ASM Press; 1992:11.2.1.

43. Master RN, Sautter RL, Brown WJ, et al. Comparison of the microbial identification system with commercially available systems for the identification of pink pigmented oxidase positive bacteria. In: *Abstracts of the Annual Meeting.* Washington, DC: American Society for Microbiology; 1991:C-218.

44. Bennett ME, Thurn JR, Klicker R, Williams CO, Weiler M. Recommendations from a Minnesota task force for the management of persons with methicillin-resistant *Staphylococcus aureus. Am J Infect Control.* 1992;20:42–48.

45. Mulligan ME, Murray-Leisure KA, Ribner BS, et al. Methicillin-resistant *Staphylococcus aureus*: a consensus review of the microbiology, pathogenesis, and epidemiology with implications for prevention and management. *Am J Med.* 1993;94:313–328.

46. Wenzel RP, Reagan DR, Bertino JS, Baron EJ, Arias K. Methicillin-resistant *Staphyllococcus aureus* outbreak: a consensus panel's definition and management guidelines. *Am J Infect Control.* 1998;26:102–110.

47. Gorss EB. Focused surveillance for oxacillin-resistant *Staphylococcus aureus.* In: Isenberg H, ed. *Clinical Microbiology Procedure Manual.* Washington, DC: ASM Press; 1992:11.15.

48. Tenover FC. Laboratory methods for surveillance of vancomycin-resistant *Enterococci. Clin Microbiol Newsl.* 1998;20:1–5.

49. Miller JM, Holmes HT. Specimen collection, transport, and storage. In: Murray PR, Baron EJ, Pfaller MA, Tenover FC, Yolken RH, eds. *Manual of Clinical Microbiology.* 6th ed. Washington, DC: ASM Press; 1995:19–32.

50. Centers for Disease Control. Laboratory practices for prenatal Group B streptococcal screening and reporting. *MMWR.* 1999;48:426–428.

51. Centers for Disease Control. Recommendations for collection of laboratory specimens associated with outbreaks of gastroenteritis. *MMWR.* 1990;39:RR-14.

52. Kyne L, Merry C, O'Connell B, Harrington P, Keane C, O'Neill. Simultaneous outbreaks of two strains of toxigenic *Clostridium difficile* in a general hospital. *J Hosp Infect.* 1998;38:101–112.

53. McFarland LV, Mulligan ME, Kwok RYY, Stamm WE. Nosocomial acquisition of *Clostridium difficile* infection. *N Engl J Med.* 1989;320:204–210.

54. LaBaron CW, Furutan NP, Lew JF, et al. Viral agents of gastroenteritis—public health importance and outbreak management. *MMWR.* 1990;39(RR-5):1–24.

55. Macone AB. Prospective, focused surveillance for high-level aminoglycoside-resistant gram-negative bacilli. In: Isenberg H, ed. *Clinical Microbiology Procedure Manual.* Washington, DC: ASM Press; 1992:11.17.

56. Isenberg H, ed. *Clinical Microbiology Procedure Manual.* Washington, DC: ASM Press; 1992.

57. Bond WW, Hedrick ER. Microbiological culturing of environmental and medical-device surfaces. In: Isenberg H, ed. *Clinical Microbiology Procedure Manual.* Washington, DC: ASM Press; 1992:11.10.

58. Sautter RL, Brown WJ, Mattman LH. The use of a selective staphylococcal broth versus direct plating for the recovery of *Staphylococcus aureus. Infect Control Hosp Epidemiol.* 1988;9:204–205.

59. Streifel AJ. Air cultures for fungi. In: Isenberg H, ed. *Clinical Microbiology Procedure Manual.* Washington DC: ASM Press; 1992:11.8.

60. Hall NH. Culture of hospital water for members of the family Legionellaceae. In: Isenberg H, ed. *Clinical Microbiology Procedure Manual.* Washington, DC: ASM Press; 1992:11.3.

61. Smith JP. Culture and endotoxin assay of hemodialysis water. In: Isenberg H., ed. *Clinical Microbiology Procedure Manual.* Washington DC: ASM Press; 1992:11.4.

62. Holloway PM, Platt JH, Reybrouck G, Lilly HA, Mehtar S, Drabu Y. A multi-centre evaluation of two chlorhexidine-containing formulations for surgical hand disinfection. *J Hosp Infect.* 1990;16:151–159.

63. Moland ES, Sanders CC, Thomson KS. Can results obtained with commercially available Microscan microdilution panels serve as an indicator of beta-lactamase production among *Escherichia coli* and *Klebsiella* isolates with hidden resistance to expanded-spectrum cephalosporins and aztreonam. *J Clin Microbiol.* 1998;36:2575–2579.

64. Jacoby GA. Extended-spectrum beta-lactamases and other enzymes providing resistance to oxyimino-beta-lactams. *Infect Dis Clin N Am.* 1997;11:875–887.

65. Pool EJ, Joharr G, Janes S, Peterson I, Baric P. Differentiation between endotoxin and non-endotoxin pyrogens in human albumin solutions using an ex vivo whole blood culture assay. *J Immunoassay.* 1999;20:79–89.

66. Tenover FC, Arbeit RD, Goering RV, and the Molecular Typing Working Group of the Society for Healthcare Epidemiology of America. How to select and interpret molecular typing methods for epidemiological studies of bacterial infections: a review for healthcare epidemiologists. *Infect Control Hosp Epidemiol.* 1991;18:426–439.

67. Maslow J, Mulligan ME. Epidemiologic typing systems. *Infect Control Hosp Epidemiol.* 1996;17:595–604.

68. Bingen E. Applications of molecular methods to epidemiologic investigations of nosocomial infections in a pediatric hospital. *Infect Control Hosp Epidemiol.* 1994;15:488–493.

69. Olive DM, Bean P. Principles and applications of methods for DNA-based typing microbial organisms. *J Clin Microbiol.* 1999;37:1661–1669.

70. Stone A, Shaffer M, Sautter RL. *Salmonella poona* infection and surveillance in a neonatal nursery. *Am J Infect Control.* 1993;21:270–273.

71. Baddour LM, Robinson VL, Baselski V. Pseudoepidemic of salmonellosis in a nursery: importance of isolate serotyping. *Am J Infect Control.* 1987;15:79–80.

72. Sader HS, Hollis RJ, Pfaller MA. The use of molecular techniques in the epidemiology and control of infectious diseases. *Clin Lab Med.* 1995;15:407–431.

73. Miller, JM. Molecular technology for hospital epidemiology. *Diag Microbiol Infect Dis.* 1993;16:153–157.

74. Struelens MJ, De Gheldre Y, Deplano A. Comparative and library epidemiological typing systems: outbreak investigations versus surveillance systems. *Infect Control Hosp Epidemiol.* 1998;19:565–569.

75. Streulens MJ, and the Members of the European Study Group on Epidemiological Markers (ESGEM) of the European Society for Clinical Microbiology and Infectious Diseases (ESCMID). Consensus guidelines for appropriate use and evaluation of microbial epidemiologic typing systems. *Clin Microbiol Infect.* 1996;2:2–11.

76. Cockerill FR III. Genetic methods for assessing antimicrobial resistance. *Antimicrob Agents Chemother.* 1999;43:199–212.

77. Wurtz R, Demarais P, Trainor W, et al. Specimen contamination in mycobacteriology laboratory detected by pseudo-outbreak of multidrug-resistant tuberculosis: analysis by routine epidemiology and confirmation by molecular technique. *J Clin Microbiol.* 1996;34:1017–1019.

78. Campbell JR, Zaccaria E, Mason EO Jr, Baker CJ. Epidemiological analysis defining concurrent outbreaks of *Serratia marcescens* and methicillin-resistant *Staphylococcus aureus* in a neonatal intensive care unit. *Infect Control Hosp Epidemiol.* 1998;19:924–928.

79. Kluytmans J, Berg H, Steegh P, Vandenesch F, Etienne J, van Belkum A. Outbreak of *Staphylococcus schleiferi* wound infections: strain characterization by randomly amplified polymorphic DNA analysis, PCR ribotyping conventional ribotyping, and pulsed-field gel electrophoresis. *J Clin Microbiol.* 1998;36:2214–2219.

80. Fowler SL, Rhoton B, Springer SC, Messer SA, Hollis RJ, Pfaller MA. Evidence for person-to-person transmission of *Candida lusitaniae* in a neonatal intensive-care unit. *Infect Control Hosp Epidemiol.* 1998;19:343–345.

81. Louie L, Louie M, Simor AE. Investigation of a pseudo-outbreak of *Nocardia asteroides* infection by pulsed-field gel electrophoresis and randomly amplified polymorphic DNA PCR. *J Clin Microbiol.* 1997;35:1582–1584.

82. Blanc DS, Parret T, Janin B, Raselli P, Francioli P. Nosocomial infections and pseudoinfections from contaminated bronchoscopes: two-year follow up using molecular markers. *Infect Control Hosp Epidemiol.* 1997;18:134–136..

83. DeGheldre Y, Maes N, Rost F, et al. Molecular epidemiology of an outbreak of multidrug-resistant *Enterobacter aerogenes* infections and in vivo emergence of imipenem resistance. *J Clin Microbiol.* 1997;35:152–160.

84. Cimolai N, Trombley C, Wensley D, LeBlanc J. Heterogeneous *Serratia marcescens* genotypes from a nosocomial pediatric outbreak. *Chest.* 1997;111:194–197.

85. Welbel SF, McNeil MM, Kuykendall RJ, et al. *Candida parapsilosis* bloodstream infections in neonatal intensive care unit patients: epidemiologic and laboratory confirmation of common source outbreak. *Pediatr Infect Dis J.* 1996;15:998–1002.

86. Ruef C, Fanconi S, Nadal D. Sternal wound infection after heart operations in pediatric patients associated with nasal carriage of *Staphylococcus aureus. J Thor Cardiovasc Surg.* 1996;112:681–686.

87. Sheretz RJ, Reagan DR, Hampton KD, et al. A cloud adult: the *Staphylococcus aureus*-virus interaction revisited. *Ann Intern Med.* 1996;124:539–547.

88. Marx A, Shay DK, Noel JS, et al. An outbreak of acute gastroenteritis in a geriatric long-term-care facility: combined application of epide-

miological and molecular diagnostic methods. *Infect Control Hosp Epidemiol*. 1999;20:306–311.

89. Noel GJ, Kreiswirth BN, Edelson PF, et al. Multiple methicillin-resistant *Staphylococcus aureus* strains as a cause for a single outbreak of severe disease in hospital neonates. *Pediatr Infect Dis J*. 1992;11:184–188.

90. Gross CM, Stamillio C, Sautter RL, et al. Pseudo-outbreak of *Mycobacterium tuberculosis* associated with laboratory processing contamination. Abstracts from: Proceedings of the Eighth Annual Meeting of the Society for Healthcare Epidemiology of America. *Infect Control Hosp Epidemiol*. 1998;19:681.

91. Burman WJ, Stone BL, Reves RR, et al. The incidence of false-positive cultures for *Mycobacterium tuberculosis*. *Am J Respir Crit Care Med*. 1997;155:321–326.

92. Panlilio AL, Beck-Sague CM, Siegel JD, et al. Infections and pseudoinfections due to povidone-iodine solution contaminated with *Pseudomonas cepacia*. *Clin Infect Dis*. 1992;14:1078–1083.

93. Farmer JJ 3d, Davis BR, Hickman FW, et al. Detection of *Serratia* outbreaks in hospital. *Lancet*. 1976;2:455–459.

94. Budnick LD, Moll ME, Hull HF, Mann JM, Kendal AP. A pseudo-outbreak of influenza A associated with use of laboratory stock strain. *Am J Public Health*. 1984;74:607–609.

95. Burman WJ, Wilson ML, Reves RR. Specimen contamination in mycobacteriology laboratory detected by pseudo-outbreak of multidrug-resistant tuberculosis: analysis by routine epidemiology and confirmation by molecular technique. *J Clin Microbiol*. 1996;34:3257.

96. Morris T, Brecher SM, Fitzimmons D, Durbin A, Arbeit RD, Maslow JN. A pseudoepidemic due to laboratory contamination deciphered by molecular analysis. *Infect Control Hosp Epidemiol*. 1995;16:82–87.

97. Wallace RJ, Brown BA, Griffith DE. Nosocomial outbreaks/pseudo-outbreaks due to nontuberculous *Mycobacteria*. *Ann Rev Microbiol*. 1998;52:453–490.

98. Snyder JW. Infectious disease associated with Operation Desert Storm. *Clin Microbiol Newsl*. 1993;15:161–163.

99. Oldfield EC III, Rodier GR, Gray GC. Endemic infectious diseases of the Middle East. *Rev Infect Dis*. 1991;3:5199–5217.

100. Snyder JW. Responding to bioterrorism: the role of the microbiology laboratory. *ASM News*. 1999;65:524–525.

101. Ruoff KL. Biological warfare. *Clin Microbiol Newsl*. 1998;20:173–176.

102. Centers for Disease Control and Prevention. Bioterrorism alleging use of Anthrax and interim guidelines for management—United States, 1998. *MMWR*. 1999;48:69–74.

103. Henderson DA. Bioterrorism as a public health threat. *Emerg Infect Dis*. 1998;4:489–492.

104. McDade JE, Frantz D. Bioterrorism as a public health threat. *Emerg Infect Dis*. 1998;4:493–494.

CHAPTER 12

Collecting, Organizing, and Displaying Epidemiologic Data

Kathleen Meehan Arias

Excellence in statistical graphics consists of complex ideas communicated with clarity, precision, and efficiency.

Edward R. Tufte[1(p.13)]

Surveillance is an integral part of any health care facility's infection control and quality management programs. Because surveillance involves the ongoing collection, analysis, interpretation, and dissemination of large amounts of data, infection control and quality management personnel should be familiar with the tools and methods used to process this data and communicate their findings to others. The purpose of this chapter is to discuss practical tools that can be used to collect, organize, and display epidemiologic data:

- Forms and databases to collect and organize data
- Tables, graphs, and charts to organize and display data
- Computers to manage data

COLLECTING AND ORGANIZING EPIDEMIOLOGIC DATA

Using Forms and Databases

In order to detect an outbreak or a cluster of events, data must be compared over time; therefore the data must be collected accurately and consistently and then collated. This can be accomplished by creating data collection forms and simple databases tailored to fit individual needs, as discussed in Chapter 2. Forms and databases should be used for routine surveillance ac-

tivities, special studies, and outbreak investigations. These forms and databases should be carefully designed to include only those data points that are likely to be used in the final analysis so that the user does not waste valuable time and resources collecting unnecessary information.

One of the most common methods used to store and collate epidemiologic data is a rectangular database that consists of rows and columns. Each row contains information on one individual and each column contains information on one characteristic or variable. The first two columns usually contain the case's name or initials and a medical record number or other unique identifier since two cases may have the same name. The size of the database depends on the number of individuals (or cases) and variables being studied (e.g., age, sex, location, surgery, procedures, symptoms, medications, food eaten, and other exposures).

The Line-List

One of the initial steps in investigating a possible outbreak or a cluster of events is the creation of a rectangular database known as a line-list. Whether created by hand or on a computer, each row in a line-list represents a case, usually a person with a disease or an adverse outcome, and each column contains information on variables relevant to the event being studied. A line-list allows data to be visually inspected to see if any one factor stands out. When conducting an outbreak investigation, a data collection form should be created and used for recording information on each case. This allows information to be collected consistently and efficiently. The information on the data collection form is then entered on to the line-list for inspection. Examples of a data collection form and its corresponding line-list are shown in Exhibits 12–1 and 12–2, respectively. Information on creating line-lists and data collection forms can be found in Chapter 2.

Using Computers

Hospitals and other health care facilities have various computer systems for managing client information such as demographics, billing, diagnostic test results, and treatment provided. These systems should be used

Exhibit 12–1 Data Collection Form: Necrotizing Enterocolitis (NEC) Surveillance

Name _____	Unit # _____
DOB _____	weight _____
gestation _____	APGAR _____

NEC	Confirmatory test(s)	Hemorrhagic gastroenteritis (if not NEC)	Date onset	Outcome
yes no	____ clinical ____ histopathic ____ roentgenographic	yes no		resolved fatal

C. difficile		Rotavirus	
pos neg not done		pos neg not done	

Culture data for the week prior to NEC

Date	Source	Organism(s) isolated

Procedures, treatment, etc. prior to NEC

transfusions	yes	no
PDA diagnosed	yes	no
type feeding	breastmilk	formula

Medications

indocin	yes	no
theophylline	yes	no
furosemide	yes	no

Feeding (in the 5 days prior to NEC)

Date	Feeding	cc/kg/day

DOB = date of birth; PDA = patent ductus arteriosis.

Courtesy of Infection Control Department, Sinai Hospital of Baltimore, Baltimore, Maryland.

Exhibit 12–2 Patients with Necrotizing Enterocolitis (NEC)

Name	Medical Record #	DOB	Weight	Apgar	Gestation (wks)	C. difficile		Rotavirus		Other infectious agent	Transfusion		PDA		Type feeding		indocin		theoph.		furosemide	
						y	n	y	n		y	n	y	n	b	f	y	n	y	n	y	n

Note: DOB, date of birth; PDA, patent ductus arteriosis; b, breastmilk; f, formula; theoph., theophylline; y, yes; n, no.

Courtesy of Infection Control Department, Sinai Hospital of Baltimore, Baltimore, Maryland.

whenever possible to access data needed for surveillance (e.g., client names, age, sex, admission and discharge dates, diagnosis, and diagnostic test results, and medications given). Some microbiology laboratories use systems that can provide epidemiologic reports, such as the names or numbers of patients on a specific nursing unit from whom a particular organism was isolated over a specified period of time. Some programs can provide lists of names and locations of individuals for whom isolation precautions were ordered or lists of patients or residents and their admission diagnoses. These pieces of information can be used to identify clusters of infection or colonization; persons admitted with infections that can be transmitted to others, such as tuberculosis; or patients re-admitted with infections that were acquired from a previous hospitalization, such as surgical site infections.

The various computer programs and systems used in an institution are frequently incompatible and do not share data over a network. This often hinders the seamless flow of data and exchange of information between departments. Infection control and quality management personnel should discuss their data management needs with personnel who are familiar with the information systems in their facility. This will help to identify the following:

- Reports generated for other departments that could also be useful for the infection control or quality management programs, such as lists of admission diagnoses or surgical procedures.
- Reports produced specifically for the infection control or quality management departments (such as positive microbiology culture reports, positive and negative wound culture reports, viral hepatitis serology results, and *Clostridium difficile* toxin results).
- Mainframe systems containing patient or resident data and how to obtain access to that data.
- Programs that search medical literature databases and the Internet and information on how to obtain access to them.
- Information on how to obtain access to a personal computer if one is not readily available.

Infection control and quality management personnel in many health care facilities in the United States use a personal computer (PC). Some have found portable notebook or palmtop computers to be a valuable tool

for collecting and storing epidemiologic data as these computers allow the user to enter data while making rounds anywhere in a facility, thus eliminating the need for paper forms. Although a PC allows large amounts of information to be processed quickly, it is important to keep in mind that it is only a tool. The user, not the computer, should determine how to manage the data. In many cases, surveillance data can be managed easily by using paper forms to collect data, and spreadsheets or simple databases to store, sort, and report it. There are many word processing, spreadsheet, statistics, database, and graphics programs from which to choose. To avoid costly mistakes, it is important to identify the needs of the facility before purchasing a software system.[2]

Much has been written about using computers and choosing software for hospital surveillance. Since a detailed discussion on this topic is beyond the scope of this chapter, the interested reader should refer to the references.[2-8] One very useful program that should be mentioned here is *Epi Info*, from the Centers for Disease Control and Prevention (CDC). This program can store data and perform the advanced statistical analyses needed when investigating an outbreak. *Epi Info* is also used by some infection control professionals to manage routine surveillance data. It can be downloaded to a personal computer through the Internet from the CDC's web site (http://www.cdc.gov) and the *Epi Info* user's manual can be either purchased or copied since it is in the public domain.[9]

DISPLAYING EPIDEMIOLOGIC DATA

Using Tables, Graphs, and Charts

Tables, graphs, and charts can be used to organize, summarize, and visually display epidemiologic data. While computers have certainly made it easier to prepare these visual displays, it is still necessary to understand their proper design and function in order to use them appropriately and effectively. This section defines and describes the features of tables, graphs, and charts; demonstrates how to correctly construct a table, graph, or chart; and explains when to use each of these tools.

Once data has been collected and checked for accuracy and completeness, it should be collated and analyzed to identify the frequency of occurrence of disease and any patterns, trends, and relationships. The findings must then be communicated to others. Although line-lists and other databases are indispensable tools for collating and examining raw data, they usually contain too much information to be useful for presenting it to others. Therefore, tables, graphs, and charts are usually used to illustrate data.

Tables

A table is a display of data that is arranged in rows and columns. In health care epidemiology, tables are frequently used to present quantitative data, such as the rates of infection on patient care units. The information in a table is often used to prepare a graph or chart. Figure 12–1 shows the features of a properly constructed table used to present epidemiologic data. The first column shows the classes into which the data are grouped (here it is age group in years) and the second column lists the frequencies of events in each class (here it is the number of cases of tuberculosis).

Each table should be self-explanatory (i.e., it should contain all of the information needed for the reader to understand what is being presented) and should contain the following features:[10(p.207)]

- A clear title that describes the data presented: what, where, and when. The title is generally

placed at the top of the table. When showing more than one table, each title should be preceded with a table number (e.g., Table 1, Table 2).
- A label for each row and column. The units of measurement should be included (e.g., age in years; percent; rate per 1,000 device-days; number of cases; number of records reviewed; number of incidents).
- Totals for rows and columns, as appropriate.
- Footnotes to explain any abbreviations, codes or explanations (e.g., SSI = surgical site infection; percentages do not add up to 100 percent due to rounding) or any exclusions (e.g., three patients excluded because charts not available).

The one-variable table. The most basic table shows data distributed by one variable, as shown in Figure 12–1. In this type of table, known as a simple frequency distribution, the first column shows the categories of the data being displayed, and the second column lists the number, or frequency, of persons or events in each category. Additional columns can be added to show the numbers of the population at risk and the incidence

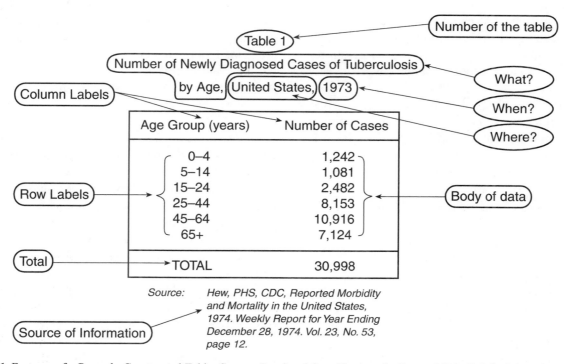

Figure 12–1 Features of a Properly Constructed Table. *Source:* Reprinted from Homestudy Course 3030–G: Principles of Epidemiology, Manual 4, *Methods for Organizing Epidemiologic Data*, p. 3, 1977, Centers for Disease Control and Prevention, Department of Health and Human Services.

rates in each category. Data such as this can be used to identify potential problems and to target areas for improvement.

For example, Table 12–1 displays a simple frequency distribution in which the category (column 1) is the residential units in the Greentree Nursing Home and the variable, or event, being studied (column 2) is the number of residents who sustained a fall. Column 3 displays the resident-days for the population at risk, and column 4 shows the incidence rate. The data displayed in Table 12–1 suggests a possible problem on 1 East, where the incidence rate of 17.5 falls per 1,000 resident-days is considerably higher than any other unit. A review of the resident population in each unit shows that 1 East contains a unit for residents with Alzheimer's disease and other dementias that may put this population at higher risk for falls than the residents of the other units. This information could possibly be used to target 1 East for a falls risk-reduction program.

Two- and three-variable tables. Data can also be cross-tabulated to show numbers distributed by a second or third variable. Table 12–2 shows the same data as in Table 12–1 except that it is cross-tabulated by a second variable, age. The data in Table 12–2 illustrates that the incidence of falls in those over 70 years of age is three times greater (7.5 versus 2.3) than the incidence of falls in those equal to or less than 70 years of age. This information could be used to focus efforts on reducing the risk of falls on those residents over 70 years of age.

The data in Table 12–2 data could also be shown distributed by a third variable, such as sex. The maximum number of variables that should be used in a table is three, so that it does not appear too busy.[10(p.210)] It is better to use several small tables than to try to compress data into one large table.

The two-by-two table. This type of table is used to study the association between two variables. In an outbreak investigation the two-by-two table is used to study the association between an exposure to a risk factor and the presence or absence of a disease. It is called a "two-by-two" table because it contains two variables that are cross-tabulated into two categories. Exhibit 12–3 is an illustration of the usual format of a two-by-two table. The use of these tables is explained in Chapter 10.

Although tables are excellent tools for showing quantitative data, they are frequently not useful for identifying trends and showing comparisons. Graphs and charts are better suited for this purpose. Graphs and charts are frequently used to display the data that is organized in tables. Many computer programs, especially spreadsheet programs, allow the user to generate graphs and charts from the data in tables without having to re-enter the data.

Graphs

A graph is a method used for visually displaying quantitative data. The types of graphs explained here are arithmetic-scale line graphs and histograms. Both of these graphs are rectangular coordinate graphs that are made by drawing two lines, one horizontal and one vertical, that intersect at a right angle. The horizontal line is known as the x-axis and the vertical line is known as the y-axis.

Arithmetic-scale line graphs. In health care epidemiology, the arithmetic-scale line graph is commonly used to show trends, patterns, or differences over time, as shown in Figure 12–2. Time is shown on the x-axis, and the frequency of the event monitored, such as rate, percent, or numbers of cases, is shown on the y-axis. An arithmetic-scale line graph has equal intervals (tick marks) along each axis. This type of graph can be used to show one series of data or to compare several series, such as in Figure 12–2. Each series of data is plotted as a line. An arithmetic-scale line graph should be used when illustrating trends in numbers or rates over time.[10(p.227)]

Histograms. A histogram is used to graph a frequency distribution of a set of continuous data (ie, the number of times an event occurs in each interval).[10(p.236)] A continu-

Table 12–1 Incidence of Resident Falls, by Unit, in January 1999, Greentree Nursing Home

Unit	No. Residents Experiencing a Fall	No. Resident-Days	Fall Rate (No. Falls per 1,000 Resident-Days)
1 East	6	342	17.5
1 West	1	465	2.2
1 North	2	644	3.1
2 East	3	450	6.7
2 West	2	330	6.1
2 North	3	620	4.8
Total	17	2851	6.0

Table 12–2 Incidence of Resident Falls, by Unit and Age, in January 1999, Greentree Nursing Home

Unit	≤70 Years			>70 Years		
	No. Residents Experiencing a Fall	No. Resident-Days	Fall Rate (No. Falls per 1,000 Resident-Days)	No. Residents Experiencing a Fall	No. Resident-Days	Rate (No. Falls per 1,000 Resident-Days)
1 East	1	54	18.5	5	288	17.4
1 West	0	87	0	1	378	2.6
1 North	0	343	0	2	301	6.6
2 East	1	150	6.7	2	300	6.7
2 West	0	112	0	2	218	9.2
2 North	0	117	0	3	503	6.0
Total	2	863	2.3	15	1988	7.5

ous data set consists of a series of measurements for which there are an infinite number of possible values between the lowest value and the highest value in the set (such as time, weight, age, volume, or concentration). When plotted on a histogram, the data should appear as adjoining columns with the height of each column being proportional to the frequency of events in that interval (Figure 12–3). A histogram should be used to display the number of cases (not rates) over time.

When conducting an outbreak investigation, one of the initial steps is to create an epidemic curve. The epidemic curve is actually a histogram that shows the number of cases of disease in an outbreak on the y-axis and the time of onset on the x-axis. The time interval on the x-axis should be appropriate for the disease or event being depicted. The interval may be hours for diseases with a short incubation period, such as staphylococcal food poisoning, or weeks for those with a long incubation period, such as hepatitis A. When drawing an epidemic curve, the columns may be shown as stacks of squares, with each square representing one case, as shown in Figure 12–3, although many computer programs will not construct this type of graph. It is also

perfectly acceptable to omit the horizontal lines between each of the cases, as shown in Figure 12–4.

The following guidelines should be used when constructing a graph:

- The title should clearly describe the data being presented: what, where, and when. The title can be placed at the top or bottom of the graph.
- The graph should be kept simple—it will be easier to read and will present the data more effectively.
- The independent variable (the method of classification), such as time, should be plotted on the x-axis (horizontal).

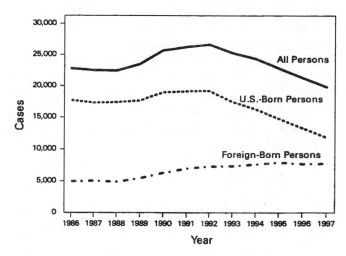

Figure 12–2 Number of Persons with Reported Cases of Tuberculosis, by Country of Birth—United States, 1986–1997. *Source:* Reprinted from Tuberculosis Morbidity—United States, 1997, *MMWR,* Vol. 47, No. 13, p. 255, 1998, Centers for Disease Control and Prevention.

Exhibit 12–3 General Format for a Two-by-Two Table

	Disease	No Disease	Total
Exposed	a	b	a + b
Unexposed	c	d	c + d
Total	a + c	b + d	a + b + c + d

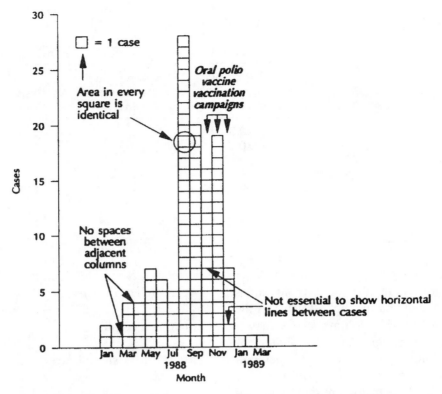

Figure 12–3 Example of Histogram. Reported cases of paralytic poliomyelitis by month of occurrence. Oman, January 1988–March 1989. *Source:* Reprinted from *Principles of Epidemiology: An Introduction to Applied Epidemiology and Biostatistics,* 2nd ed., p. 236, 1992, Centers for Disease Control and Prevention, Department of Health and Human Services.

- The dependent variable should be plotted on the y-axis (vertical). This variable is usually a measure of frequency, such as the number of incidents, rate of disease, or number of cases.
- When plotting more than one variable, each should be clearly differentiated by using a legend or key. If black and white copies of the report are likely to be made, the lines or the areas representing the different variables on a graph should be made sufficiently dissimilar so that the reader can tell them apart. For example, lines should be solid, dotted, etc., as shown in Figure 12–2, and columns should be solid, shaded, hatched, etc., as shown in Figure 12–5.
- The x- and y-axes should be labeled with the appropriate units of measurement.
- Each graph should be self-explanatory and should contain all of the information needed for the reader to understand what is being presented.

- The y-axis should begin with 0. The largest value to appear on the y-axis is selected by identifying the largest value in the set and rounding up to a slightly higher number. For instance, in Figure 12–2, the cases are shown in intervals of 5,000, and the highest value in the set of numbers plotted on the graph is slightly more than 25,000; therefore, 30,000 was chosen as the highest value in the range shown on the y-axis.
- The date of preparation should be noted because the data may change over time. For instance, when an arithmetic-scale line graph is used to display surgical site infection rates, the data may change as new cases are reported, and when drawing a histogram for an epidemic curve, the data may change as new cases are identified during the course of an outbreak investigation.
- The source of the data should be placed in a footnote, especially if the data are not original.

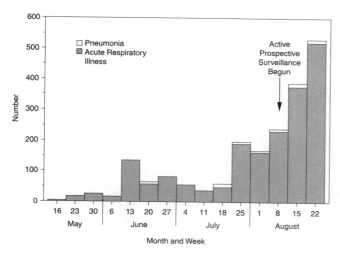

Figure 12–4 A Histogram Displaying the Number of Cases of Acute Respiratory Illness and Pneumonia in Tourists (*n* = 1778), Residents (*n* = 46), and Tourism Workers (*n* = 375), by Week of Presentation—Alaska and Yukon Territory, Weeks Ending May 16–August 22, 1998. Dates of presentation to a health care provider were known for 1538 cases, were estimated for 475 cases based on dates of travel, and could not be estimated for 186 cases. *Source:* Reprinted from Outbreak of Influenza A Infection—Alaska and the Yukon Territory, July–August 1998, *MMWR,* Vol. 47, No. 33, p. 686, 1998, Centers for Disease Control and Prevention.

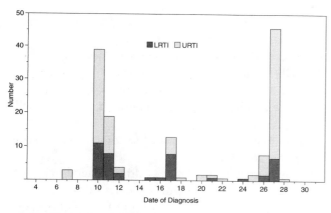

Figure 12–5 A Histogram Displaying the Number of Cases of Lower Respiratory Tract Infection (LRTI) and Upper Respiratory Tract Infection (URTI) among Students at a Job-Training Facility, by Date of Diagnosis—South Dakota, March 4–31, 1997. A case of LRTI was defined as physician-diagnosed pneumonia, an abnormal chest radiograph, or rales or wheezing on pulmonary ascultation in any student. A case of URTI was defined as coryza and sore throat without LRTI in any student. *Source:* Reprinted from Civilian Outbreak of Adenovirus Acute Respiratory Disease—South Dakota, 1997, *MMWR,* Vol. 47, No. 27, p. 568, 1998, Centers for Disease Control and Prevention.

Charts

Three types of charts used in health care epidemiology are bar charts, pie charts, and maps (geographic coordinate charts).

Bar charts. Figure 12–6 shows the components of a bar chart.

Bar charts can be used to show frequency distributions of a set of discrete data, as in Figure 12–7, or to compare magnitudes of several sets of data, as in Figure 12–8. In these charts, each category of a variable is represented by a bar, which may be displayed either vertically, as in Figures 12–7 and 12–8, or horizontally, as in Figure 12–9. The height or length of the bar is proportional to the values in that category. A stacked bar chart can be used to show the categories of a second variable, as in Figure 12–10.

Vertical bar charts (Figures 12–7 and 12–8) differ from histograms (Figures 12–4 and 12–5) in that each bar or cell in a vertical bar chart is separated by a space, whereas in a histogram the bars are adjoining. A bar chart is used to display information that is discrete and noncontinuous, such as sex, race, job category or

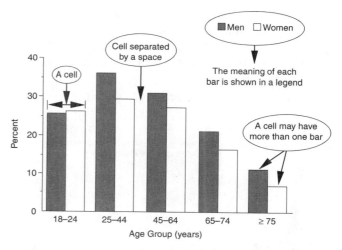

Figure 12–6 Example of a Vertical Bar Chart with Annotation. Percentage of adults who were current cigarette smokers (persons ≥ 18 years of age who reported having smoked at least 100 cigarettes and who were currently smoking) by sex and age, United States, 1988. *Source:* Reprinted from *Principles of Epidemiology: An Introduction to Applied Epidemiology and Biostatistics,* 2nd ed., p. 248, 1992, Centers for Disease Control and Prevention, Department of Health and Human Services.

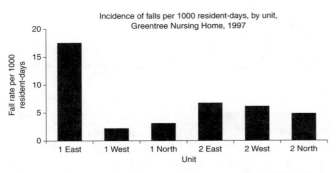

Figure 12–7 Frequency Distribution Shown as a Bar Chart. Incidence of falls per 1000 resident-days, by unit, Greentree Nursing Home, 1997.

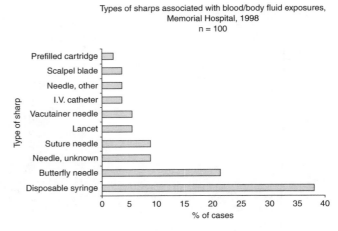

Figure 12–9 Frequency Distribution Shown as a Horizontal Bar Chart. Types of sharps associated with blood/body fluid exposures, Memorial Hospital, 1998.

location, or that is shown as being discrete and noncontinuous, such as age groups, as shown in Figure 12–6. By contrast, a histogram is used to display the frequency distribution of a set of continuous data (such as time or age).

The following guidelines should be used when constructing a bar chart:

- The title should clearly describe the data presented: what, where, and when. In an epidemiological report, the title is placed at the top of the chart.
- When creating a chart that has more than one bar in a cell, each bar should be clearly differentiated by using a legend or key as in Figure 12–8.
- The categories in a stacked bar chart should be clearly differentiated by using a legend or key, as in Figure 12–10. If black and white copies of the

report are likely to be made, the areas representing each bar or each component should have clearly discernible shades or patterns.

- When possible, the categories that define the bars should be positioned in such a way that the length or height of the bars is in ascending or descending order.
- All of the bars should be the same width.
- The length or height of each bar should be proportional to the values in each category.
- There should be a space between each bar or each cell (group of bars).
- The x- and y-axes should be labeled.
- As in a table or a graph, a bar chart should be self-explanatory and should contain all of the information needed for the reader to understand what is being presented.
- The source of the data should be placed in a footnote, especially if the data are not original.

Pie charts. Pie charts are used for showing the component parts of a set of data, as in Figure 12–11. Each slice of the pie represents a proportion of the whole. The following guidelines should be used when constructing a pie chart:

- The title should clearly describe the data presented: what, where and when. The title may be placed at the top or the bottom of the chart.
- Each slice should be labeled with the percentage that it represents. The label can be placed either inside the slice or outside and next to it.

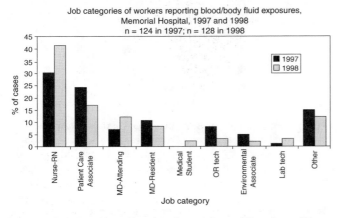

Figure 12–8 Bar Chart Showing Comparison of Two Sets of Data. Job categories of workers reporting blood/body fluid exposures, Memorial Hospital, 1997 and 1998.

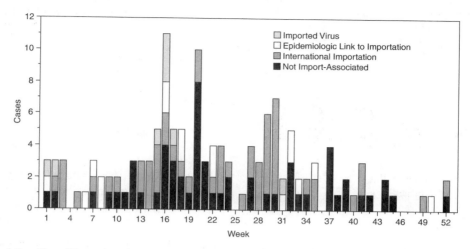

Figure 12–10 Stacked Bar Chart Illustrating the Number of Reported Measles Cases (*n* = 138) by Importation Status and Week of Rash Onset—United States, 1997. *Source:* Reprinted from Measles—United States, 1997, *MMWR,* Vol. 47, No. 14, p. 275, 1998, Centers for Disease Control and Prevention.

- Each piece of the pie should be differentiated clearly by using a legend or key. The chart is easier to read if the components are different colors or, when using black and white, clearly discernible shades or patterns.
- The total number of cases or events (the number that represents 100 percent) should be noted somewhere on the chart.
- The chart should be self-explanatory and should contain all of the information needed for the reader to understand what is being presented.
- The source of the data should be placed in a footnote, especially if the data are not original.

Maps

Maps can be used to show where a disease or event occurred. Two types of maps used to display epidemiological data are spot maps and area maps.

Spot maps. Spot maps are constructed by drawing a dot or some other symbol at each location where an event occurred, as in Figure 12–12. When investigating an outbreak or a cluster of infections, a spot map can be used to illustrate the geographic distribution of the cases and may be useful in forming a hypothesis on how a disease may have spread.

Area maps. Area maps are used to show the geographic distribution of a disease or an event. The distribution can be shown as a rate, such as the incidence of

a disease, or as the number of events or cases. Figure 12–13 shows both the number of reported cases and the average annual incidence rates of tetanus, by state, in the United States from 1995 to 1997. Area maps are frequently used by health departments to show patterns

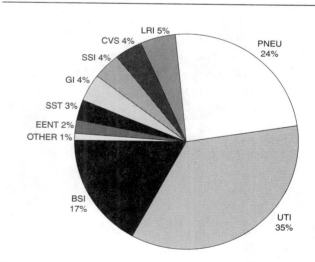

Figure 12–11 Site Distribution of 2,321 Nosocomial Infections in Coronary Care Units, NNIS System, 1992–1997. PNEU, pneumonia; UTI, urinary tract infection; BSI, primary bloodstream infection; EENT, eye, ear, nose, and throat infection; SST, skin and soft tissue infection; GI, gastrointestinal infection; SSI, surgical site infection; CVS, cardiovascular system infection; LRI, lower respiratory tract infection other than pneumonia; OTHER, other. *Source:* Reprinted from *National Nosocomial Infections Surveillance (NNIS) System Report,* Data Summary from October 1986–April 1998, Issued June 1998, Centers for Disease Control and Prevention.

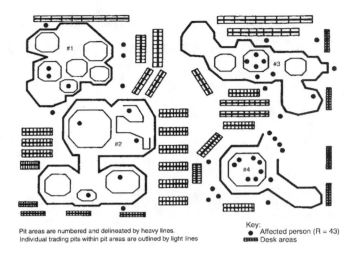

Pit areas are numbered and delineated by heavy lines.
Individual trading pits within pit areas are outlined by light lines

Key:
● Affected person (R = 43)
▦ Desk areas

Figure 12–12 Spot Map Illustrating the Occurrence of Mumps Cases in Trading Pits of Exchange A, Chicago, Illinois, August 18–December 25, 1987. *Source:* Reprinted from *Principles of Epidemiology: An Introduction to Applied Epidemiology and Biostatistics,* 2nd ed., p. 23, 1992, Centers for Disease Control and Prevention, Department of Health and Human Services.

of infectious diseases and are useful for evaluating the occurrence of a specific disease, such as tuberculosis or influenza, in a community.

Using Computers To Create Graphs and Charts

Histograms versus Bar Charts

Computers are generally used to prepare reports of outbreak investigations. When choosing a software program, it is important to select one that can create the types of charts and graphs that are needed for preparing epidemiology reports. When constructing an epidemic curve (the number of cases occurring over time in an outbreak), one should use a histogram—a graph that has adjoining columns, rather than a bar chart that has spaces between each column. Some commonly used spreadsheet and graphics programs can be used to produce bar charts, but cannot be used to create a histogram.

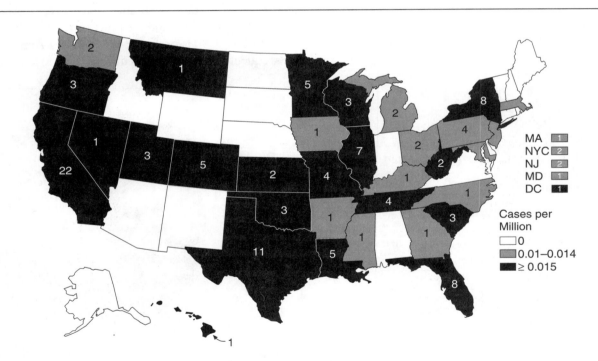

Figure 12–13 Area Map Illustrating the Reported Number of Tetanus Cases (Cases Were Reported from 33 States, the District of Columbia, and New York City) and Average Annual Incidence Rates, by State—United States, 1995–1997. *Source:* Reprinted from Tetanus Surveillance—United States, 1995–1997, *MMWR,* Vol. 47, No. SS–2, p. 4, 1998, Centers for Disease Control and Prevention.

Table 12–3 Guideline for Selecting a Graph or Chart to Illustrate Epidemiologic Data

Type of Graph or Chart	When To Use
Arithmetic-scale line graph	Display trends in numbers or rates over time
Histogram	1. Show frequency distribution of a continuous variable 2. Show number of cases over time during an epidemic (epidemic curve)
Simple bar chart	Compare size or frequency of different categories of a single variable
Grouped bar chart	Compare size or frequency of different categories of 2 to 4 series of data
Stacked bar chart	Compare totals and illustrate component parts of the total among different groups
Pie chart	Show components of a whole
Spot map	Show locations of cases or events
Area map	Display events or rates geographically

Source: Adapted from *Principles of Epidemiology: An Introduction to Applied Epidemiology and Biostatistics,* 2nd ed., p. 263, 1992, Centers for Disease Control and Prevention, Department of Health and Human Services.

Selecting the Best Method To Illustrate Data

It is important to choose the method of illustrating epidemiologic data that is best suited for conveying that particular data easily and quickly. Table 12–3 provides a guideline for selecting a graph or chart to illustrate epidemiologic data.

Avoiding Chartjunk

Many computer programs produce three-dimensional bar charts and pie charts. Which is really better—a three-dimensional or a two-dimensional graphic? The pie charts in Figure 12–14 display the same information; however, one chart is two dimensional and the other is three dimensional. As a rule, a two-dimensional chart should be used, especially when information must be communicated quickly in a short presentation, because it is easier to judge the relative sizes of the component parts in the two-dimensional version of the pie than in the three-dimensional version.

The bar charts in Figure 12–15 contain the same data, a comparison of rates in two different years; however, one is two-dimensional and the other contains gridlines and

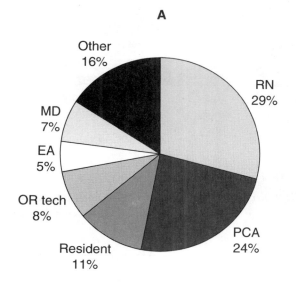
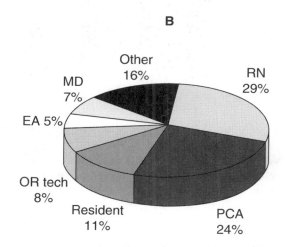

Figure 12–14 Job Category Distribution of 58 Personnel with Needlesticks, St. Anne's Hospital, 1998. Boths parts contain the same information; however, one (**A**) is shown as a two-dimensional pie chart and the other (**B**) is shown as a three-dimensional pie chart. PCA, patient care associate; EA, environmental associate.

A

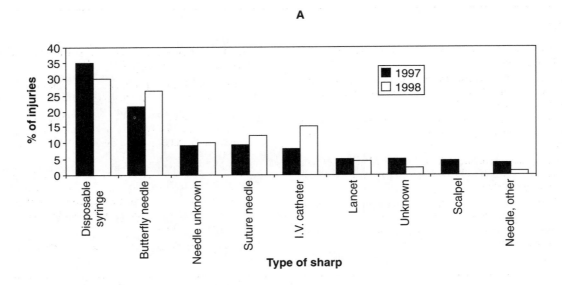

B

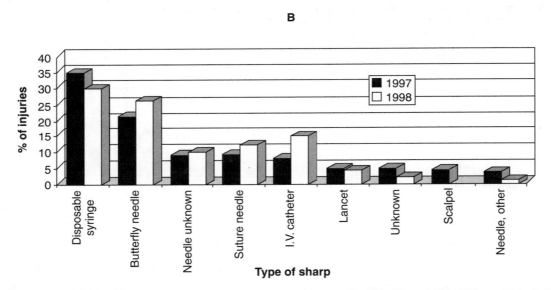

Figure 12–15 Types of Sharps Associated with Injuries, Community Hospital, 1997 and 1998; $n = 95$ in 1997, $n = 90$ in 1998. Both parts contain the same information; however, one (**A**) is shown as a two-dimensional bar chart and the other (**B**) is shown as a three-dimensional bar chart.

three-dimensional bars. Which chart gets the message across more quickly? Graphs and charts are used to communicate information to others—it is important to keep them simple and avoid the glitter.[11] The "third dimension" in three-dimensional charts contains no additional information. Graphic activity that is unrelated to data informa-

tion, such as three-dimensional graphics, gridlines, and excessive cross-hatching, has been called "chartjunk"[1] and should be avoided. As stated by Tufte, "Graphical excellence is that which gives to the viewer the greatest number of ideas in the shortest time with the least ink in the smallest space."[1(p.51)]

REFERENCES

1. Tufte ER. *The Visual Display of Quantitative Information*. Cheshire, CT: Graphics Press; 1983.

2. Freeman, J. The use of computerized systems in hospital epidemiology. In: Bennett JV, Brachman PS, eds. *Hospital Infections*. 3rd ed. Boston: Little, Brown and Company; 1992:161–185.

3. Gaynes R, et al. Methodology to evaluate a computer-based system for surveillance of hospital-acquired infections. *Am J Infect Control*. 1990;18:40–46.

4. La Haise S. A comparison of infection control software for use by hospital epidemiologists in meeting the new JCAHO standards. *Infect Control Hosp Epidemiol*. 1990;11:185–190.

5. Reagan DR. The choice of microcomputer software for infection control. *Infect Control Hosp Epidemiol*. 1990;11:178–179.

6. Zellner S, Polley N. Infection control software. *Infect Control Hosp Epidemiol*. 1990;11:400–401.

7. Barr RL, Gerzoff RB. Controlling urges and infections. *Infect Control Hosp Epidemiol*. 1985;6:317–322.

8. Reagan DR. Microcomputers in hospital epidemiology. *Infect Control Hosp Epidemiol*. 1997;18:440–448.

9. Dean, AG, Dean JA, Columbier D, et al. *Epi Info, Version 6.02: A Word Processing Database and Statistics Program for Epidemiology on Microcomputers*. Atlanta, GA: Centers for Disease Control and Prevention; 1994.

10. Centers for Disease Control and Prevention. *Principles of Epidemiology: An Introduction to Applied Epidemiology and Biostatistics*. 2nd ed. Atlanta, GA: US Dept of Health and Human Services, Public Health Service, Centers for Disease Control and Prevention, Epidemiology Program Office; 1992.

11. Jolley D. The glitter of the t table. *Lancet*. 1993;342:27–29.

SUGGESTED READING

Centers for Disease Control and Prevention. *Principles of Epidemiology: An Introduction to Applied Epidemiology and Biostatistics*. 2nd ed. Atlanta, GA: US Dept of Health and Human Services, Public Health Service, Centers for Disease Control and Prevention, Epidemiology Program Office; 1992.

Tufte ER. The *Visual Display of Quantitative Information*. Cheshire, CT: Graphics Press; 1983.

Glossary

The terms in this glossary have been adapted for use in the health care setting. Many of the definitions are taken or adapted from the glossaries in (1) the CDC Homestudy Course 3030-G, Principles of Epidemiology, *US Department of Health and Human Services, Centers for Disease Control, Atlanta, GA, 1985, and (2) the Centers for Disease Control and Prevention,* Principles of Epidemiology: An Introduction to Applied Epidemiology and Biostatistics, *2nd ed., US Department of Health and Human Services, Centers for Disease Control and Prevention, Atlanta, GA, 1992.*

agent—a biological, physical, or chemical entity capable of causing disease.

antiseptic—a chemical germicide formulated to inactivate microbial agents on skin or tissue.

attack rate—a measure of the frequency of new cases of a disease or condition in a specified population during a specified period of time; usually expressed as a percent.

bar chart—a visual display of quantitative data in which each category or value of a variable is represented by a bar.

bias—deviation of results from the truth.

baseline—a number or value used as a base for measurement or comparison.

carrier—a person who has no apparent clinical disease but harbors a specific infectious agent and is capable of transmitting the agent to others; a carrier is a potential source of infection.

case—a person who has a particular disease or condition under investigation.

case control study—a type of observational analytic study. Enrollment into the study is based on presence ("case") or absence ("control") of a particular disease or condition. Characteristics such as previous exposure to particular agents are then compared between cases and controls.

case definition—standard criteria used for deciding whether or not a person has a particular disease or condition, by specifying clinical, laboratory and epidemiologic characteristics such as time, place, and person.

chain of infection—a process that begins when an agent leaves its reservoir or host through a portal of exit and is conveyed by some mode of transmission and then enters through an appropriate portal of entry to infect a susceptible host.

cleaning—the process of physically removing foreign material, such as dirt, blood, microorganisms, and body fluids, from a surface.

cluster—a group of cases of a disease or other health-related event that occurs closely related in time and place. The number of cases may or may not exceed the expected number; frequently the expected number is not known.

cohort—a well-defined group of persons selected for a study. Persons in the group have had a common exposure and are then followed up for the occurrence of disease.

cohort study—a type of observational analytic study. Also known as a prospective study.

colonization—presence and growth of a microorganism on a host that has no symptoms or cellular injury. A colonized host may serve as a source of infection.

common source outbreak—an outbreak that results from a group of persons being exposed to a common noxious influence, such as an infectious agent or toxin. If the group is exposed over a relatively brief period of time, so that all cases occur within one incubation period, then the common source outbreak is further classified as a point source outbreak. In some common source outbreaks, persons may be exposed over a period of days, weeks, or longer, with the exposure being either intermittent or continuous.

communicable—may be transmitted directly or indirectly from one person to another.

contact—(1) exposure to a source of infection; (2) a person who has been exposed to a source of infection.

contagious—able to easily transmit an infectious agent from one person to another.

contingency table—a two-variable table with cross-tabulated data.

control—in a case-control study, the person or group of persons without the disease or condition being studied; the group to which the cases (those with the disease or condition) are compared.

data, continuous—data consisting of measurements of things for which there are an infinite number of possible values between the minimum and the maximum values in the data set (e.g., age, weight, height, and temperature).

data, discrete—data consisting of measurements of things that can be counted or measured only in whole units (e.g., the number of persons with a specific disease or condition).

demographic information—those characteristics of persons, such as age, sex, and race, that are used in descriptive epidemiology to characterize the population at risk.

denominator—the lower portion of a fraction; contains the data used to calculate a rate or ratio. In a rate, the denominator is usually the population at risk.

dependent variable—in a statistical analysis, the outcome variable(s), or the variable(s) whose values are a function of other variable(s) called independent variable(s) in the relationship under study.

descriptive epidemiology—the aspect of epidemiology concerned with organizing and summarizing health-related data according to time, place, and person.

direct transmission—the immediate transfer of an agent from a reservoir to a susceptible host by direct contact or droplet spread.

disease—a condition that represents a deviation from normal health and is associated with characteristic signs and symptoms.

disinfectant—a chemical germicide formulated to inactivate microbial agents on inanimate surfaces.

disinfection—a process that eliminates pathogenic microorganisms, except bacterial spores, from a surface.

droplets—liquid particles expelled into the air when a person talks, sings, coughs, or sneezes.

droplet nuclei—the residue of dried droplets that may remain suspended in the air for long periods, may be carried over great distances, and are easily inhaled into the lungs.

droplet spread—the direct transmission of an infectious agent from a reservoir to a susceptible host by spray with relatively large, short-ranged aerosols produced by sneezing, coughing, or talking.

endemic—the usual presence of a disease or infectious agent within a given geographic area or population group.

endogenous—originating or growing from within.

environmental factor—an extrinsic factor (geology, climate, insects, sanitation, health services, etc.) that affects the agent and the opportunity for exposure.

epidemic—the occurrence of more cases of a disease or event than expected during a specified period of time in a given area or among a specific group of people.

epidemic curve—a histogram that shows the course of a disease outbreak or epidemic by plotting the number of cases by time of onset.

epidemic period—a time period when the number of cases of disease or events reported is greater than expected.

epidemiology—the study of the distribution and determinants of health-related states or events in specified populations and the application of this study to the control of health problems.

experimental study—a study in which the investigator specifies the exposure category for each individual in the study and then follows the individual to determine the effects of the exposure (e.g., a clinical trial).

etiology—the cause of a specific disease.

etiologic agent—an agent that causes a specific disease.

exogenous—originating from an external source.

fomite—an inanimate object that can become contaminated and can transmit infectious agents.

frequency distribution—a tabulation of the number of times an event occurs in each class interval or category; often displayed in a two-column table in which the left column lists the individual values or categories and the right column indicates the number of events in each category.

graph—a visual display of quantitative data that uses a system of coordinates.

histogram—a graph that displays the frequency distribution of a continuous variable. Rectangles are drawn in such a way that their bases lie on a linear scale representing different intervals, and their heights are proportional to the frequencies of the values within each of the intervals.

host—a person or animal that can be infected by an infectious agent under natural conditions.

hypothesis—a supposition, arrived at from observation or reflection, that leads to refutable predictions. Any conjecture cast in a form that will allow it to be tested and refuted.

hypothesis, null—the first step in testing for statistical significance in which it is assumed that an exposure is not related to a disease or other health-related event.

iatrogenic—related to a medical intervention.

immunity, active—resistance developed in response to stimulus by an antigen (infecting agent or vaccine) and usually characterized by the presence of antibody produced by the host.

immunity, herd—the resistance of a group to invasion and spread of an infectious agent, based on the resistance to infection of a high proportion of individual members of the group. The resistance is a product of the number of susceptible persons and the probability that those who are susceptible will come into contact with an infected person.

immunity, passive—immunity conferred by an antibody produced in another host and acquired either naturally by an infant from its mother or artificially by administration of an antibody-containing preparation (antiserum or immune globulin).

incidence rate—a measure of the frequency with which an event, such as a new case of illness, occurs in a population over a period of time. When calculating an incidence rate, the numerator is the number of new cases occurring during a given time period and the denominator is the population at risk during that time period.

incubation period—the interval between the effective exposure of a susceptible host to an infectious agent and the onset of signs and symptoms of disease.

independent variable—an exposure, risk factor, or other characteristic being observed or measured that is hypothesized to influence an event or manifestation (i.e., the dependent variable).

index case—the first recognized case having a specific disease or attribute.

indirect transmission—the transmission of an agent carried from a reservoir to a susceptible host either by suspended air particles or by an animate (vector) or inanimate (vehicle) intermediary.

infection—the entry and multiplication of an infectious agent into the body, resulting in a reaction.

infectivity—the ability of an agent to infect a host.

infestation—the lodgment, development, and reproduction of arthropods on the body or in the clothes.

isolation—the separation of infected persons from those who are not infected for the purpose of preventing the spread of an infectious agent to others.

line-listing—a rectangular database in which each row represents a case, usually a person with a disease or health-related condition, and each column contains information on variables relevant to the event being studied.

mean, arithmetic—the measure of central location commonly called the average; it is calculated by adding together all of the individual values in a data set and dividing by the number of values in the set.

measure of association—a quantified relationship between exposure and disease; examples of measures of association include relative risk, rate ratio, and odds ratio.

measure of central location—a measure of central tendency; a central value that represents a distribution of data. Measures of central location include the mean, median, and mode.

measure of dispersion—a measure of the spread of a distribution out from its central value. Measures of dispersion used in epidemiology include the variance and the standard deviation.

median—the measure of central location that divides a set of data into two equal parts.

mode—a measure of central location; the value that occurs most frequently in a set of observations.

mode of transmission—the mechanism by which an agent is spread from person to person.

morbidity—any departure, subjective or objective, from a state of physiological or psychological well-being.

natural history of disease—the temporal course of disease from onset (inception) to resolution.

necessary cause—a causal factor whose presence is required for the occurrence of a disease or health-related event.

normal curve—a bell-shaped curve that results when a normal distribution is graphed.

normal distribution—the symmetrical clustering of values around a central location. The properties of a normal distribution include the following—(1) it is a continuous, symmetrical distribution in which both tails extend to infinity; (2) the arithmetic mean, median, and mode are identical; and (3) its shape is determined by the mean and standard deviation.

nosocomial infection—an infection resulting from exposure to a source within a health care facility; may occur in patients, personnel, or visitors.

numerator—the upper portion of a fraction. In epidemiology, it is usually the number of cases of a disease or event being studied.

observational study—an epidemiological study in which nature is allowed to take its course. Changes or differences in one characteristic are studied in relation to changes or differences in others, without the intervention of the investigator.

odds ratio—a measure of association that quantifies the relationship between an exposure and health outcome from a comparative study.

outbreak—synonymous with epidemic.

pandemic—an epidemic that occurs over a very wide area, such as several countries or continents, and that usually affects a large proportion of the population.

pathogenicity—the capacity of an agent to cause disease.

pie chart—a circular chart in which the size of each slice of the pie is proportional to the frequency of each category of a variable.

population—the total number of persons in a specified place or area.

prevalence—the number or proportion of cases or events in a given population.

prevalence rate—the proportion of persons in a population who have a particular disease or attribute at a given point in time (i.e., point prevalence) or over a given time interval (i.e., period prevalence).

propagated outbreak—an outbreak that spreads from person to person rather than originating from a common source.

proportion—a type of ratio in which the numerator is included in the denominator.

pseudoepidemic—a real cluster or increase in false infections or an artificial cluster or increase in true infections.

pseudo-outbreak—see pseudoepidemic.

random sample—a sample derived by selecting individuals such that each individual has the same probability of being selected.

range—in statistics, the difference between the largest and the smallest values in a distribution. In common use, the span of values from smallest to largest.

rate—an expression of the frequency with which an illness or event occurs in a defined population.

ratio—the value obtained by dividing one quantity by another.

relative risk—a comparison of the risk of some health-related event, such as disease, in two groups.

reservoir—the habitat in which an infectious agent normally lives, grows, and multiplies; reservoirs may be human, animal, or environmental.

risk—the probability that an event will occur (e.g., that a person will develop a specific disease).

risk factor—a characteristic that is associated with an increased occurrence of disease or other health-related event (e.g., exposure to a therapeutic or diagnostic procedure).

risk ratio—a comparison of the risk of some health-related event, such as disease, in two groups.

sample—a selected subset of a population.

secondary attack rate—a measure of the frequency of new cases of a disease among the contacts of known cases.

sensitivity—the ability of a system to detect epidemics and other changes in disease occurrence. The proportion of persons with disease who are correctly identified by a screening test or case definition as having disease.

skewed—a distribution that is asymmetrical.

source of infection—a person, animal, or inanimate object from which an infectious agent is transmitted to a host.

specificity—the proportion of persons without disease who are correctly identified by a screening test or case definition as not having disease.

sporadic—a disease that occurs infrequently and irregularly.

spot map—a map that indicates the location of each case of a disease or event.

standard deviation—the most widely used measure of dispersion of a frequency distribution, equal to the positive square root of the variance.

standard error of the mean—the standard deviation of a theoretical distribution of sample means about the true population mean.

standard precautions—an infection control strategy designed to reduce the risk of transmission of microorganisms from both recognized and unrecognized sources of infection in hospitals. These precautions are applied to all patients regardless of their diagnosis or presumed infection status.

sterilization—a process that eliminates or destroys all forms of microorganisms.

surveillance—the systematic collection, analysis, interpretation, and dissemination of data on an ongoing basis, to gain knowledge of the pattern of disease or event occurrence in a population in order to control and prevent disease in that population.

susceptible—a person who does not have sufficient resistance to an infectious agent to prevent infection if exposure occurs.

validity—the degree to which a measurement actually measures or detects what it is supposed to measure.

variable—any characteristic or attribute that can be measured.

variance—a measure of the dispersion shown by a set of observations, defined by the sum of the squares of deviations from the mean, divided by the number of degrees of freedom in the set of observations.

vector—an animate intermediary, frequently an arthropod or insect, that is involved in the indirect transmission of an agent by carrying the agent from a reservoir to a susceptible host.

vehicle—an inanimate intermediary that is involved in the indirect transmission of an agent by carrying the agent from a reservoir to a susceptible host.

virulence—the degree of pathogenicity of an infectious agent.

zoonoses—an infectious disease that is transmissible under normal conditions from animals to humans.

Sample Data Collection Forms for Routine Surveillance and Outbreak Investigation in Health Care Facilities

Infection Control Surveillance Worksheet

MR no:_____ DOB: _____

Last name: _____

First name: _____ Sex:_____M_____F

Comments: _____

ADMISSION

Account no: _____

Admission date: _____/_____/_____   Type admission: IP OP OPS SNF

Discharge date: _____/_____/_____   Disposition: DIS EXP SNF TRN

Previous facility: _____

INFECTION

Infection type: N C U _____ Culture no: _____

General site: SSI OPSI CVS GI SYS GU _____ Culture date:_____/_____/_____

                Pneum OTH_____CNS _____ Specimen: _____

Surgical site: SUPERFICIAL, DEEP, ORGAN/SPACE

Onset date:_____/_____/_____
              (within report quarter)   Sternal: Donor site:
                                                   ___Yes   ___Yes
                                                   ___No   ___No

Notes: _____

_____

_____

continues

continued

PATHOGEN

Pathogen: _____

_____

HOST RISK

Host risks: _____

_____

SYMPTOMS

Symptoms: _____

_____

DIAGNOSIS

Diagnosis: _____

_____

LOCATION

Unit code: _____   Start date: _____/_____/_____

Room/bed: _____   Stop date: _____/_____/_____

Unit code: _____   Start date: _____/_____/_____

Room/bed: _____   Stop date: _____/_____/_____

Unit code: _____   Start date: _____/_____/_____

Room/bed: _____   Stop date: _____/_____/_____

PROCEDURE/SURGERY

General site code: _____   Room: _____

Surgery: _____   Class: _____

Surgery date: _____/_____/_____   ASA: _____

                                              Implant ___Yes ___No

Start time: _____   Physician #1: _____

Stop time: _____   Physician #2: _____

Redo:	Laparoscopy:	Antibiotics:	30 minutes pre-incision:	Flow:
___Yes	___Yes	___Yes	___Yes	___Yes
___No	___No	___No	___No	___No

Comments: _____

_____

_____

continues

continued

RISK FACTOR/DEVICES

Device: _____   Staff: _____

Device site: _____

Start date:_____/_____/_____

Stop date:_____/_____/_____

Device: _____   Staff: _____

Device site: _____

Start date:_____/_____/_____

Stop date:_____/_____/_____

Device: _____   Staff: _____

Device site: _____

Start date:_____/_____/_____

Stop date:_____/_____/_____

Comments: _____

_____

_____

_____

_____

_____

_____

_____

Note: MR no, medical record number; DOB, date of birth; IP, inpatient; OP, outpatient; OPS, outpatient surgery; SNF, skilled nursing facility; DIS, discharged; EXP, expired; TRN, transferred; N, nosocomial; C, community-acquired; U, undetermined; SSI, surgical site infection; OPSI, outpatient surgical infection; CVS, cardiovascular system; GI, gastrointestinal; SYS, systemic; GU, genitourinary; Pneum, pneumonia; OTH, other; CNS, central nervous system; ASA, American Society of Anesthesiologists score.

Nosocomial Infection Surveillance

Month/Year:_____

Name_____ Medical Record #_____ Age_____ Sex_____

Admit Date_____ Disch/Transfer/Expire Date _____   Unit_____ Room_____ Date_____

Diagnosis _____   Unit_____ Room_____ Date_____

Attending _____ Service _____   Unit_____ Room_____ Date_____

PROCEDURE/SURGERY

Date	Type	Physician/Surgeon	Prophylaxis

CENTRAL LINES

Type	Site	Date inserted	Date removed	Comments

VENTILATOR: From _____ to _____   **Chest X-ray:**   Date_____ Results _____

From _____ to _____   Date_____ Results _____

CULTURES

Date	Unit	Source	Smear	Organism	Con/Col	CA	NI	Comments

NI #1   NI #2   NI #3

Date_____   Date_____   Date_____

Unit_____   Unit_____   Unit_____

Site_____   Site_____   Site_____

Organism_____   Organism_____   Organism_____

Linked_____   Linked_____   Linked_____

Note: Disch, discharged; Con/Col, contaminated or colonized; CA, community acquired; NI, nosocomial infection.

Courtesy of the Infection Control Department, Sinai Hospital of Baltimore, Baltimore, Maryland.

Infection Control Department
Nosocomial Pathogens Report

Month/Year:_____

PATHOGEN	PBSI	YTD PBSI	SBSI	YTD SBSI	SSI	YTD SSI
GRAM POSITIVE COCCI/RODS						
Bacillus species						
Colstridium perfringens						
Corynebacterium JK						
Corynebacterium species						
Lactobacillus species						
Propionibacterium species						
Streptococcus, Group A						
Streptococcus, Group B						
Streptococcus, Group C						
Streptococcus mitis						
Streptococcus pneumoniae						
Streptococcus viridans						
Subtotal—Gram positive cocci/rods						
E. faecalis (vanc-S)						
E. faecalis (vanc-R)						
E. faecium (vanc-S)						
E. faecium (vanc-R)						
Enterococcus species, other						
Subtotal—Enterococcus						
Staph coagulase negative (ox-S)						
Staph coagulase negative (ox-R)						
Staph simulans (ox-S)						
Subtotal—Staph coagulase negative						
S. aureus (ox-S)						
S. aureus (ox-R)						
Subtotal—S aureus						
TOTAL GRAM POSITIVE						

Note: PBSI, primary bloodstream infection; SBSI, secondary bloodstream infection; SSI, surgical site infection; YTD, year-to-date; vanc, vancomycin; ox, oxacillin; S, sensitive; R, resistant; Staph, staphylococcus.

Courtesy of the Infection Control Department, Sinai Hospital of Baltimore, Baltimore, Maryland.

Infection Control Department
Nosocomial Pathogens Report

Month/Year:_____

PATHOGEN	PBSI	YTD PBSI	SBSI	YTD SBSI	SSI	YTD SSI
GRAM NEGATIVE COCCI						
Veillonella species						
GRAM NEGATIVE RODS						
Acinetobacter anitratus						
Alcaligenes xylosoxidans						
Bacteroides fragilis						
Bacteroides species						
Burkholderia cepacia						
Citrobacter freundii						
Citrobacter koseri						
E. coli						
Enterobacter aerogenes						
Enterobacter cloacae						
Hafnia alvei						
Klebsiella pneumoniae						
Klebsiella oxytoca						
Morganella morganii						
Proteus mirabilis						
Providencia stuartii						
Pseudomonas aeruginosa						
Serratia marcescens						
Stenotrophomonas maltophilia						
TOTAL GRAM NEGATIVE RODS						
FUNGI						
Aspergillus fumigatus						
Candida albicans						
Candida glabrata						
Candida guilliermondi						
Candida parapsilosis						
Candida tropicalis						
TOTAL FUNGI						

Note: PBSI, primary bloodstream infection; SBSI, secondary bloodstream infection; SSI, surgical site infection; YTD, year-to-date; vanc, vancomycin; ox, oxacillin; S, sensitive; R, resistant; Staph, staphylococcus.

Courtesy of the Infection Control Department, Sinai Hospital of Baltimore, Baltimore, Maryland.

Nosocomial Infection Surveillance: Line-List of Nosocomial Infections

Month/Year: _____

Name	Med Rec #	Room/ Unit	Adm Date	Cult Date	Org	BSI	CVC BSI	Pneu	VAP	UTI	CUTI	SSI	C dif	Rota	RSV

Note: Med Rec #, medical record number; Adm Date, admission date; Cult Date, culture date; Org, organism isolated; BSI, bloodstream infection; CVC BSI, central line–associated bloodstream infection; Pneu, pneumonia; VAP, ventilator-associated pneumonia; UTI, urinary tract infection; CUTI, catheter-associated urinary tract infection; SSI, surgical site infection; C dif, *Clostridium difficile* infection; Rota, rotavirus infection; RSV, respiratory syncytial virus infection.

Courtesy of the Infection Control Department, Sinai Hospital of Baltimore, Baltimore, Maryland.

Surgical Site Infection Surveillance

Pt. Name _____ Medical Record #: _____

Procedure: _____

Date operation: _____

O.R. Room #: _____

Personnel

Surgeon: _____ Anesthesiologist: _____

Surgeon Assistant: _____ Other (names & titles): _____

Circulator: _____ _____

Scrub: _____ _____

Wound Class: Clean   Clean-contaminated   Contaminated   Dirty/infected

ASA Class: 1   2   3   4   5   Repeat Procedure: no   yes

Duration   incision open:_____   NNIS SSI Risk
operation: incision closed: _____   Index Category: 0   1   2   3
                duration:_____

SSI Onset date:_____   NNIS SSI Category: Superficial/Incisional

                                                                        Deep Incisional

                                                                        Organ/Space

Readmitted for SSI: no   yes   Date of readmission: _____

Risk factors (medical, etc.): _____

Surgical Prophylaxis

Antibiotic:_____ Pre-op time given: _____

Intra-op time given: _____ Post-op times given: _____

Comments: _____

_____

_____

_____

_____

_____

Note: ASA, American Society of Anesthesiologists; NNIS, National Nosocomial Infections Surveillance; SSI, surgical site infection.
Courtesy of the Infection Control Department, Sinai Hospital of Baltimore, Baltimore, Maryland.

Surgical Joint Replacement Surveillance Report

Month: _____

Name	MRN	Date Surg	Age	Sex	Duration	WND CLS	GA	ASA CLS	EM/TR E	EM/TR T	Surgeon	1 PRO	2 DO	3 CO	4 P	Surg Time	Prophylactic Antibiotic	Comments

Note: MRN, medical record number; WND CLS, wound classification; GA, general anesthesia (Y/N); ASA CLS, anesthesia scoring guide; EM, emergency; TR, trauma; PRO, specific procedure (TH, TK, etc.); DO, disoriented; CO, continent; P, number of previous joints done; Surg, surgery.

Neonatal Infections/Colonizations Report

Month: _____

	Sex	Race	PMD	DEL V/CS	DOB/TIME	DOD	NSY	Onset Date Time	S/S or Site	Date, Spec, Result	Comments	CAI MAI HAI COL
Name_____ Mom_____ Hosp #_____												
Name_____ Mom_____ Hosp #_____												
Name_____ Mom_____ Hosp #_____												
Name_____ Mom_____ Hosp #_____												
Name_____ Mom_____ Hosp #_____												
Name_____ Mom_____ Hosp #_____												
Name_____ Mom_____ Hosp #_____												
Name_____ Mom_____ Hosp #_____												

Note: PMD, primary medical doctor; DEL V/CS, delivery by vaginal or C-section; DOB, date of birth; DOD, date of discharge; NSY, nursery; S/S, signs/symptoms; Spec, specimen type; CAI, community-acquired infection; MAI, maternally acquired infection; HAI, hospital-acquired infection; COL, colonized.

Vancomycin-Resistant Enterococcus Report

	Room	DOA	DOD	Adm Dx	PMD	Site VRE +	Date +	Prev Med Care	Previous Antibiotics	Current Antibiotics	Significant History	COL CAI HAI
Name ___ MRN ___												
Name ___ MRN ___												
Name ___ MRN ___												
Name ___ MRN ___												
Name ___ MRN ___												
Name ___ MRN ___												
Name ___ MRN ___												
Name ___ MRN ___												
Name ___ MRN ___												
Name ___ MRN ___												
Name ___ MRN ___												

Note: DOA, date of admission; DOD, date of discharge; MRN, medical record number; Adm Dx, admission diagnosis; VRE, vancomycin-resistant enterococcus; PMD, primary medical doctor; Prev Med, previous medical; COL, colonized; CAI, community-acquired infection; HAI, hospital-acquired infection.

Methicillin-Resistant *Staphylococcus aureus* Report

	Room/ Bed	DOA ICU	DOD to:	Attending PMD	Adm Dx	Prev Med Care	Date and Site MRSA +	Days Positive	Org. Sens.	1	2	3	4	5	Other Comments	COL CAI HAI
Name _____ MRN _____																
Name _____ MRN _____																
Name _____ MRN _____																
Name _____ MRN _____																
Name _____ MRN _____																
Name _____ MRN _____																
Name _____ MRN _____																
Name _____ MRN _____																
Name _____ MRN _____																
Name _____ MRN _____																
Name _____ MRN _____																

Note: DOA ICU, date of admission to intensive care unit; DOD, date of discharge (to other unit); MRN, medical record number; PMD, primary medical doctor; Adm Dx, admission diagnosis; Prev Med, previous medical; Org. Sens., organism antibiotic sensitivity; COL, colonized; CAI, community-acquired infection; HAI, hospital-acquired infection; 1, trach; 2, vent; 3, other respiratory support; 4, respiratory treatments; 5, infected site.

Mycobacterium tuberculosis and Other Mycobacteria Report

	Room	ISO	DOA	DOD	Adm Diagnosis	PPD	X-ray (N/A)	Cgh	Pre TB	Date/ Spec/Result	Anti-TB Meds	HD Rpt	CL (I, II, III, IV)	Comments
Name ___ MRN ___ PMD ___														
Name ___ MRN ___ PMD ___														
Name ___ MRN ___ PMD ___														
Name ___ MRN ___ PMD ___														
Name ___ MRN ___ PMD ___														
Name ___ MRN ___ PMD ___														
Name ___ MRN ___ PMD ___														
Name ___ MRN ___ PMD ___														

Note: MRN, medical record number; X-ray (N/A), chest film normal/abnormal; Cgh, cough; Pre TB, history of tuberculosis in past; PPD, purified protein derivative result in mm; ISO, dates in isolation; DOA, date of admission; DOD, date of discharge; Spec/Result, specimen/results; HD Rpt, date reported to health department; CL, Classification; I, TB suspect; II, TB infection, no disease; III, TB disease, infectious; IV, TB disease, noninfectious.

Clostridium difficile Surveillance Report

Month: _____

Room Assignment	Name/MRN	DOA	DOT	Physician Name/Code	TOX ASY	CLN DIS	HAI (Y/N)	Antibiotics Prior to Test	Treatment

Note: MRN, medical record number; DOA, date of admission; DOT, date of test; TOX ASY, toxin assay result; CLIN DIS, clinical disease; HAI, hospital-acquired infection (yes or no).

Line-List of Personnel Exposed to Patient with Scabies

Name of Source Patient: _____

Patient Room: _____

Patient Unit:_____

Patient Medical Record Number: _____

Probable Period of Communicability: _____

Name	Title	Phone	Date(s) Exposed	Type of Contact	Prophylaxis indicated		Date prophylaxis received
					yes	no	
					yes	no	
					yes	no	
					yes	no	
					yes	no	
					yes	no	
					yes	no	
					yes	no	
					yes	no	
					yes	no	
					yes	no	
					yes	no	
					yes	no	
					yes	no	
					yes	no	
					yes	no	
					yes	no	
					yes	no	
					yes	no	
					yes	no	
					yes	no	

Courtesy of the Infection Control Department, Sinai Hospital of Baltimore, Baltimore, Maryland.

Evaluation of Peripheral Line Sites (Current or Past Symptomatic Patients)

Unit: _____

Name	Rm	ADM	S/S (R, P, T, D)	Date & Time of Insertion		Site/DR Dated & Timed		Line Placed By (Name)	Where Placed (Location)	Site of IV	Type/Gauge (P, L, TL, S)		Long-Term		Purpose of Line (A, PPN, C, F, M, O)	Dwell Time (Days)	Comments
				D	T	Yes	No				T	G	Yes	No			

Note: ADM, admission date; DR, dressing; S/S, clinical signs or symptoms; R, red; P, phlebitis (red streak along vein); T, tenderness; D, drainage; P, PICC; L, landmark; TL, triple lumen; S, standard; A, antibiotics; PPN, parenteral nutrition; C, chemotherapy; F, fluid replacement; M, other intravenous meds; O, other. Allow one row for each peripheral line.

Case Definitions for Infectious Conditions Under Public Health Surveillance

NOTE: This appendix includes the complete Summary, Introduction, Definition of Terms, and Tables from the following report: Centers for Disease Control and Prevention. Case definitions for infectious conditions under public health surveillance. MMWR 1997;46(No.RR-10):1–55. However, only the definitions for diseases with the potential to cause outbreaks in the health care setting have been included. The complete report can be purchased from the Superintendent of Documents, U.S. Government Printing Office, Washington, D.C. 20402-9325. Telephone: 202-783-3238 or it can be downloaded from the CDC's Web site at http://www.cdc.gov/epo/mmwr/other/case_def/about.html.

This report provides updated uniform criteria for state health department personnel to use when reporting the nationally notifiable infectious diseases listed in Part 1 of this report. A revision date is listed for each case definition that has been revised. Newly generated case definitions that have not been published previously are designated as "adopted" on the specified date. Case definitions for some infectious conditions not designated as nationally notifiable are included in Part 2 of this report. Some of these conditions may have been nationally notifiable or may become so; definitions are included here to facilitate interpretation of data for these diseases. These conditions may be reportable in some states.

SUMMARY

State and local public health officials rely on health care providers, laboratories, and other public health personnel to report the occurrence of notifiable diseases to state and local health departments. Without such data, trends cannot be accurately monitored, unusual occurrences of diseases might not be detected, and the effectiveness of intervention activities cannot be easily evaluated.

In the United States, requirements for reporting diseases are mandated by state laws or regulations and the list of reportable diseases in each state differs. In October 1990, in collaboration with the Council of State and Territorial Epidemiologists, CDC published Case Definitions for Public Health Surveillance (MMWR 1990;39[No. RR-13]), which, for the first time, provided uniform criteria for reporting cases.

INTRODUCTION

State and local public health officials rely on health care providers, laboratories, and other public health personnel to report the occurrence of notifiable diseases to state and local health departments. Without such data, trends cannot be accurately monitored, unusual occurrences of diseases might not be detected, and the effectiveness of intervention activities cannot be easily evaluated.

In the United States, requirements for reporting diseases are mandated by state laws or regulations and the list of reportable diseases in each state differs. CDC and the Council of State and Territorial Epidemiologists (CSTE) have established a policy that requires state health departments to report cases of selected diseases (Table 1) to CDC's National Notifiable

Table C–1 Infectious Diseases Designated as Notifiable at the National Level—United States, 1997

Acquired immunodeficiency syndrome (AIDS)	Encephalitis, western equine	Malaria	Shigellosis
Anthrax	Escherichia coli O157:H7	Measles	Streptococcal disease, invasive Group A
Botulism	Gonorrhea	Meningococcal disease	Streptococcus pneumoniae, drug-resistant invasive disease
Brucellosis	Haemophilus influenzae, invasive disease	Mumps	
Chancroid	Hansen disease (leprosy)	Pertussis	
Chlamydia trachomatis, genital infections	Hantavirus pulmonary syndrome	Plague	Streptococcal toxic-shock syndrome
Cholera	Hemolytic uremic syndrome, postdiarrheal	Poliomyelitis, paralytic	Syphilis
Coccidioidomycosis	Hepatitis A	Psittacosis	Syphilis, congenital
Cryptosporidiosis	Hepatitis B	Rabies, animal	Tetanus
Diphtheria	Hepatitis, C/non-A, non-B	Rabies, human	Toxic-shock syndrome
Encephalitis, California serogroup	HIV infection, pediatric	Rocky Mountain spotted fever	Trichinosis
Encephalitis, eastern equine	Legionellosis	Rubella	Tuberculosis
Encephalitis, St. Louis	Lyme disease	Rubella, congenital syndrome	Typhoid fever
		Salmonellosis	Yellow fever

Diseases Surveillance System (NNDSS).[1,2] However, before 1990, the usefulness of such data was limited by the lack of uniform case definitions for public health surveillance. Without explicit criteria for identifying cases for public health surveillance purposes, state health departments and individual practitioners often applied different criteria for reporting similar cases.[3]

In October 1990, in collaboration with CSTE, CDC published Case Definitions for Public Health Surveillance,[4] which, for the first time, provided uniform criteria for reporting cases to increase the specificity of reporting and improve the comparability of diseases reported from different geographic areas. This report supersedes the 1990 report, which included infectious diseases and one noninfectious condition (i.e., spinal cord injury). The CDC Surveillance Coordination Group has established a steering committee that is charged with the development of a broad range of case definitions for noninfectious conditions (e.g., environmental or occupational conditions, chronic diseases, adverse reproductive health events, and injuries). This report provides updated uniform criteria for public health professionals to use when reporting the nationally notifiable infectious diseases listed in Part 1. A revision date is included for each case definition that has been revised. Newly generated case definitions that have not been previously published are designated as "adopted" on the specified date.

Data for nationally notifiable diseases reported by the 50 states, New York City, the District of Columbia, and the U.S. territories are collated and published weekly in the *Morbidity and Mortality Weekly Report* (MMWR). Cases reported by state health departments to the NNDSS for weekly publication are provisional because of ongoing revision of information and delayed reporting; thus, these numbers may change. Updated final reports are published annually in CDC's Summary of Notifiable Diseases, United States.[1]

The CDC/CSTE surveillance case definitions included in this report differ in their use of clinical, laboratory, and epidemiologic criteria to define cases. Some clinical syndromes do not have confirmatory laboratory tests; however, laboratory evidence may be one component of a clinical definition (e.g., toxic-shock syndrome). Most case definitions include a brief clinical description; however, unless this description is explicitly cited in the case classification section, it is included only as background information.

Some diseases require laboratory confirmation for diagnosis regardless of clinical symptoms, whereas others are diagnosed based on epidemiologic data. Many case definitions for the childhood vaccine-preventable diseases and foodborne diseases include epidemiologic criteria (e.g., exposure to probable or confirmed cases of disease or to a point source of infection [i.e., a single source of infection, such as an event resulting in a foodborne-disease outbreak, to which all confirmed case-patients were exposed]). In some instances, the anatomic site of infection may be important; for example, respiratory diphtheria is notifiable, whereas cutaneous diphtheria is not.

Substantial amounts of information, including results of laboratory tests, must be collected for many diseases before a final case classification is possible. State health departments should continue prompt reporting of provisional cases to CDC, and records should be updated with the appropriate classification status when additional surveillance information becomes available. Cases should be categorized as laboratory-confirmed (a subset of all confirmed cases) only if they meet the laboratory criteria specified. For additional information about procedures for reporting diseases to CDC, see the Manual of Procedures for the Reporting of Nationally Notifiable Diseases to CDC.[5]

Case definitions for some infectious conditions not considered nationally notifiable also are included in this report. Some of these conditions may have been nationally reportable or may become so; definitions are included here to facilitate interpretation of data for these diseases (Table 2). State health departments also provide CDC with information regarding certain conditions of public health interest, whether nationally reportable, through supplementary surveillance systems that collect more detailed, condition-specific information.[5]

The usefulness of public health surveillance data depends on its uniformity, simplicity, and timeliness. The case definitions contained in this report establish uniform criteria for disease reporting and should not be used as the sole criteria for establishing clinical diagnoses, determining the standard of care necessary for a particular patient, setting guidelines for quality assurance, or providing standards for reimbursement. Use of additional clinical, epidemiologic, and laboratory data may enable a physician to diagnose a disease even though the formal surveillance case definition may not be met.

The list of nationally reportable infectious diseases changes periodically. Diseases may be added to the list as new pathogens emerge or deleted as their incidence declines. Public health officials at state health departments and CDC collaborate in determining which diseases should be nationally notifiable; CSTE, in conjunction with CDC, makes recommendations annually for additions and deletions to the list of nationally notifiable diseases.[1,2] As knowledge increases and diagnostic technology improves, some definitions will change to reflect those trends. Thus, future revisions can be expected. This report also is available in Adobe™ Acrobat™ portable document format (.pdf) through the World Wide Web at http://www.cdc.gov/epo/mmwr/other/case_def/about.html. Future changes to the case definitions for nationally notifiable infectious diseases will be announced in the MMWR and made available in the electronic version.

Table C–2 Infectious Diseases and Conditions Not Nationally Notifiable but with Case Definitions Useful for Surveillance*

Amebiasis	*Granuloma inguinale*
Aseptic meningitis	Leptospirosis
Bacterial meningitis, other	Listeriosis
Campylobacter infection	*Lymphogranulmoa venereum*
Cyclospora infection	Mucopurulent cervicitis
Dengue fever	Nongonococcal urethritis
Ehrlichiosis	Pelvic inflammatory disease
Genital herpes (herpes	Rheumatic fever
simplex virus)	Tularemia
Genital warts	Varicella (chickenpox)
Giardiasis	

*This list includes only the diseases and conditions that are not nationally notifiable for which case definitions are provided in this report; it is not a complete list of such diseases for which CDC and state and territorial health departments maintain surveillance systems.

HOW TO USE INFORMATION IN THIS REPORT

Terms that are used in case classifications for both Parts 1 and 2 are defined (see Definition of Terms Used in Case Classification). Because each case definition in Parts 1 and 2 is intended to stand alone, abbreviations are defined the first time they appear in each case definition section and abbreviated throughout the rest of that section. A publications list is included only for the section on acquired immunodeficiency syndrome (AIDS); this list provides further sources regarding AIDS.

These case definitions are to be used for identifying and classifying cases, both of which are often done retrospectively, for national reporting purposes. They should not be used as criteria for public health action. For many conditions of public health importance, action to contain disease should be initiated as soon as a problem is identified; in many circumstances, appropriate public health action should be undertaken even though insufficient information is available to determine whether cases meet the case definition.

DEFINITION OF TERMS USED IN CASE CLASSIFICATION

Clinically compatible case: a clinical syndrome generally compatible with the disease, as described in the clinical description.

Confirmed case: a case that is classified as confirmed for reporting purposes.

Epidemiologically linked case: a case in which a) the patient has had contact with one or more persons who either have/had the disease or have been exposed to a point source of infection (i.e., a single source of infection, such as an event leading to a foodborne-disease outbreak, to which all confirmed case-patients were exposed) and b) transmission of the agent by the usual modes of transmission is plausible. A case may be considered epidemiologically linked to a laboratory-confirmed case if at least one case in the chain of transmission is laboratory confirmed.

Laboratory-confirmed case: a case that is confirmed by one or more of the laboratory methods listed in the case definition under Laboratory Criteria for Diagnosis. Although other laboratory methods can be used in clinical diagnosis, only those listed are accepted as laboratory confirmation for national reporting purposes.

Probable case: a case that is classified as probable for reporting purposes.

Supportive or presumptive laboratory results: specified laboratory results that are consistent with the diagnosis, yet do not meet the criteria for laboratory confirmation.

Suspected case: a case that is classified as suspected for reporting purposes.

PART 1. CASE DEFINITIONS FOR NATIONALLY NOTIFIABLE INFECTIOUS DISEASES

Botulism, Foodborne (Revised September 1996)

Clinical description: Ingestion of botulinum toxin results in an illness of variable severity. Common symptoms are diplopia, blurred vision, and bulbar weakness. Symmetric paralysis may progress rapidly.

Laboratory criteria for diagnosis: Detection of botulinum toxin in serum, stool, or patient's food or isolation of *Clostridium botulinum* from stool.

Case classification: Probable—a clinically compatible case with an epidemiologic link (e.g., ingestion of a home-canned food within the previous 48 hours). Confirmed—a clinically compatible case that is laboratory confirmed or that occurs among persons who ate the same food as persons who have laboratory-confirmed botulism.

Botulism, Infant (Revised September 1996)

Clinical description: An illness of infants, characterized by constipation, poor feeding, and "failure to thrive" that may be followed by progressive weakness, impaired respiration, and death.

Laboratory criteria for diagnosis: Detection of botulinum toxin in stool or serum or isolation of *Clostridium botulinum* from stool.

Case classification: Confirmed—a clinically compatible case that is laboratory confirmed occurring in a child aged less than one year.

Cryptosporidiosis (Adopted March 1995)

Clinical description: An illness caused by the protozoan *Cryptosporidium parvum* and characterized by diarrhea, abdominal cramps, loss of appetite, low-grade fever, nausea, and vomiting. Infected persons may be asymptomatic. The disease can be prolonged and life-threatening in severely immunocompromised persons.

Laboratory criteria for diagnosis: Demonstration of Cryptosporidium oocysts in stool, demonstration of Cryptosporidium in intestinal fluid or small-bowel biopsy specimens, or demonstration of Cryptosporidium antigen in stool by a specific immunodiagnostic test (e.g., enzyme-linked immunosorbent assay).

Case classification: Probable—a clinically compatible case that is epidemiologically linked to a confirmed case. Confirmed—a case that is laboratory confirmed.

Diphtheria (Revised March 1995)

Clinical description: An upper respiratory tract illness characterized by sore throat, low-grade fever, and an adherent membrane of the tonsil(s), pharynx, and/or nose.

Laboratory criteria for diagnosis: Isolation of *Corynebacterium diphtheriae* from a clinical specimen or histopathologic diagnosis of diphtheria.

Case classification: Probable—a clinically compatible case that is not laboratory confirmed and is not epidemiologically linked to a laboratory-confirmed case. Confirmed—a clinically compatible case that is either laboratory confirmed or epidemiologically linked to a laboratory-confirmed case.

Comment: Cutaneous diphtheria should not be reported. Respiratory disease caused by nontoxigenic *C. diphtheriae* should be reported as diphtheria. All diphtheria isolates, regardless of association with disease, should be sent to the Diphtheria Laboratory, National Center for Infectious Diseases, CDC.

Escherichia coli O157:H7 (Adopted March 1995)

Clinical description: An infection of variable severity characterized by diarrhea (often bloody) and abdominal cramps. Illness may be complicated by hemolytic uremic syndrome (HUS) or thrombotic thrombocytopenic purpura (TTP); asymptomatic infections may also occur.

Laboratory criteria for diagnosis: Isolation of *E. coli* O157:H7 from a specimen or isolation of Shiga-like toxin-producing *E. coli* O157:NM from a clinical specimen. (Strains of *E. coli* O157:H7 that have lost the flagellar "H" antigen become nonmotile and are designated "NM.")

Case classification: Suspect—a case of post-diarrheal HUS or TTP (see HUS case definition). Probable—isolation of *E. coli* O157 from a clinical specimen, pending confirmation of H7 or Shiga-like toxin or bloody diarrhea, HUS, or TTP that is epidemiologically linked to a confirmed or probable case. Confirmed—a case that is laboratory confirmed.

Comment: Confirmation is based on laboratory findings, and clinical illness is not required. Suspect, probable, and confirmed cases should be reported to local or state health departments. Only confirmed cases are reported nationally.

Haemophilus influenzae (Invasive Disease)

Clinical description: Invasive disease caused by *Haemophilus influenzae* may produce any of several clinical syndromes, including meningitis, bacteremia, epiglottitis, or pneumonia.

Laboratory criteria for diagnosis: Isolation of *H. influenzae* from a normally sterile site (e.g., blood or cerebrospinal fluid [CSF] or, less commonly, joint, pleural, or pericardial fluid).

Case classification: Probable—a clinically compatible case with detection of *H. influenzae* type b antigen in CSF. Confirmed—a clinically compatible case that is laboratory confirmed.

Comment: Positive antigen test results from urine or serum samples are unreliable for diagnosis of *H. influenzae* disease.

Hepatitis, Viral, Acute (Revised September 1996)

Clinical case definition: An acute illness with a) discrete onset of symptoms and b) jaundice or elevated serum aminotransferase levels.

Laboratory criteria for diagnosis: Hepatitis A— immunoglobulin M (IgM) antibody to hepatitis A virus (anti-HAV) positive. Hepatitis B—IgM antibody to hepatitis B core antigen (anti-HBc) positive or hepatitis B surface antigen (HBsAg) positive; and IgM anti-HAV negative (if done). Hepatitis C—Serum aminotransferase levels greater than 2.5 times the upper limit of normal, and IgM anti-HAV negative, and IgM anti-HBc negative (if done) or HBsAg negative, and antibody to hepatitis C virus (anti-HCV) positive, verified by a supplemental test. Non-A, Non-B hepatitis— Serum aminotransferase levels greater than times the upper limit of normal, and IgM anti-HAV negative, and IgM anti-HBc negative (if done) or HBsAg negative, and anti-HCV negative (if done). Delta hepatitis—HBsAg or IgM anti-HBc positive and antibody to hepatitis delta virus positive (Delta Hepatitis is not a nationally notifiable disease).

Case classification: Confirmed—a case that meets the clinical case definition and is laboratory confirmed or, for hepatitis A, a case that meets the clinical case definition and occurs in a person who has an epidemiologic link with a person who has laboratory-confirmed hepatitis A (i.e., household or sexual contact with an infected person during the 15–50 days before the onset of symptoms).

Comment: Persons who have chronic hepatitis or persons identified as HBsAg positive or anti-HCV positive should not be reported as having acute viral hepatitis unless they have evidence of an acute illness compatible with viral hepatitis (with the exception of perinatal hepatitis B infection). Up to 20 percent of acute hepatitis C cases will be anti-HCV negative when reported and will be classified as non-A, non-B hepatitis because some (5–10%) have not yet seroconverted and others (5–10%) remain negative even with prolonged follow-up. Available serologic tests for anti-HCV do not distinguish between acute and chronic or past infection. Thus, other causes of acute hepatitis should be excluded for anti-HCV positive patients who have an acute illness compatible with viral hepatitis.

Legionellosis (Revised September 1996)

Clinical description: Legionellosis is associated with two clinically and epidemiologically distinct illnesses: Legionnaires' disease, which is characterized by fever, myalgia, cough, pneumonia, and Pontiac fever, a milder illness without pneumonia.

Laboratory criteria for diagnosis: Isolation of Legionella from respiratory secretions, lung tissue, pleural fluid, or other normally sterile fluids; demonstration of a fourfold or greater rise in the reciprocal immunofluorescence antibody (IFA) titer to greater than or equal to 128 against *Legionella pneumophila* serogroup 1 between paired acute- and convalescent-phase serum specimens; or detection of L. pneumophila serogroup 1 in respiratory secretions, lung tissue, or pleural fluid by direct fluorescent antibody testing or demonstration of *L. pneumophila* serogroup 1 antigens in urine by radioimmunoassay or enzyme-linked immunosorbent assay.

Case classification: Confirmed—a clinically compatible case that is laboratory confirmed.

Comment: The previously used category of "probable case," which was based on a single IFA titer, lacks specificity for surveillance and is no longer used.

Measles (Revised September 1996)

Clinical case definition: An illness characterized by all the following: a generalized rash lasting greater than or equal to 3 days, a temperature greater than or equal to 101.0 F (greater than or equal to 38.3 C), and cough, coryza, or conjunctivitis.

Laboratory criteria for diagnosis: Positive serologic test for measles immunoglobulin M antibody, or significant rise in measles antibody level by any standard serologic assay, or isolation of measles virus from a clinical specimen.

Case classification: Suspected—any febrile illness accompanied by rash. Probable—a case that meets the clinical case definition, has noncontributory or no serologic or virologic testing, and is not epidemiologically linked to a confirmed case. Confirmed—a case that is laboratory confirmed or that meets the clinical case definition and is epidemiologically linked to a confirmed case. A laboratory-confirmed case does not need to meet the clinical case definition.

Comment: Confirmed cases should be reported to NNDSS. An imported case has its source outside the country or state. Rash onset occurs within 18 days after entering the jurisdiction, and illness cannot be linked to local transmission. Imported cases should be classified as international (a case that is imported from another country) or out-of-state (a case that is imported from another state in the United States). The possibility that a patient was exposed within his or her state of residence should be excluded; therefore, the patient either must have been out of state continuously for the entire period of possible exposure (at least 7–18 days before onset of rash) or have had one of the following types of exposure while out of state: (1) face-to-face contact with a person who had either a probable or confirmed case or (2) attendance in the same institution as a person who had a case of measles (e.g., in a school, classroom, or day care center).

An indigenous case is defined as a case of measles that is not imported. Cases that are linked to imported cases should be classified as indigenous if the exposure to the imported case occurred in the reporting state. Any case that cannot be proved to be imported should be classified as indigenous.

Meningococcal Disease

Clinical description: Meningococcal disease manifests most commonly as meningitis and/or meningococcemia that may progress rapidly to purpura fulminans, shock, and death. However, other manifestations might be observed.

Laboratory criteria for diagnosis: Isolation of *Neisseria meningitidis* from a normally sterile site (e.g., blood or cerebrospinal fluid [CSF] or, less commonly, joint, pleural, or pericardial fluid).

Case classification: Probable—a case with a positive antigen test in CSF or clinical purpura fulminans in the absence of a positive blood culture. Confirmed—a clinically compatible case that is laboratory confirmed.

Comment: Positive antigen test results from urine or serum samples are unreliable for diagnosing meningococcal disease.

Pertussis (Revised November 1997)

Clinical Case Definition: A cough illness lasting at least two weeks with one of the following: paroxysms of coughing, inspiratory "whoop," or post-tussive

vomiting, without other apparent cause (as reported by a health professional).

Laboratory criteria for diagnosis: Isolation of *Bordetella pertussis* from clinical specimen or positive polymerase chain reaction (PCR) for *B. pertussis*.

Case classification: Probable—meets the clinical case definition, is not laboratory confirmed, and is not epidemiologically linked to a laboratory-confirmed case. Confirmed—a case that is culture positive and in which an acute cough illness of any duration is present; or a case that meets the clinical case definition and is confirmed by positive PCR; or a case that meets the clinical case definition and is epidemiologically linked directly to a case confirmed by either culture or PCR.

Comment: The clinical case definition above is appropriate for endemic or sporadic cases. In outbreak settings, a case may be defined as a cough illness lasting at least two weeks (as reported by a health professional). Because direct fluorescent antibody testing of nasopharyngeal secretions has been demonstrated in some studies to have low sensitivity and variable specificity, such testing should not be relied on as a criterion for laboratory confirmation. Serologic testing for pertussis is available in some areas but is not standardized and, therefore, should not be relied on as a criterion for laboratory confirmation. Both probable and confirmed cases should be reported nationally.

Rubella (Revised September 1996)

Clinical case definition: An illness that has all the following characteristics: acute onset of generalized maculopapular rash, temperature greater than 99.0 F (greater than 37.2 C), if measured, and arthralgia/arthritis, lymphadenopathy, or conjunctivitis.

Laboratory critera for diagnosis: Isolation of rubella virus, or significant rise between acute- and convalescent-phase titers in serum rubella immunoglobulin G antibody level by any standard serologic assay, or positive serologic test for rubella immunoglobulin M (IgM) antibody.

Case classification: Suspected—any generalized rash illness of acute onset. Probable—a case that meets the clinical case definition, has no or noncontributory serologic or virologic testing, and is not epidemiologically linked to a laboratory-confirmed case. Confirmed—a case that is laboratory confirmed or that meets the clinical case definition and is epidemiologically linked to a laboratory-confirmed case.

Comments: Serum rubella IgM test results that are false positives have been reported in persons with other viral infections (e.g., acute infection with Epstein-Barr virus [infectious mononucleosis], recent cytomegalovirus infection, and parvovirus infection) or in the presence of rheumatoid factor. Patients who have laboratory evidence of recent measles infection are excluded.

Salmonellosis

Clinical description: An illness of variable severity commonly manifested by diarrhea, abdominal pain, nausea, and sometimes vomiting. Asymptomatic infections may occur, and the organism may cause extraintestinal infections.

Laboratory criteria for diagnosis: Isolation of *Salmonella* from a clinical specimen.

Case classification: Probable—a clinically compatible case that is epidemiologically linked to a confirmed case. Confirmed—a case that is laboratory confirmed.

Comment: Laboratory-confirmed isolates are reported to CDC via the Public Health Laboratory Information System (PHLIS), which is managed by the Foodborne and Diarrheal Diseases Branch, Division of Bacterial and Mycotic Diseases, National Center for Infectious Diseases, CDC. Both probable and confirmed cases are reported to the National Notifiable Diseases Surveillance System, but only confirmed cases are reported to PHLIS. Both asymptomatic infections and infections at sites other than the gastrointestinal tract, if laboratory confirmed, are considered confirmed cases that should be reported to PHLIS.

Shigellosis

Clinical description: An illness of variable severity characterized by diarrhea, fever, nausea, cramps, and tenesmus. Asymptomatic infections may occur.

Laboratory criteria for diagnosis: Isolation of *Shigella* from a clinical specimen.

Case classification: Probable—a clinically compatible case that is epidemiologically linked to a confirmed case. Confirmed—a case that is laboratory confirmed.

Comment: Laboratory-confirmed isolates are reported to CDC via the Public Health Laboratory Information System (PHLIS), which is managed by the Foodborne and Diarrheal Diseases Branch, Division of Bacterial and Mycotic Diseases, National Center for Infectious Diseases, CDC. Both probable and confirmed cases are reported to the National Notifiable Diseases Surveillance System, but only confirmed cases are reported to PHLIS. Confirmation is based on laboratory findings, and clinical illness is not required.

Streptococcal Disease, Invasive, Group A (Adopted March 1995)

Clinical description: Invasive group A streptococcal infections may manifest as any of several clinical syndromes, including pneumonia, bacteremia in association with cutaneous infection (e.g., cellulitis, erysipelas, or infection of a surgical or nonsurgical wound), deep soft-tissue infection (e.g., myositis or necrotizing fasciitis), meningitis, peritonitis, osteomyelitis, septic arthritis, postpartum sepsis (i.e., puerperal fever), neonatal sepsis, and nonfocal bacteremia.

Laboratory criteria for diagnosis: Isolation of group A Streptococcus (*Streptococcus pyogenes*) by culture from a normally sterile site (e.g., blood or cerebrospinal fluid, or, less commonly, joint, pleural, or pericardial fluid).

Case classification: Confirmed—a case that is laboratory confirmed.

Comment: *See also* Streptococcal Toxic-Shock Syndrome.

Streptococcal Toxic-Shock Syndrome (Revised September 1996)

Clinical description: Streptococcal toxic-shock syndrome (STSS) is a severe illness associated with invasive or noninvasive group A Streptococcal (*Streptococcus pyogenes*) infection. STSS may occur with infection at any site but most often occurs in association with infection of a cutaneous lesion. Signs of toxicity and a rapidly progressive clinical course are characteristic, and the case-fatality rate may exceed 50 percent.

Clinical case definition: An illness with the following clinical manifestations occurring within the first 48 hours of hospitalization or, for a nosocomial case, within the first 48 hours of illness:

- Hypotension defined by a systolic blood pressure less than or equal to 90 mmHg for adults or less than the fifth percentile by age for children aged less than 16 years.
- Multi-organ involvement characterized by two or more of the following:
  1. Renal impairment: Creatinine greater than or equal to 2 mg/dL (greater than or equal to 177 μmol/L) for adults or greater than or equal to twice the upper limit of normal for age. In patients with preexisting renal disease, a greater than twofold elevation over the baseline level.
  2. Coagulopathy: Platelets less than or equal to $100,000/mm^3$ (less than or equal to $100 \times 10^6/L$) or disseminated intravascular coagulation, defined by prolonged clotting times, low fibrinogen level, and the presence of fibrin degradation products.
  3. Liver involvement: Alanine aminotransferase, aspartate aminotransferase, or total bilirubin levels greater than or equal to twice the upper limit of normal for the patient's age. In patients with preexisting liver disease, a greater than twofold increase over the baseline level.
  4. Acute respiratory distress syndrome: defined by acute onset of diffuse pulmonary infiltrates and hypoxemia in the absence of cardiac failure or by evidence of diffuse capillary leak manifested by acute onset of generalized edema, or pleural or peritoneal effusions with hypoalbuminemia.
  5. A generalized erythematous macular rash that may desquamate.
  6. Soft-tissue necrosis, including necrotizing fasciitis or myositis, or gangrene.

Laboratory criteria for diagnosis: Isolation of group A Streptococcus.

Case classification: Probable—a case that meets the clinical case definition in the absence of another identified etiology for the illness and with isolation of group A Streptococcus from a nonsterile site. Confirmed—a case that meets the clinical case definition and with isolation of group A Streptococcus from a normally sterile site (e.g., blood or cerebrospinal fluid or, less commonly, joint, pleural, or pericardial fluid).

Tuberculosis (Revised September 1996)

Clinical description: A chronic bacterial infection caused by *Mycobacterium tuberculosis*, characterized pathologically by the formation of granulomas. The most common site of infection is the lung, but other organs may be involved.

Clinical case definition: A case that meets the following criteria: (1) a positive tuberculin skin test, (2) other signs and symptoms compatible with tuberculosis (e.g., an abnormal, unstable [i.e., worsening or improving] chest radiograph, or clinical evidence of current disease), (3) treatment with two or more antituberculosis medications, and (4) completed diagnostic evaluation.

Laboratory criteria for diagnosis: Isolation of *M. tuberculosis* from a clinical specimen (use of rapid identification techniques for *M. tuberculosis* [e.g., DNA probes and mycolic acids high-pressure liquid chromatography performed on a culture from a clinical specimen] are acceptable under this criterion); or demonstration of *M. tuberculosis* from a clinical specimen by nucleic acid amplification test (nucleic acid amplification [NAA] tests must be accompanied by culture for mycobacteria species; however, for surveillance purposes, CDC will accept results obtained from NAA tests approved by the Food and Drug Administration [FDA] and used according to the approved product labeling on the package insert. Current FDA-approved NAA tests are only approved for smear-positive respiratory specimens.); or demonstration of acid-fast bacilli in a clinical specimen when a culture has not been or cannot be obtained.

Case classification: Confirmed—a case that meets the clinical case definition or is laboratory confirmed.

Comment: A case should not be counted twice within any consecutive 12-month period. However, cases in which the patients had previously had verified disease should be reported again if the patients were discharged from treatment. Cases also should be reported again if patients were lost to supervision for greater than 12 months and disease can be verified again. Mycobacterial diseases, other than those caused by *M. tuberculosis* complex, should not be counted in tuberculosis morbidity statistics unless there is concurrent tuberculosis.

Typhoid Fever

Clinical description: An illness caused by *Salmonella typhi* that is often characterized by insidious onset of sustained fever, headache, malaise, anorexia, relative bradycardia, constipation or diarrhea, and nonproductive cough. However, many mild and atypical infections occur. Carriage of *S. typhi* may be prolonged.

Laboratory criteria for diagnosis: Isolation of *S. typhi* from blood, stool, or other clinical specimen.

Case classification: Probable—a clinically compatible case that is epidemiologically linked to a confirmed case in an outbreak. Confirmed—a clinically compatible case that is laboratory confirmed.

Comment: Isolation of the organism is required for confirmation. Serologic evidence alone is not sufficient for diagnosis. Asymptomatic carriage should not be reported as typhoid fever. Isolates of *S. typhi* are reported to the Foodborne and Diarrheal Diseases Branch, Division of Bacterial and Mycotic Diseases, National Center for Infectious Diseases, CDC, through the Public Health Laboratory Information System (see Salmonellosis).

PART 2. CASE DEFINITIONS FOR NON-NOTIFIABLE DISEASES

Campylobacter Infection

Clinical description: An infection that may result in diarrheal illness of variable severity.

Laboratory criteria for diagnosis: Isolation of Campylobacter from any clinical specimen.

Case classification: Probable—a clinically compatible case that is epidemiologically linked to a confirmed case. Confirmed—a case that is laboratory confirmed.

Comment: Only confirmed cases are reported to the laboratory-based surveillance system managed by the Foodborne and Diarrheal Diseases Branch, Division of Bacterial and Mycotic Diseases, National Center for Infectious Diseases, CDC.

Varicella (Chickenpox) (Revised September 1996)

Clinical case definition: An illness with acute onset of diffuse (generalized) papulovesicular rash without other apparent cause.

Laboratory criteria for diagnosis: Isolation of varicella virus from a clinical specimen or significant rise in serum varicella immunoglobulin G antibody level by any standard serologic assay.

Case classification: Probable—a case that meets the clinical case definition, is not laboratory confirmed, and is not epidemiologically linked to another probable or confirmed case. Confirmed—a case that is laboratory confirmed or that meets the clinical case definition and is epidemiologically linked to a confirmed or probable case.

Comment: Two probable cases that are epidemiologically linked would be considered confirmed, even in the absence of laboratory confirmation.

Foodborne Disease Outbreak

From: CDC. Case definitions for public health surveillance. MMWR 1990;39(No. RR-13):13.

Clinical description: Symptoms of illness depend upon etiologic agent.

Laboratory criteria for diagnosis: Depends upon etiologic agent.

Definition: An incident in which two or more persons experience a similar illness after ingestion of a common food, and epidemiologic analysis implicates the food as the source of the illness.

Comment: There are two exceptions: one case of botulism or chemical poisoning constitutes an outbreak.

Waterborne Disease Outbreak

From: CDC. Case definitions for public health surveillance. MMWR 1990;39(No. RR-13):33.

Clinical description: Symptoms of illness depend upon etiologic agent.

Laboratory criteria for diagnosis: Depends upon etiologic agent.

Definition: An incident in which two or more persons experience a similar illness after consumption or use of water intended for drinking, and epidemiologic evidence implicates the water as the source of the illness.

Comment: In addition, a single case of chemical poisoning constitutes an outbreak if laboratory studies indicate that the water has been contaminated by the chemical. Other outbreaks that should be reported include (1) epidemiologic investigations of outbreaks of gastroenteritis (even if not waterborne) on ocean-going passenger vessels that call on U.S. ports, and (2) outbreaks of illness associated with exposure to recreational water. Disease outbreaks associated with water used for recreational purposes should meet the same criteria used for waterborne outbreaks associated with drinking water. However, outbreaks associated with recreational water involve exposure to or unintentional ingestion of fresh or marine water, excluding wound infections caused by water-related organisms.

REFERENCES

1. CDC. Summary of notifiable diseases, United States, 1995. *MMWR.* 1995;44(No. 53).
2. Koo D, Wetterhall SF. History and current status of the National Notifiable Diseases Surveillance System. *J Public Health Manage Pract.* 1996;2:4–10.
3. Sacks JJ. Utilization of case definitions and laboratory reporting in the surveillance of notifiable communicable diseases in the United States. *Am J Public Health.* 1985;75:1420–2.
4. CDC. Case definitions for public health surveillance, 1990. *MMWR.* 1990;39(No. RR-13).
5. CDC. *Manual of procedures for the reporting of nationally notifiable diseases to CDC.* Atlanta: US Department of Health and Human Services, Public Health Service, CDC, 1995.

Guidelines for Measles Case Investigation and Outbreak Control

Excerpted from: Centers for Disease Control and Prevention (CDC). Measles, Mumps, and Rubella—Vaccine Use and Strategies for Elimination of Measles, Rubella, and Congenital Rubella Syndrome and Control of Mumps: Recommendations of the Advisory Committee on Immunization Practices (ACIP). MMWR. 1998; 47 (RR-8):1–57. This document can be downloaded from the CDC Web site (http://www.cdc.gov/epo/mmwr).

Measles should be suspected in any person who has a febrile illness accompanied by a rash. Hospital personnel and other health care providers should immediately report suspected and known cases of measles to the local or state health department. These guidelines outline strategies for investigating cases of measles and for preventing the transmission of measles. In addition to excerpts from the MMWR, this appendix contains a measles exposure contact follow-up form that can be used when performing contact tracing following exposure to measles (see Exhibit D–1).

DOCUMENTATION OF IMMUNITY

"Persons generally can be presumed immune to measles (Table D–1) if they have documentation of adequate vaccination, laboratory evidence of immunity to measles, documentation of physician-diagnosed measles, or were born before 1957. Criteria for adequate vaccination currently vary depending on state and local vaccination policy because of differences in the way states have implemented the two-dose measles vaccination schedule. All states are strongly encouraged to take immediate steps to implement the two-

dose MMR vaccination schedule so that, by 2001, adequate vaccination of children will be defined in all 50 states as follows:

- For preschool-aged children: documentation of at least one dose of MMR vaccine administered on or after the first birthday.
- For children in kindergarten through grade 12: documentation of two doses of MMR vaccine separated by at least 28 days (i.e., 1 month), with the first dose administered no earlier than the first birthday.
- Doses of MMR and other measles-containing vaccines administered before the first birthday should not be counted when determining adequacy of measles vaccination.

When measles virus is introduced into a community, persons who work in health care facilities are at greater risk for acquiring measles than the general population. Because persons working in medical settings have been infected with and have transmitted measles to patients and coworkers, rigorous criteria for immunity among health care workers have been established. For persons born during or after 1957 who work in health care facilities, adequate vaccination consists of two doses of MMR or other live measles-containing vaccine separated by at least 28 days, with the first dose administered no earlier than the first birthday (Table D–1). In addition, although birth before 1957 is generally considered acceptable evidence of measles immunity (Table D–1), measles has occurred in some unvaccinated persons born before 1957 who worked in health

Exhibit D–1 Measles Exposure Contact Follow-Up Form

Case Patient Name: _____   Medical record #: _____

Date of rash onset: _____

Infectious period (from 4 days prior to rash onset to 4 days after rash onset): _____ to _____

Exposed Patients

Name	Record #	Room	Date of birth	Date & time exposed[1]	Phone number, if discharged	Immune[2] yes	Immune[2] no	If not immune, date vaccine provided

Exposed Personnel

Name	Unit	Phone number	Date of birth	Date & time exposed[1]	Immune[2] yes	Immune[2] no	If not immune, dates of work restriction[3] 5th day	If not immune, dates of work restriction[3] 21st day	If not immune, date vaccine provided

1. Exposure is defined as being in the same room (or area supplied by the same recirculating air-handling system) at the same time as the patient or for up to one hour after the patient left the room/area.
2. A person born before 1957 is generally considered immune. Persons born on or after January 1, 1957 are considered immune if they have one of the following:
   - documentation of physician-diagnosed measles
   - documentation of two doses of live measles vaccine on or after their first birthday
   - serologic evidence of measles immunity.
3. Exposed non-immune personnel should be restricted from work from 5th day after the first exposure through 21st day after the last exposure.

Courtesy of Infection Control Department, Sinai Hospital of Baltimore, Baltimore, Maryland.

Table D–1 Acceptable Presumptive Evidence of Immunity to Measles, Rubella, and Mumps

	Routine	*Persons Who Work in Health Care Facilities*	*International Travelers*	*Students at Post-High School Educational Institutions*
Measles	1. documentation of adequate vaccination+: preschool-aged children and adults not a high risk—1 dose; school-aged children (grades K–12)—2 doses, OR 2. laboratory evidence of immunity, OR 3. born before 1957, OR 4. documentation of physician-diagnosed measles	1. documented administration of 2 doses of live measles virus vaccine,+@ OR 2. laboratory evidence of immunity, OR 3. born before 1957,& OR 4. documentation of physician-diagnosed measles	1. documented administration of 2 doses of live measles virus vaccine,+** OR 2. laboratory evidence of immunity, OR 3. born before 1957, OR 4. documentation of physician-diagnosed measles	1. documented administration of 2 doses of live measles virus vaccine,+ OR 2. laboratory evidence of immunity, OR 3. born before 1957, OR 4. documentation of physician-diagnosed measles
Rubella	1. documented administration of 1 dose of live rubella virus vaccine,+ OR 2. laboratory evidence of immunity, OR 3. born before 1957 (except women of childbearing age who could become pregnant)++	1. documented administration of 1 dose of live rubella virus vaccine,+ OR 2. laboratory evidence of immunity, OR 3. born before 1957 (except women of childbearing age who could become pregnant)++	1. documented administration of 1 dose of live rubella virus vaccine,+ OR 2. laboratory evidence of immunity, OR 3. born before 1957 (except women of childbearing age who could become pregnant)++	1. documented administration of 1 dose of live rubella virus vaccine,+ OR 2. laboratory evidence of immunity, OR 3. born before 1957 (except women of childbearing age who could become pregnant)++
Mumps	1. documented administration of 1 dose of live mumps virus vaccine,+ OR 2. laboratory evidence of immunity, OR 3. born before 1957, OR 4. documentation of physician-diagnosed mumps	1. documented administration of 1 dose of live mumps virus vaccine,+ OR 2. laboratory evidence of immunity, OR 3. born before 1957, OR 4. documentation of physician-diagnosed mumps	1. documented administration of 1 dose of live mumps virus vaccine,+ OR 2. laboratory evidence of immunity, OR 3. born before 1957, OR 4. documentation of physician-diagnosed mumps	1. documented administration of 1 dose of live mumps virus vaccine,+ OR 2. laboratory evidence of immunity, OR 3. born before 1957, OR 4. documentation of physician-diagnosed mumps

*Health care workers include all persons (i.e., medical or nonmedical, paid or volunteer, full- or part-time, student or nonstudent, with or without patient-care responsibilities) who work in facilities that provide health care to patients (i.e., inpatient and outpatient, private and public). Facilities that provide care exclusively for elderly patients who are at minimal risk for measles and rubella and complications of these diseases are a possible exception.

+The first dose should be administered on or after the first birthday; the second dose of measles-containing vaccine should be administered no earlier than one month (i.e., minimum of 28 days) after the first dose. Combined measles-mumps-rubella (MMR) vaccine generally should be used whenever any of its component vaccines is indicated.

&May vary depending on current state or local requirements.

@Health care facilities should consider recommending a dose of MMR vaccine for unvaccinated workers born before 1957 who are at risk for occupational exposure to measles and who do not have a history of measles disease or laboratory evidence of measles immunity.

**Children aged 6–11 months should receive a dose of monovalent measles vaccine (or MMR, if monovalent vaccine is not available) before departure. Children who receive a dose of measles-containing vaccine before their first birthdays should be revaccinated with two doses of MMR vaccine, the first of which should be administered when the child is aged 12–15 months (12 months if the child remains in a high-risk area) and the second at least 28 days later.

++Women of childbearing age are adolescent girls and premenopausal adult women. Because rubella can occur in some persons born before 1957 and because congenital rubella and congenital rubella syndrome can occur in the offspring of women infected with rubella virus during pregnancy, birth before 1957 is not acceptable evidence of rubella immunity for women who could become pregnant.

Source: Reprinted from http://www.cdc.gov/epo/mmwr/preview/mmwrhtml/00053391.htm.

care facilities. Therefore, health care facilities should consider recommending a dose of MMR vaccine for unvaccinated workers born before 1957 who lack a history of measles disease or laboratory evidence of measles immunity (see Health Care Facilities).

The previously described criteria apply only to routine vaccination. During measles outbreaks, evidence of adequate vaccination for school-aged children, adolescents, and adults born during or after 1957 who are at risk for measles exposure and infection consists of two doses of measles-containing vaccine separated by at least 28 days, with the first dose administered no earlier than the first birthday (see Measles Outbreak Control)."[1(pg12–13)]

HEALTH CARE FACILITIES

"When measles virus is introduced into a community, persons who work in health care facilities are at increased risk for acquiring measles compared with the general population. During 1985–1991, at least 795 measles cases (1.1% of all reported cases) occurred among adult health care workers. Of these, 29 percent occurred among nurses, 15 percent among physicians, 11 percent among persons in other health care occupations (e.g., laboratory and radiology technicians, etc.), 11 percent among clerks, 4 percent among nursing assistants, and 4 percent among medical and nursing students (CDC, unpublished data). A general decline in measles incidence occurred after 1991. However, 15 of the 75 measles outbreaks reported during 1993–1996 involved transmission in a medical facility, and a total of 36 measles cases (1.8% of all reported cases) occurred among persons working in health care facilities (CDC, unpublished data). Although similar surveillance data are not available for rubella, outbreaks have occurred in health care settings, and health care workers have transmitted rubella to patients (CDC, unpublished data).

All persons who work in health care facilities should be immune to measles and rubella (Table D–1). Because any health care worker (i.e., medical or nonmedical, paid or volunteer, full- or part-time, student or nonstudent, with or without patient-care responsibilities) who is not immune to measles and rubella can contract and transmit these diseases, all health care facilities (i.e., inpatient and outpatient, private and public)

should ensure that those who work in their facilities are immune to measles and rubella (Table D–1).

Health care workers have a responsibility to avoid transmitting these diseases and thereby causing harm to patients. Adequate vaccination for health care workers born during or after 1957 consists of two doses of a live measles-containing vaccine and at least one dose of a live rubella-containing vaccine (Table D–1). Health care workers who need a second dose of measles-containing vaccine should be revaccinated one month (at least 28 days) after their first dose."[1(pg18–19)]

MEASLES CASE INVESTIGATION AND OUTBREAK CONTROL

Case Definition

"A *suspected* measles case is defined as any febrile illness accompanied by rash. Suspected and known cases of measles should be reported immediately to the local or state health department. The designated public health authorities should quickly initiate an investigation of the reported case. Rapid case reporting and investigation can help limit further transmission.

A *clinical* case of measles is defined as an illness characterized by

- a generalized rash lasting greater than or equal to three days, and
- a temperature of greater than or equal to 38.3 C (greater than or equal to 101 F), and
- cough, coryza, or conjunctivitis

A *probable* case of measles

- meets the clinical case definition for measles, and
- is not epidemiologically linked to a confirmed case, and
- has not been serologically or virologically tested or has noncontributory serologic or virologic results

A *confirmed* case of measles

- meets the laboratory criteria for measles, or
- meets the clinical case definition and is epidemiologically linked to a confirmed case

Confirmed measles cases are routinely reported to CDC by state health departments.

Laboratory Diagnosis

The laboratory criteria for measles diagnosis are

- a positive serologic test for measles IgM antibody, or
- a significant rise in measles antibody level by any standard serologic assay, or
- isolation of measles virus from a clinical specimen

A laboratory-confirmed case need not meet the clinical case definition. Serologic confirmation should be attempted for every suspected case of measles and is particularly important for any case that cannot be epidemiologically linked through a chain of transmission to a confirmed case. However, reporting of suspected or probable cases, investigation of cases, and the implementation of control activities should not be delayed pending laboratory results.

Blood for serologic testing should be collected during the first clinical encounter with a person who has suspected or probable measles. The serum should be tested for measles IgM antibody as soon as possible using an assay that is both sensitive and specific (e.g., direct-capture IgM EIA method). Correct interpretation of serologic data depends on the timing of specimen collection in relation to rash onset and on the characteristics of the antibody assay used. This timing is especially important for interpreting negative results because IgM antibody may not be detectable with some less sensitive assays until at least 72 hours after rash onset. Measles IgM may be detectable at the time of rash onset, peaks approximately 10 days after rash onset, and is usually undetectable 30–60 days after rash onset. In general, if measles IgM is not detected in a serum specimen obtained in the first 72 hours after rash onset from a person whose illness meets the clinical case definition for measles, another specimen should be obtained at least 72 hours after rash onset and tested for measles IgM antibody. Measles IgM is detectable for at least 1 month after rash onset. Persons with febrile rash illnesses who are seronegative for measles should be tested for rubella.

As measles becomes rare in the United States, the likelihood of obtaining false positive serologic results from measles IgM antibody testing increases. False positive results have been obtained by using a commercially available ELISA assay for measles IgM in persons with parvovirus infection (fifth disease). Confirmatory testing by using an assay that is both sensitive and specific (e.g., direct-capture IgM EIA method) should be considered when IgM is detected in a patient with suspected measles who has no identified source of infection and no epidemiologic linkage to another confirmed case. The Measles Virus Laboratory of CDC's National Center for Infectious Diseases has provided training to all state public health laboratories to perform such testing.

Serologic diagnosis of measles can also be confirmed by a significant rise in antibody titer between acute- and convalescent-phase serum specimens. Typically, the acute-phase serum specimen is obtained within 1–3 days after rash onset and the convalescent-phase specimen is obtained approximately 2–4 weeks later. This method has been largely supplanted by IgM assays which can be done on a single serum specimen obtained soon after rash onset.

Asymptomatic measles reinfection can occur among persons who have previously developed antibodies from vaccination or from natural disease. Symptomatic reinfections accompanied by rises in measles antibody titers are rare, and those resulting in detectable measles IgM antibody occur even more rarely.

Molecular characterization of measles virus isolates has become an important tool for defining the epidemiologic features of measles during periods of low disease incidence and for documenting the impact of measles elimination efforts. In addition to serologic confirmation, a specimen (e.g., urine or nasopharyngeal mucus) for measles virus isolation and genetic characterization should be collected as close to the time of rash onset as possible. Delay in collection of these clinical specimens reduces the chance of isolating measles virus. Clinicians who have a patient with suspected measles should immediately contact their local or state health departments concerning additional information about collecting and shipping urine and nasal specimens for measles virus isolation."[1(pg38–40)]

Measles Outbreak Control

"Because of the potential for rapid spread of the disease, one confirmed case of measles in a community is an urgent public health situation. Health care personnel should immediately report suspect and confirmed cases to the local or state health department.

Once a case is confirmed, prompt vaccination of susceptible persons at risk for exposure may help prevent dissemination of measles. Control activities should not be delayed pending the return of laboratory results from persons with suspected or probable cases. Persons who cannot readily provide acceptable evidence of measles immunity (Table D–1) should be vaccinated or excluded from the setting of the outbreak (e.g., school, day care facility, hospital, clinic). Almost all persons who are excluded from an outbreak area because they lack acceptable evidence of immunity quickly comply with vaccination requirements. Persons exempted from measles vaccination for medical, religious, or other reasons should be excluded from involved institutions in the outbreak area until 21 days after the onset of rash in the last case of measles."[1](pg40)

Measles Outbreaks in Health Care Settings

"If a measles outbreak occurs within a health care facility (e.g., hospital, clinic, physician office) or in the areas served by the facility, all persons working at the facility who cannot provide documentation of two doses of measles-containing vaccine separated by at least 28 days with the first dose administered on or after the first birthday, or who do not have other evidence of measles immunity (Table D–1), should receive a dose of MMR vaccine. If indicated, health care workers born during or after 1957 should receive a second dose of MMR vaccine at least 28 days after the previous dose (see Documentation of Immunity). Some health care workers born before 1957 have acquired measles in health care facilities and have transmitted the disease to patients or coworkers. Therefore, during outbreaks, health care facilities also should strongly consider recommending a dose of MMR vaccine to unvaccinated health care workers born before 1957 who do not have serologic evidence of immunity or a history of measles disease.

Serologic testing of health care workers before vaccination is not generally recommended during an outbreak because arresting measles transmission requires rapid vaccination of susceptible health care workers. The need to screen, wait for results, and then contact and vaccinate susceptible persons can impede the rapid vaccination needed to curb the outbreak.

Susceptible health care workers (Table D–1) exposed to measles should receive a dose of MMR vaccine and should be removed from all patient contact and excluded from the facility from the fifth to the 21st day after the exposure. They may return to work on the 22nd day after exposure. However, susceptible health care workers who are not vaccinated after exposure should be removed from all patient contact and excluded from the facility from the fifth day after their first exposure to the 21st day after the last exposure, even if they receive postexposure IG. Personnel who become ill with prodromal symptoms or rash should be removed from all patient contact and excluded immediately from the facility until four days after the onset of their rash."[1](pg42)

REFERENCE

1. Centers for Disease Control and Prevention. Measles, Mumps, and Rubella—Vaccine Use and Strategies for Elimination of Measles, Rubella, and Congenital Rubella Syndrome and Control of Mumps: Recommendations of the Advisory Committee on Immunization Practices (ACIP). *MMWR*. 1998; 47 (RR-8):1–57.

Immunization of Health Care Workers

Recommendations for Immunization Practices and Use of Immunobiologics Applicable to Disease Prevention among Health Care Workers—Advisory Committee on Immunization Practices Statements Published as of September 1, 1997

Subject	MMWR Publication
General recommendations on immunization	1994;43(RR-1):1–39
Adult immunization	1991;40(RR-12):1–94
Altered immunocompetence	1993;42(RR-4):1–18
Adverse reactions, contraindications, and precautions	1996;45(RR-12):1–35
Bacille Calmette-Guerin vaccine	1996;45(RR-4):1–18
Diphtheria, tetanus, and pertussis	1991;40(RR-10):1–28 1997;46(RR-7)
Hepatitis B	1991;40(RR-13):1–25
Hepatitis A	1996;45(RR-15):1–30
Influenza*	1997;46(RR-9):1–25
Japanese encephalitis	1993;42(RR-1):1–15
Measles, mumps, rubella (MMR)	1998;47(RR-8):1–57
Meningococcal disease and outbreaks	1997;46(RR-5):1–21

Pertussis, acellular
  (see also Diphtheria above)
  (supplementary statements)
	1992;41(RR-1):1–10
	1992;41(RR-15):1–5
	1997;46(RR-7):1–25

Pneumococcal	1997;46(RR-8):1–24
Poliomyelitis	1997;46(RR-3):1–25
Rabies	1991;40(RR-3):1–19
Typhoid	1994;43(RR-14):1–7
Vaccinia (smallpox)	1991;40(RR-14):1–10
Varicella	1996;45(RR-11):1–36

*Each year influenze vaccine recommendations are reviewed and amended to reflect updated information concerning influenza activity in the United States for the preceding influenza season and to provide information on the vaccine available for the upcoming influenza season. These recommendations are published annually in the MMWR, usually during May or June.

Source: Adapted from Immunization of Health Care Workers: Recommendations of the Advisory Committee on Immunization Practices (ACIP) and the Hospital Infection Control Practices Advisory Committee (HICPAC), MMWR, 1997, 46(RR-18):1–42, Centers for Disease Control and Prevention.

Immunizing Agents and Immunization Schedules for Health Care Workers (HCWs)*

Generic Name	Primary Schedule and Booster(s)	Indications	Major Precautions and Contraindications	Special Considerations
IMMUNIZING AGENTS STRONGLY RECOMMENDED FOR HEALTH CARE WORKERS				
Hepatitis B (HB) recombinant vaccine	Two doses IM 4 weeks apart; third dose 5 months after second; booster doses not necessary.	**Preexposure:** HCWs at risk for exposure to blood or body fluids.	On the basis of limited data, no risk of adverse effects to developing fetuses is apparent. Pregnancy should *not* be considered a contraindication to vaccination of women. Previous anaphylactic reactions to common baker's yeast is a contraindication to vaccination.	The vaccine produces neither therapeutic nor adverse effects on HBV-infected persons. Prevaccination serologic screening is not indicated for persons being vaccinated because of occupational risk. HCWs who have contact with patients or blood should be tested 1 to 2 months after vaccination to determine serologic response.
Hepatitis B immune globulin (HBIG)	0.06 mL/kg IM as soon as possible after exposure. A second dose of HBIG should be administered 1 month later if the HB vaccine series has not been started.	**Postexposure** prophylaxis: For persons exposed to blood or body fluids containing HBsAg and who are not immune to HBV infection—0.06 mL/kg IM as soon as possible (but no later than 7 days after exposure).		
Influenza vaccine (inactivated whole-virus and split-virus vaccines)	Annual vaccination with current vaccine. Administered IM.	HCWs who have contact with patients at high risk for influenza or its complications; HCWs who work in chronic care facilities; HCWs with high-risk medical conditions or who are aged ≥65 years.	History of anaphylactic hypersensitivity to egg ingestion.	No evidence exists of risk to mother or fetus when the whole-virus and vaccine is administered to a pregnant woman with an underlying high-risk condition. Influenza vaccination is recommended during second and third trimesters of pregnancy because of increased risk for hospitalization.
Measles live-virus vaccine	One dose SC; second dose at least 1 month later.	HSWs[†] born during or after 1957 who do not have documentation of having received 2 doses of live vaccine on or after the first birthday or a history of physician-diagnosed measles or serologic evidence of immunity. Vaccination should be considered for all HCWs who lack proof of immunity, including those born before 1957.	Pregnancy; immunocompromised persons[§], including HIV-infected persons who have evidence of severe immunosuppression; anaphylaxis after gelatin ingestion or administration of neomycin; recent administration of immune globulin.	MMR is the vaccine of choice if vaccine recipients are likely to be susceptible to rubella and/or mumps as well as to measles. Persons vaccinated from 1963 to 1967 with a killed measles vaccine alone, killed vaccine followed by live vaccine, or with a vaccine of unknown type should be revaccinated with 2 doses of live measles virus vaccine.

Generic Name	Primary Schedule and Booster(s)	Indications	Major Precautions and Contraindications	Special Considerations
Mumps live-virus vaccine	One dose SC; no booster.	HCWs[†] believed to be susceptible can be vaccinated. Adults born before 1957 can be considered immune.	Pregnancy; immuno-compromised persons[§]; history of anaphylactic reaction after gelatin ingestion or administration of neomycin.	MMR is the vaccine of choice if vaccine recipients are likely to be susceptible to measles and rubella as well as to mumps.
Rubella live-virus vaccine	One dose SC; no booster	Indicated for HCWs,[†] both men and women, who do not have documentation of having received live vaccine on or after their first birthday or laboratory evidence of immunity. Adults born before 1957, **except women who can become pregnant,** can be considered immune.	Pregnancy; immuno-compromised persons[†]; history of anaphylactic reaction after administration of neomycin.	The risk for rubella vaccine-associated malformations in the offspring of women pregnant when vaccinated or who became pregnant within 3 months after vaccination is negligible. Such women should be counseled regarding the theoretical basis of concern for the fetus. MMR is the vaccine of choice if recipients are likely to be susceptible to measles or mumps, as well as to rubella.
Varicella zoster live-virus vaccine	Two 0.5 mL doses SC 4–8 weeks apart if ≥13 years of age.	Indicated for HCWs[†] who do not have either a reliable history of varicella or serologic evidence of immunity.	Pregnancy, immuno-compromised persons,[§] history of anaphylactic reaction following receipt of neomycin or gelatin. Avoid salicylate use for 6 weeks after vaccination.	Vaccine is available from the live-virus vaccine manufacturer for certain patients with acute lymphocytic leukemia (ALL) in remission. Because 71–93% of persons without a history of varicella are immune serologic testing before vaccination is likely to be cost effective.
Varicella-zoster immune globulin (VZIG)	Persons <50 kg: 120 u/10 kg IM; persons ≥50 kg: 625 u.[¶]	Persons known or likely to be susceptible (particularly those at high risk for complications, e.g., pregnant women) who have close and prolonged exposure to a contact case or an infectious hospital staff worker or patient.		Serologic testing may help in assessing whether to administer VZIG. If use of VZIG prevents varicella disease, patient should be vaccinated subsequently.

BCG VACCINATION

Generic Name	Primary Schedule and Booster(s)	Indications	Major Precautions and Contraindications	Special Considerations
Bacille Calmette Guerin (BCG) Vaccine (Tuberculosis)	One percutaneous dose of 0.3 mL; no booster dose recommended.	Should be considered only for HCWs in areas where multi-drug tuberculosis is prevalent, a strong likelihood of infection exists, and where comprehensive infection control precautions have failed to prevent TB transmission to HCWs.	Should not be administered to immunocompromised persons,[§] and pregnant women.	In the United States, tuberculosis-control efforts are directed towards early (Tuberculosis) identification, treatment of cases, and preventive therapy with isoniazid.

Generic Name	Primary Schedule and Booster(s)	Indications	Major Precautions and Contraindications	Special Considerations
OTHER IMMUNOBIOLOGICS THAT ARE OR MAY BE INDICATED FOR HEALTH CARE WORKERS				
Immune globulin (Hepatitis A)	**Postexposure**—One IM dose of 0.02 mL/kg administered ≤2 weeks after exposure.	Indicated for HCWs exposed to feces of infectious patients.	Contraindicated in persons with IgA deficiency; do not administered within 2 weeks after MMR vaccine, or 3 weeks after varicella vaccine. Delay administration of MMR vaccine for ≥3 months and varicella vaccine ≥5 months after administration of IG.	Administer in large muscle mass (deltoid, gluteal).
Hepatitis A vaccine	Two doses of vaccine either 6–12 months apart (HAVRIX®), or 6 months apart (VAQTA®).	Not routinely indicated for HCWs in the United States. Persons who work with HAV-infected primates or with HAV in a research laboratory setting should be vaccinated.	History of anaphylactic hypersensitivity to alum or, for HAVRIX®, the preservative 2-phenoxyethanol. The safety of the vaccine in pregnant women has not been determined; the risk associated with vaccination should be weighed agasint the risk for hepatitis A in women who may be at high risk for exposure to HAV.	
Meningococcal polysaccharide vaccine (tetravalent A, C, W135, and Y)	One dose in volume and by route specified by manufacturer; need for boosters unknown.	Not routinely indicated for HCWs in the United States.	The safety of the vaccine in pregnant women has not been evaluated; it should not be administered during pregnancy unless the risk for infection is high.	
Tyhpoid vaccine, IM, SC, and oral	*IM vaccine:* One 0.5 mL dose, booster 0.5 mL every 2 years. *SC vaccine:* two 0.5 mL doses, ≥4 weeks apart, booster 0.5 mL SC or 0.1 ID every 3 years if exposure continues. *Oral vaccine:* Four doses on alternate days. The manufacturer recommends revaccination with the entire four-dose series every 5 years.	Workers in microbiology laboratories who frequently work with *Salmonella typhi*.	Severe local or systemic reaction to a previous dose. Ty21a (oral) vaccine should not be administered to immunocompromised persons§ or to persons receiving antimicrobial agents.	Vaccination should not be considered an alternative to the use of proper procedures when handling specimens and cultures in the laboratory.
Vaccinia vaccine (smallpox)	One dose administered with a bifurcated needle; boosters administered every 10 years.	Laboratory workers who directly handle cultures with vaccinia, recombinant vaccinia viruses, or orthopox viruses that infect humans.	The vaccine is contraindicated in pregnancy, in persons with eczema or a history of eczema, and in immunocompromised persons[†] and their household contacts.	Vaccination may be considered for HCWs who have direct contact with contaminated dressings or other infectious material from volunteers in clinical studies involving recombinant vaccinia virus.

Generic Name	Primary Schedule and Booster(s)	Indications	Major Precautions and Contraindications	Special Considerations
OTHER VACCINE-PREVENTABLE DISEASES				
Tetanus and diphtheria (toxoids [Td])	Two IM doses 4 weeks apart; third dose 6–12 months after second dose; booster every 10 years.	All adults.	Except in the first trimester, pregnancy is not a precaution. History of a neurologic reaction or immediate hypersensitivity reaction after a previous dose. History of severe local (Arthus-type) reaction after a previous dose. Such persons should not receive further routine or emergency doses of Td for 10 years.	Tetanus prophylaxis in wound management.**
Pneumococcal polysaccharide vaccine (23 valent).	One dose, 0.5 mL, IM or SC; revaccination recommended for those at highest risk ≥5 years after the first dose.	Adults who are at increased risk of pneumococcal disease and its complications because of underlying health conditions; older adults, especially those age ≥65 who are healthy.	The safety of vaccine in pregnant women has not been evaluated; it should not be administered during pregnancy unless the risk for infection is high. Previous recipients of any type of pneumococcal polysaccharide vaccine who are at highest risk for fatal infection or antibody loss may be revaccinated ≥5 years after the first dose.	

*Persons who provide health care to patients or work in institutions that provide patient care, e.g., physicians, nurses, emergency medical personnel, dental professionals and students, medical and nursing students, laboratory technicians, hospital volunteers, and administrative and support staff in health-care institutions.

†All HCWs (i.e., medical or nonmedical, paid or volunteer, full time or part time, student or non-student, with or without patient-care responsibilities) who work in health-care institutions (e.g., inpatient and outpatient, public and private) should be immune to measles, rubella, and varicella.

§Persons immunocompromised because of immune deficiency diseases, HIV infection (who should primarily not receive BCG, OPV, and yellow fever vaccine), leukemia, lymphoa or generalized malignancy or immunosuppressed as a result of therapy with corticosteroids, alkylating drugs, antimetabolites, or radiation.

¶Some experts recommend 125 u/10 kg regardless of total body weight.

**See (15) CDC. Update on adult immunization: recommendations of the Advisory Committee on Immunization Practices (ACIP). MMWR 1991:40(No. RR-12):1–94.

Abbreviations: IM, intramuscular; HBV, hepatitis B virus; HBsAg, hepatitis B surface antigen; SC, subcutaneous; HIV, human immunodeficiency virus; MMR, measles, mumps, rubella vaccine; HCW, health-care worker; TB, tuberculosis; HAV, hepatitis A virus; IgA, immune globulin A, ID, intradermal.

Source: Reprinted from Immunization of Health-Care Workers: Recommendations of the Advisory Committee of Immunization Practices (ACIP) and the Hospital Infection Control Practices Advisory Committee (HICPAC). MMWR, 1997; 46(RR-18):1–42, Centers for Disease Control.

APPENDIX F

Suggested Work Restrictions for Personnel

Summary of Suggested Work Restrictions for Health Care Personnel Exposed to or Infected with Infectious Diseases of Concern in Health Care Settings, in the Absence of State and Local Regulations (Modified from ACIP Recommendations*)

Disease/Problem	Work Restriction	Duration	Category
Conjunctivitis	Restrict from patient contact and contact with the patient's environment	Until discharge ceases	II
Cytomegalovirus infections	No restriction		II
Diarrheal diseases			
Acute stage (diarrhea with other symptoms)	Restrict from patient contact, contact with the patient's environment, or food handling	Until symptoms resolve	IB
Convalescent stage, *Salmonella* spp.	Restrict from care of high-risk patients	Until symptoms resolve; consult with local and state health authorities regarding need for negative stool cultures	IB
Diphtheria	Exclude from duty	Until antimicrobial therapy completed and 2 cultures obtained ≥24 hours apart are negative	IB
Enteroviral infections	Restrict from care of infants, neonates, and immunocompromised patients and their environments	Until symptoms resolve	II
Hepatitis A	Restrict from patient contact, contact with patient's environment, and food handling	Until 7 days after onset of jaundice	IB
Hepatitis B			
Personnel with acute or chronic hepatitis B surface antigemia who do not perform exposure-prone procedures	No restriction*; refer to state regulations; standard precautions should always be observed		II

Disease/Problem	Work Restriction	Duration	Category
Personnel with acute or chronic hepatitis B e antigenemia who perform exposure-prone procedures	Do not perform exposure-prone invasive procedures until counsel from an expert review panel has been sought; panel should review and recommend procedures the worker can perform, taking into account specific procedure as well as skill and technique of worker; refer to state regulations	Until hepatitis B e antigen is negative	II
Hepatitis C	No recommendation		Unresolved issue
Herpes simplex Genital	No restriction		II
Hands (herpetic whitlow)	Restrict from patient contact and contact with the patient's environment	Until lesions heal	IA
Orofacial	Evaluate for need to restrict from care of high-risk patients		II
Human immuno-deficiency virus	Do not perform exposure-prone invasive procedures until counsel from an expert review panel has been sought; panel should review and recommend procedures the worker can perform, taking into account specific procedure as well as skill and technique of the worker; standard precautions should always be observed; refer to state regulations		II
Measles Active	Exclude from duty	Until 7 days after the rash appears	IA
Postexposure (susceptible personnel)	Exclude from duty	From 5th day after 1st exposure through 21st day after last exposure and/or 4 days after rash appears	IB
Meningococcal infections	Exclude from duty	Until 24 hours after start of effective therapy	IA
Mumps Active	Exclude from duty	Until 9 days after onset of parotitis	IB
Postexposure (susceptible personnel)	Exclude from duty	From 12th day after 1st exposure through 26th day after last exposure or until 9 days after onset of parotitis	II
Pediculosis	Restrict from patient contact	Until treated and observed to be free of adult and immature lice	IB
Pertussis Active	Exclude from duty	From beginning of catarrhal stage through 3rd wk after onset of paroxysms or until 5 days after start of effective antimicrobial therapy	IB
Postexposure (asymptomatic personnel)	No restriction, prophylaxis recommended		II
Postexposure (symptomatic personnel)	Exclude from duty	Until 5 days after start of effective antimicrobial therapy	IB

Disease/Problem	Work Restriction	Duration	Category
Rubella			
Active	Exclude from duty	Until 5 days after rash appears	IA
Postexposure (susceptible personnel)	Exclude from duty	From 7th day after 1st exposure through 21st day after last exposure	IB
Scabies *Staphylococcus aureau* infection	Restrict from patient contact	Until cleared by medical evaluation	IB
Active, draining skin lesions	Restrict from contact with patients and patient's environment or food handling	Until lesions have resolved	IB
Carrier state	No restriction, unless personnel are epidemiologically linked to transmission of the organism		IB
Streptococcal infection, group A	Restrict from patient care, contact with patient's environment, or food handling	Until 24 hours after adequate treatment started	IB
Tuberculosis			
Active disease	Exclude from duty	Until proved noninfectious	IA
PPD converter	No restriction		IA
Varicella			
Active	Exclude from duty	Until all lesions dry and crust	IA
Postexposure (susceptible personnel)	Exclude from duty	From 10th day after 1st exposure through 21st day (28th day if VZIG given) after last exposure	IA
Zoster			
Localized, in healthy person	Cover lesions; restrict from care of high-risk patients[†]	Until all lesions dry and crust	II
Generalized or localized in immunosuppressed person	Restrict from patient contact	Until all lesions dry and crust	IB
Postexposure (susceptible personnel)	Restrict from patient contact	From 10th day after 1st exposure through 21st day (28th day if VZIG given) after last exposure or, if varicella occurs, until all lesions dry and crust	IA
Viral respiratory infection, acute febrile	Consider excluding from the care of high-risk patients[‡] or contact with their environment during community outbreak of RSV and influenza	Until acute symptoms resolve	IB

*Unless epidemiology linked to transmission of infection.
†Those susceptible to varicella and who are at increased risk of complications of varicella, such as neonates and immunocompromised persons of any age.
‡High-risk patients as defined by the ACIP for complications of influenza.
Category IA: Strongly recommended for all hospitals and strongly supported by well-designed experimental or epidemiologic studies. Category IB: Strongly recommended for all hospitals and reviewed as effective by experts in the field and a consensus of Hospital Infection Control Practices Advisory Committee members on the basis of strong rationale and suggestive evidence, even through definitive scientific studies have not been done. Category II. Suggested for implementation in many hospitals. Recommendations may be supported by suggestive clinical or epidemiologic studies, a strong theoretic rationale, or definitive studies applicable to some but not all hospitals.
Source: Adapted from www.cdc.gov/ncidod/hip/guide.

Recommendations for Infection Control Precautions and Hepatitis B Vaccination and Serologic Surveillance for Dialysis Units

PART I: INFECTION CONTROL PRECAUTIONS FOR DIALYSIS UNITS

Dialysis Unit Precautions

In 1977, CDC published precautions to prevent transmission of HBV in dialysis centers.[1] In 1987, universal precautions were developed to prevent transmission of all bloodborne pathogens, including HBV and HIV, in health care and other settings.[2] In 1996, an updated system of precautions, termed standard precautions, was published to replace universal precautions for the hospital and most health care settings.[3] The infection control measures currently recommended for dialysis units incorporate features of each of these guidelines. These measures are effective against HBV, the most highly transmissible organism in hemodialysis units; therefore, they should also be effective against other viruses (e.g., HCV) and bacteria (e.g., VRE).

Note that dialysis unit precautions are more stringent than universal or standard precautions. For example, standard precautions require the use of gloves only when touching blood, body fluids, secretions, excretions, or contaminated items. In contrast, dialysis unit precautions require glove use whenever patients or hemodialysis equipment is touched. Standard precautions do not restrict the use of supplies, instruments, and medications to a single patient; dialysis unit precautions specify that none of these be shared between any patients.

Since dialysis patients may, known or unknown to the staff, be infected or colonized with a variety of bacteria and viruses, the following precautions should be used during care of *all dialysis patients at all times.*

Assign each patient (1) a dialysis chair or bed and machine; and (2) a supply tray (tourniquet, antiseptics, if possible blood pressure cuff). Avoid sharing these items.

Do not share clamps, scissors, or other nondisposable items unless sterilized or disinfected between patients.

Prepare and distribute medications from a centralized area. Medication carts should not be used. Separate clean and contaminated areas; for example, handling and storage of medications and hand washing should not be done in the same or adjacent area to that where blood samples or used equipment are handled.

Disposable gloves should be worn by staff members for their own protection when handling patients or dialysis equipment and accessories. Gloves should be worn when taking blood pressure, injecting saline or heparin, or touching dialysis machine knobs to adjust flow rates. For the patient's protection, the staff member should use a fresh pair of gloves with each patient to prevent cross-contamination. Gloves should also be used when handling blood specimens. Staff members should wash their hands after each patient contact.

Avoid touching surfaces with gloved hands that will subsequently be touched with ungloved hands before being disinfected.

Staff members may wish to wear protective eyeglasses and masks for procedures in which spurting or spattering of blood may occur, such as cleaning of dialyzers and centrifugation of blood.

Staff members should wear gowns, scrub suits, or the equivalent while working in the unit and should change out of this clothing at the end of each day.

After each dialysis, (1) change linen; (2) clean and disinfect the dialysis bed/chair and nondisposable equipment (especially control knobs and other surfaces touched by gloved hands).

Crowding patients or overtaxing staff may facilitate cross-transmission. Avoid clutter and allocate adequate space to facilitate cleaning and housekeeping.

Staff members should not smoke, eat, or drink in the dialysis treatment area or in the laboratory. There should be a separate lounge for this purpose. However, all patients may be served meals. The glasses, dishes, and other utensils may be cleaned in the usual manner by the hospital staff. No special care of these items is needed.

Hepatitis B Virus (HBV)

Because HBV is so highly transmissible in hemodialysis centers, several precautions in addition to those outlined above have been recommended specifically to deal with this pathogen.

Patients and staff should be vaccinated and screened as per Part II.

HBsAg-positive patients should undergo dialysis in a separate room designated only for HBsAg-positive patients. They should use separate machines, equipment, and supplies, and most importantly, staff members should not care for both HBsAg-positive and susceptible patients on the same shift or at the same time. If a separate room is not possible, they should be separated from HBV susceptible patients in an area removed from the mainstream of activity and should undergo dialysis on dedicated machines. Anti-HBs-positive patients may undergo dialysis in the same area as HBsAg-positive patients, or they may serve as a geo-

graphic buffer between HBsAg-positive and HBV susceptible patients; in either instance they may be cared for by the same staff member. When the use of separate machines is not possible, the machines can be disinfected by using conventional protocols, and the external surfaces can be cleaned or disinfected with soap and water or a detergent germicide.

Although there is no evidence that patients or staff members in centers that reuse dialyzers are at greater risk of acquiring HBV infection, it might be prudent that HBsAg-positive patients not participate in dialyzer reuse programs. HBV can occur in high concentration in blood, and handling dialyzers used on HBsAg-positive patients during the reprocessing procedures might place staff members at risk for HBV infection.

MRSA and VRE

CDC recommends contact precautions for care of hospitalized patients infected or colonized with MRSA, VRE, or certain other antimicrobial-resistant bacteria.[3,4] Dialysis unit precautions as outlined above include many of the measures recommended under contact precautions. However, under contact precautions (but not dialysis unit precautions) a private isolation room and (in certain instances) a separate gown are recommended. These measures were recommended to prevent possible transmission via contaminated environmental surfaces such as counter tops and bed rails. Hospitalized patients spend nearly 24 hours a day in their hospital, whereas dialysis patients spend only 3 to 5 hours three times a week in the dialysis unit. Note that feces are the main reservoir for VRE. The potential for bacterial contamination of environmental surfaces would appear to be much greater in hospitalized patients than in most dialysis outpatients.

Dialysis unit precautions should be used for care of all patients; at present we do not advise additional precautions for most patients with MRSA or VRE. However, additional precautions would be prudent for patients with infective material that cannot be contained (e.g., wound drainage that cannot be contained by dressings and is culture-positive for MRSA or VRE; or a positive stool culture for VRE and fecal incontinence, a colostomy, diarrhea, or poor hygiene). For these patients, if an isolation room is not available, enhanced attention to patient separation and environmental cleaning might be sufficient. Staff should wear a separate gown when caring for such patients.

Dialysis units should reevaluate their compliance with dialysis center precautions and improve precautions for care of all patients where necessary. Another approach would be cohorting—assign patients with known MRSA or VRE to certain dialysis stations at one end of the unit, use dedicated staff to care for them, and ensure that strict precautions are used at these stations.

Prudent Vancomycin Use

Prudent vancomycin use is another important issue discussed in the CDC guideline Recommendations for Preventing the Spread of Vancomycin Resistance.[4] Antibiotic use can be considered in three categories: prophylaxis given to uninfected patients in an attempt to prevent infection; empiric therapy, given to patients with signs and symptoms of infection, pending culture results; and continuing therapy, given after culture results are known.

Prophylaxis with vancomycin should not be given, other than for certain surgical procedures.[4]

Empiric treatment with vancomycin is appropriate, pending culture results, in patients with beta-lactam allergy, or in instances where serious infection with beta-lactam resistant gram-positive bacteria (i.e., MRSA or *Staphylococcus epidermidis,* which are generally beta-lactam resistent) is likely. Knowing the percent of *S aureus* that are methicillin-resistant in your area, and the percent of serious infections due to *S epidermidis,* is important in determining empiric antibiotic coverage.

Continuing treatment depends on culture results. If the patient has allergy to beta-lactam antibiotics, or if beta-lactam resistant bacteria are isolated (with the exception of single blood cultures positive for *S epidermidis*), vancomycin is appropriate. Depending on susceptibility results, alternative antibiotics (e.g., cephalosporins) with dosing intervals greater than or equal to 48 hours, which would allow postdialytic dosing, could be used. A recent study suggests that cefazolin given three times a week provides adequate blood levels.[5]

REFERENCES

1. Centers for Disease Control and Prevention. Control measures for hepatitis in dialysis centers. *Viral Hepatitis Investigations and Control Series.* November 1977.

2. Centers for Disease Control and Prevention. Recommendations for prevention of HIV transmission in health-care settings. *MMWR* 1987;36(No. 2S):3S–18S.

3. Garner JS, the Hospital Infection Control Practices Advisory Committee. Guideline for isolation precautions in hospitals. *Infect Control Hosp Epidemiol* 1996;17:53–80.

4. Centers for Disease Control and Prevention. Recommendations for preventing the spread of vancomycin resistance. *MMWR* 1995;44(No. RR-12):1–13.

5. Fogel MA. Use of cefazolin in place of vancomycin in hemodialysis patients (Abstract A0992) *J Am Soc Nephrol* 1996;7(No. 9):1446.

PART II: RECOMMENDATIONS FOR HEPATITIS B VACCINATION AND SEROLOGIC SURVEILLANCE IN CHRONIC HEMODIALYSIS PATIENTS AND STAFF

The Centers for Disease Control and Prevention (CDC) and the Immunization Practices Advisory Committee (ACIP) have published guidelines for protection against infection with hepatitis B virus.[1] This appendix is meant to collate, summarize, and update, but not replace, sections of these guidelines that deal specifically with hemodialysis patients and staff. If a patient or staff member is exposed to hepatitis B virus, the recommendations of the ACIP should be followed.[2]

Initial Testing for Hepatitis B Virus Markers

Hemodialysis patients and staff should be tested for hepatitis B surface antigen (HBsAg) and antibody to HBsAg (anti-HBs) when they begin dialysis or employment in the center. They are classified as infected if HBsAg-positive; immune if anti-HBs positive (greater than or equal to 10 milli-international units per milliliter [mIU/ml]) on at least two consecutive occasions; or susceptible if HBsAg-negative and anti-HBs negative (less than 10 mIU/ml).

For infection control purposes, testing for antibody to hepatitis B core antigen (anti-HBc) is not necessary. However, if testing is done, individuals who are HBsAg-negative and anti-HBc-positive have had past hepatitis B virus infection and are immune.

Hepatitis B Vaccination

All susceptible patients and staff should receive hepatitis B vaccine (dosage schedules in Table G–1), be tested for anti-HBs one to two months after the final dose of vaccine, and be followed up as outlined below. Vaccination of immune (anti-HBs greater than or equal to 10 mIU/ml on two consecutive occasions) persons is not necessary but also is not harmful.

Screening and Follow-Up

Screening and follow-up depends on the result of anti-HBs testing one to two months after the final dose of vaccine (Table G–2). Unvaccinated immune individuals can be screened and followed up as if they were vaccine responders.

Table G–1 Hepatitis B Vaccine Dosage Schedules

Product/Group	Dose	Schedule
Recombivax HB		
Patients	40 μg (1 ml)*	3 doses at 0, 1, and 6 months
Staff	10 μg (1 ml)	3 doses at 0, 1, and 6 months
Engerix-B		
Patients	40 μg (2 ml)†	4 doses at 0, 1, 2, and 6 months
Staff	20 μg (1 ml)	3 doses at 0, 1, and 6 months or 4 doses at 0, 1, 2, and 12 months

*Special formulation; †Two 1.0-ml doses administered at one site.

Patients, Responders. Patients who are anti-HBs positive (greater than or equal to 10 mIU/ml) after vaccination are responders. They should be tested for anti-HBs each year (Table G–2). If the level of anti-HBs falls below 10 mIU/ml, they should receive a booster dose of hepatitis B vaccine and continue to be tested for anti-HBs each year.

Patients, Nonresponders. Patients who are anti-HBs negative (less than 10 mIU/ml) after vaccination are nonresponders. They may be revaccinated with one or more doses of vaccine and retested for anti-HBs one to two months later. If they are then anti-HBs positive (greater than or equal to 10 mIU/ml), they can be reclassified and treated as responders (see above). If they continue to be nonresponders (anti-HBs less than 10 mIU/ml), they should be considered susceptible to HBV infection and tested for HBsAg every month and anti-HBs every six months (Table G–2).

Staff, Responders. Staff who are anti-HBs positive (greater than or equal to 10 mIU/ml) after vaccination are responders. They do not need any further routine anti-HBs testing (Table G–2). If exposed to blood from a patient known to be HBsAg-positive, such staff members should be tested for anti-HBs: if still anti-HBs positive (greater than or equal to 10 mIU/ml), no further action is required; however, if they have become anti-HBs negative (less than 10 mIU/ml), they should receive a booster dose of vaccine.

Staff, Nonresponders. Staff who are anti-HBs negative (less than 10 mIU/ml) after vaccination are nonresponders. At the center's discretion, they can be revaccinated with one or more doses of vaccine, and retested for anti-HBs one to two months later. If they

Table G–2 Recommendations for Serologic Surveillance for Hepatitis B Virus (HBV) among Patients and Staff of Chronic Hemodialysis Centers

Group/ Screening Test	Vaccination/Serologic Status and Frequency of Screening		
	Vaccine Nonresponder or Susceptible*	Vaccine Responder or Natural Immunity†	Chronic HBV Infection‡
Patients			
HBsAg	Every month	None	Every year
Anti-HBs	Every 6 months	Every year	If HBsAg becomes negative
Staff			
HBsAg	Every 6 months	None	Every year
Anti-HBs	Every 6 months	None	If HBsAg becomes negative

*Anti-HBs <10 mIU/ml; †Anti-HBs ≥10 mIU/ml; ‡HBsAg positive for at least 6 months; or HBsAg positive, anti-HBc positive, IgM anti-HBc negative.

then become anti-HBs positive (greater than or equal to 10 mIU/ml), they should be reclassified and treated as responders (see above). If they are not revaccinated, or are still anti-HBs negative (less than 10 mIU/ml) after vaccination, they continue to be nonresponders. Nonresponders should be considered susceptible to HBV infection and tested for HBsAg and anti-HBs every six months (Table G–1). If they are exposed to the blood of a person known to be HBsAg-positive, they should either receive two doses of hepatitis B immune globulin (HBIG), or receive one dose of HBIG and one dose of hepatitis B vaccine. They may receive similar treatment if exposed to the blood of a person known to be at high risk for hepatitis B.

REFERENCES

1. Moyer LA, Alter MJ, Favero MS. Review of hemodialysis-associated hepatitis B: revised recommendations for serologic screening. *Semin Dial* 1990;3:201–4.

2. Centers for Disease Control. Hepatitis B virus: a comprehensive strategy for eliminating transmission in the United States through universal childhood vaccination. *MMWR* 1991;40(no. RR-13).

Source: Reprinted from J.I. Tokars, E.R. Miller, M.J. Alter and M.J. Arduino, National Surveillance of Dialysis-Associated Diseases in the United States, 1996, Appendix II and Appendix III, National Center for Infectious Diseases, Centers for Disease Control and Prevention.

Maryland Department of Health and Mental Hygiene, Epidemiology and Disease Control Program. Guidelines for the Prevention and Control of Upper and Lower Acute Respiratory Illnesses (including Influenza and Pneumonia) in Long-Term Care Facilities. December 1997.

INTRODUCTION

These guidelines supersede *Guidelines for Influenza and Influenza-like Illness (ILI), 1996* and covers all long-term care facilities (LTCFs) within Maryland except those designated as assisted living centers. These guidelines, however, may be tailored for alternative settings such as assisted living centers. At this time, the Maryland Department of Health and Mental Hygiene does not recognize differences between acuity levels or units within a LTCF.

Each year outbreaks of respiratory illness, including pneumonia, occur in LTCFs such as nursing homes. Because of their underlying health status, residents in LTCFs are at high risk for developing serious complications or dying when they become ill. Historically, specific emphasis has been placed on influenza. In the United States, influenza is associated with an average of 20,000 deaths yearly and an even larger number of hospitalizations. Not only are morbidity and mortality a problem, but because people are in close proximity to one another, once the influenza virus is introduced into the LTCF, it can spread rapidly. During some nursing home outbreaks over half of the residents have been affected. In addition to the burden of influenza, other respiratory viruses that cause the "common cold" and bacterial pathogens causing respiratory illness affect residents and staff of LTCFs each year. Because infection with these agents can compromise an already poor health status of the LTCF resident, control of these agents in the LTCF is also critical.

In order to facilitate the investigation of respiratory disease outbreaks and implementation of control measures, the following guidelines have been established. These guidelines emphasize priorities regarding prevention and control of influenza and pneumococcal disease including pneumonia as follows:

- To prevent pneumococcal disease through immunization
- To prevent outbreaks through influenza immunization and antiviral drug use
- To detect the occurrence of an outbreak early
- To stop transmission of the influenza virus through control measures
- To measure the level of morbidity and mortality
- To identify the etiologic agent, e.g., the strain of influenza virus responsible for the outbreak

These guidelines are divided into seven sections plus attachments:

- Section 1 discusses prevention of influenza and pneumococcal disease.
- Section 2 provides definitions and characteristics of respiratory illnesses.
- Section 3 addresses the use of surveillance to detect cases.
- Section 4 outlines management of single cases.
- Section 5 outlines the management of respiratory illness outbreaks in LTCFs.
- Section 6 covers specimen collection including transport.

- Section 7 reviews data collection and the summary.

SECTION 1. PREVENTION

A. Influenza

Two measures are available in the United States to minimize the impact of influenza: vaccination and use of antiviral drugs. Annual vaccination before the influenza season of high risk persons and employees, volunteers, and family members in contact with those at high risk is the most important way of reducing the impact of influenza. Antiviral drugs, such as amantadine and rimantadine, are effective only against influenza type A infections and are used in both prevention and treatment. Additional information can be found in the annually updated Centers for Disease Control and Prevention (CDC), *Morbidity and Mortality Weekly Report (MMWR), Prevention and Control of Influenza.* An example of the most recent *MMWR* document is *MMWR* 1997; Vol. 46, No. RR-9.

B. Pneumococcal Pneumonia

Pneumococcal vaccine is available to prevent illness due to *Streptococcus pneumoniae*. Pneumococcal pneumonia is a common complication of influenza. Receipt of one dose of pneumococcal vaccine should be documented in the chart of each resident of a LTCF. If the vaccination status is unknown to the facility, vaccinate the resident after obtaining appropriate consent. The *Code of Maryland Regulations* (COMAR 10.06.01.12-1) puts this responsibility upon the physician in attendance for a resident of a LTCF. The physician is responsible for educating the resident or their guardian on the availability of pneumococcal vaccine and administering the vaccine to individuals who have not already been immunized with pneumococcal vaccine or referring the individual to a health care provider who will administer the vaccine. Further information regarding the vaccine can be found in the CDC *MMWR* Recommendations of the Immunization Practices Advisory Committee, *Prevention of Pneumococcal Disease* (most recent version: *MMWR* 1997; Vol. 46, No. RR-8).

Included in these Guidelines is the Vaccine Administration Record form to assist with documentation of vaccines given to LTCF residents and employees (see Exhibit H–1).

SECTION 2. CASE DEFINITIONS, CLINICAL CHARACTERISTICS, AND OUTBREAK DEFINITIONS

A. Case Definitions

A case of acute respiratory disease (ARD) is defined as a person with mild to moderate symptoms of one or more of the following: rhinitis, pharyngitis, laryngitis, bronchitis, and cough. These symptoms are usually caused by a rhinovirus, of which there are more than 100 recognized subtypes. The incubation period is between 12 hours and five days but usually two days. Getting freshly shed virus particles from one person onto the mucous membranes of another is thought to be the most important mode of transmission. Inhaling virus particles by the airborne route is another way to spread rhinoviruses. The duration of illness is normally two to seven days.

A case of acute febrile respiratory disease (ARFD) is defined as a person with one or more respiratory symptoms (rhinitis, pharyngitis, laryngitis, bronchitis, and cough) in the presence of a temperature of 37.8 degrees C (100 degrees F) or greater orally or 38.3 degrees C (101 degrees F) rectally. Acute febrile respiratory diseases are caused by numerous agents including viruses and bacteria. The incubation period is one to 10 days. While influenza is spread via airborne transmission, the chief mode of transmission for noninfluenza agents is contact with infectious secretions either directly or indirectly through contaminated hands or environmental surfaces (bed rails, telephones, etc.). A person infected with one of these agents can shed the agent from a few days prior to symptom onset and throughout the course of active disease.

A case of influence or influenza-like illness (ILI) is defined as a person with a temperature of 37.8 degrees C (100 degrees F) or greater orally or 38.3 degrees C (101 degrees F) rectally *plus* cough during the influenza season (October 1 through May 31). A person with laboratory confirmed influenza is also considered a case even if the person doesn't have all of the above symptoms and fever. The incubation period for influenza is short, usually one to three days. Communicability includes the period immediately prior to clinical onset and throughout the course of active disease.

A case of pneumonia is defined as a person with clinical symptomatology *plus* a new radiograph finding of pneumonia that is not felt to be aspiration pneumo-

Exhibit H–1 Vaccine Administration Record

Patient Name: _____   Birth date: _____/_____/_____

Address: _____   Chart #: _____

_____

_____

"I have been given a copy and have read or have had explained to me the information contained in the Vaccine Information Statement (VIS) or Important Information Statement (IIS) about the disease(s) and the vaccine(s) listed below. I have had a chance to ask questions that were answered to my satisfaction. I believe I understand the benefits and risks of these vaccines and ask that the vaccine(s) listed below be given to me or to the person named above for whom I am authorized to make this request."

	Date Given	Vaccine Manufacturer	Vaccine Lot Number	Site Given	Date of VIS/IIS	Signature and Title of Vaccine Administrator	Name of, and Signature of Person Authorized to Consent
Pneumococcal Vaccine							
Pneumococcal Booster							
Annual Influenza Vaccine							
Flu Season ____-____							
Flu Season ____-____							
Flu Season ____-____							
Flu Season ____-____							
Flu Season ____-____							
Flu Season ____-____							
Flu Season ____-____							
Flu Season ____-____							
Flu Season ____-____							
Flu Season ____-____							
Flu Season ____-____							
Tetanus-Diphtheria Vaccine							
Tetanus-Diphtheria Vaccine							
Tetanus-Diphtheria Vaccine							
Other (_____)							

Facility (Name/Address)

Maryland Department of Health and Mental Hygiene
Epidemiology and Disease Control Program
Center for Immunization

DHMH 4500B (9/97)

nia. For the purposes of these Guidelines, specific emphasis is placed on *Streptococcus pneumoniae* (the "pneumococcus"), respiratory viruses, *Haemophilus influenzae,* aerobic gram-negative bacilli, and *Staphylococcus aureus*. Pneumococcal pneumonia is characterized by fever, chills, cough, and pleuritic pain. The case-fatality rate remains 20 percent to 40 percent among patients with substantial underlying disease. The organism is spread by droplet, direct, or indirect inoculation. Person-to-person transmission is common, but illness among casual contacts and attendants is uncommon. The incubation period may be as short as one to three days. Appropriate antibiotic therapy will render patients noninfectious within one to two days.

B. Outbreak Definitions

An outbreak of acute febrile respiratory disease (AFRD), influenza, or ILI is defined as *three or more* clinically defined cases in a facility within a seven-day period or one laboratory proven case of influenza. Unless indicated by laboratory results, influenza and ILI apply only between October 1 and May 31.

An outbreak of pneumonia is defined as two or more cases of pneumonia in a ward or unit within a seven-day period.

SECTION 3. SURVEILLANCE

Each LTCF should have their designated infection control practitioner (ICP) routinely maintain records on the occurrence of fever and illness in residents and employees. Employees should report respiratory illness (as well as other acute illnesses such as diarrhea) to the appropriate staff person at the LTCF throughout the year. The one-time pneumococcal vaccination and yearly influenza vaccination status of each current resident should also be recorded in the resident's chart and employee information should be recorded in the employee record. This will enable rapid assessment of susceptible individuals in the event of an outbreak.

Influenza and/or ILI should be suspected during the influenza season from October 1 through May 31. When a person who meets the case definition is identified, the case management procedures as described below should be followed unless the fever is known to have another cause.

SECTION 4. SINGLE CASE MANAGEMENT

A stepped-care approach has been developed for case and outbreak management of respiratory illness in LTCFs. This section covers single cases among LTCF residents and employees.

Acute Respiratory Disease

A. Residents

- Observe case for signs/symptoms that suggest need for physician consult.
- Encourage the case to limit contact with other residents and others (if possible) by limiting group activities while ill, washing hands, and using tissues to cover mouth and nose while coughing and sneezing.

B. Employees

- Exclude from direct patient care (if possible) and review vigilance for hand washing and covering the mouth when coughing or sneezing.

Acute Febrile Respiratory Disease, Influenza, or ILI

A. Residents

- Observe case for signs/symptoms that suggest a need for physician consult.
- Restrict the case to his/her room as much as possible (e.g., restrict the case from participating in group activities) until the patient no longer has active symptoms.
- Consider confirmation of the diagnosis with appropriate viral throat culture and/or rapid antigen test, bacterial throat or sputum culture, or consultation with a physician.
- If between October 1 and May 31, suspect influenza or ILI.
- Give antiviral treatment to the case regardless of vaccination status within the first 48 hours of illness when a physician has a high suspicion of an influenza type A diagnosis and when the Maryland Department of Health and Mental Hygiene (DHMH) has determined that influenza type A is in the community.
- Give influenza vaccine to any unvaccinated roommates of a case and to other unvaccinated residents and staff during the influenza season.

- Observe the roommates of a case and others in the facility closely for similar signs and symptoms of influenza-like illness.

B. Employees

When a case of acute febrile respiratory disease, influenza or ILI is recognized in an employee, exclude from the facility or from clinical duties until the employee is no longer symptomatic.

Pneumonia

A. Residents

- Perform diagnostic testing to establish the diagnosis and to determine the cause of pneumonia (e.g., chest radiograph, sputum and/or throat culture).
- Consult with a resident's physician regarding appropriate antibiotic treatment.
- Restrict case to his/her room until completion of first 48 hours of antibiotic therapy if treated with antibiotics.
- Report individual case of pneumonia caused by *Legionella pneumophila* to your local health department.

B. Employees

- Exclude from the facility until completion of first 48 hours of antibiotic therapy if given and until the employee is no longer symptomatic.

SECTION 5. OUTBREAK MANAGEMENT

A. Reporting

Per the *Code of Maryland Regulations* 10.06.01, nursing homes and other LTCFs should report outbreaks of diseases of public health importance including outbreaks as defined in these guidelines. Reporting should be made within 24 hours to a local health department. Please contact your local health department for an emergency telephone number where they can be reached during weekends and after work hours in the event of an outbreak.

(Note: Acute upper respiratory disease outbreaks (i.e., colds) are *not reportable* to the local health department. The LTCF may call the local health department if consultation is needed.)

B. Outbreak Control Measures

Acute Febrile Respiratory Disease, Influenza, or ILI

When an outbreak of febrile respiratory disease, influenza, or ILI is recognized in a LTCF, the control measures for a single case should be instituted immediately on each case.

In addition, the following control measures should be implemented and maintained for the duration of the outbreak. All outbreak control measures can be lifted when no new cases have occurred for three consecutive days.

- Stop new admissions of residents after one case of lab proven influenza or three or more cases of acute febrile respiratory disease or influenza-like illness in a seven-day period; the Health Officer may allow new admissions to an unaffected ward or unit based on the progression of the outbreak.
- Allow readmissions to the facility, preferably to an unaffected ward or unit.
- Institute visitor precautions (e.g., posting a sign to alert visitors that an outbreak is occurring). A ban on visitors is not necessary.
- Assign employees to care for the same group of patients during a shift, to the extent possible.

During the influenza season (October 1 through May 31):

- Offer influenza vaccine to any unvaccinated residents and employees if appropriate.
- Consider antiviral prophylaxis (e.g., amantadine or rimantadine) for ill and well residents (regardless of vaccination status) and unvaccinated employees if influenza type A is present in the community (as determined by positive lab findings or DHMH).

Pneumonia

- During pneumonia outbreaks, in addition to the recommendations made for the management of a single case with pneumonia, follow the recommendations listed above for acute febrile respiratory disease, influenza, and ILI outbreaks.
- Also, follow the attached Recommended Diagnostic Procedures for Pneumonia Outbreaks in Long-Term Case Facilities (see Exhibit H–2).
- Consider using the attached questionnaires: Respiratory Illness Employee Questionnaire (see Ex-

Exhibit H–2 Recommended Diagnostic Procedures for Pneumonia Outbreaks in Long-Term Care Facilities

I. **For patients with respiratory illness:**

A. Bacterial sputum culture—no preservative necessary; make sure that the laboratory includes *Mycoplasma* and *Streptococcus pneumoniae* among the organisms for which they test.

    If sputum is not obtainable, collect a bacterial throat culture—tellurite tube if sent to DHMH; make sure that the laboratory includes *Streptococcus pneumoniae* among the organisms for which they test.

B. Viral throat culture:

Request that the laboratory culture for influenza, parainfluenza, adenovirus, and RSV. Specimens should be refrigerated and transported on wet ice within 72 hours of collection. The swabs must remain refrigerated or on wet ice at all times. The swabs must *not be* frozen.

C. Paired serum specimens for viral antibody titers—(red top tube):

❑ An *acute* specimen should be collected as early as possible after the onset of illness.

❑ A *convalescent* specimen should be collected three weeks later.

Ask the laboratory to hold the acute specimen until the convalescent specimen is submitted. Consult EDCP for specific tests to request.

II. **For patients with suspected or confirmed pneumonia:**

A. Chest X-ray

B. Bacterial sputum culture—no preservative necessary; make sure the laboratory includes *Mycoplasma, Legionella,* and *Streptococcus pneumoniae* among the organisms for which they test.

If sputum is not obtainable, collect the following:

1. a bacterial throat culture—tellurite tube if sent to DHMH; make sure the laboratory includes *Streptococcus pneumoniae* among the organisms for which they test

2. a throat culture for *Mycoplasma*—sucrose phosphate medium if sent to DHMH

C. Viral throat culture—viral throat swab kit.

Request that the laboratory culture for influenza, parainfluenza, adenovirus, and RSV. Specimens should be refrigerated and transported on wet ice within 72 hours of collection. The swabs must remain refrigerated or on wet ice at all times. The swabs must *not be* frozen.

D. Paired serum specimens for viral antibody titers—red top tube:

❑ An *acute* specimen should be collected as early as possible after the onset of illness.

❑ A *convalescent* specimen should be collected three weeks later.

Ask the laboratory to hold the acute specimen until the convalescent specimen is submitted. Consult EDCP for specific tests to request.

E. Blood culture (prior to antimicrobial treatment)—check with lab for collection tube

F. Urine for *Legionella* antigen—sterile container, no preservative necessary

Please note: Specimens may be sent to DHMH (except for blood cultures) or to a private laboratory. The DHMH laboratory is not open Sunday for receipt of specimens. Please plan accordingly. Specimens can be sent to: DHMH Laboratories Administration, 201 West Preston Street, Baltimore, MD 21201.

---

hibit H–3) and Respiratory Illness Resident Questionnaire (see Exhibit H–4).

• If legionellosis is diagnosed, contact your local health department for further recommendations.

SECTION 6. SPECIMEN COLLECTION

If influenza is suspected based on clinical symptoms, laboratory testing will confirm the diagnosis. A case of influenza can be laboratory confirmed by three techniques. Most commonly, a viral throat culture is used to detect influenza; however, influenza infection can be confirmed using serology, as well as a rapid antigen detection method.

A. Viral Throat Culture

A throat culture should be collected on up to 10 to 12 cases within 72 hours of illness onset (a viral throat swab kit should be used if submitting samples to the DHMH Laboratory). The following steps, from the *Procedures for Collection and Transport of Viral Throat Specimens* (from DHMH Guidelines, January 1996), should be followed closely when preparing to submit viral throat swabs for laboratory culture:

1. Obtain viral throat swab kits from DHMH Laboratories Administration, Specimen Mailing Assemblies (Outfit Room) at 410-767-6120 or your local health department.

Exhibit H–3 Respiratory Illness Employee Questionnaire

Please fill out this questionnaire as completely as possible, including negative answers where relevant.

Name of facility: _____

County: _____

Employee name: _____ Sex: _____ Age: _____

Job description: _____

_____

Work areas: _____

Have you had a flu vaccine this season?   yes ❏   no ❏

Have you had any symptoms of respiratory illness since _____?   yes ❏   no ❏   If yes,

　　　Date of onset: _____ Duration of symptoms: _____

　　　Did you miss work because of these symptoms?   yes ❏   no ❏   Dates: _____

Signs and symptoms:

Fever:	yes ❏ no ❏	GI symptoms:	yes ❏ no ❏
Highest temp. _____		(specify) _____	
Chills:	yes ❏ no ❏	Chest congestion:	yes ❏ no ❏
Headache:	yes ❏ no ❏	Sore throat:	yes ❏ no ❏
Muscle aches:	yes ❏ no ❏	SOB:	yes ❏ no ❏
Cough:	yes ❏ no ❏	Nasal congestion:	yes ❏ no ❏
Wheezing:	yes ❏ no ❏	Other:_____	

　　Did you consult a physician for these symptoms?   yes ❏   no ❏   If yes,

　　What was the physician's diagnosis? _____

　　What was the prescribed treatment? _____

　　Did you follow the prescribed treatment?   yes ❏   no ❏   If no,

　　what treatment did you follow? _____

Today's date: _____

Thank you for your cooperation.

2. Complete the accompanying Virus Throat Swab form (DHMH-72) including clinical diagnosis. Note "influenza" if influenza is suspected as the clinical diagnosis.
3. Open sterile cotton-tipped swabs. Hold two swabs together and swab the posterior pharynx and tonsillar areas vigorously with swabs.
4. Immerse swab-tips in media and break off the top portion of the wooden swab to allow the swabs to fit into the tube.
5. Refrigerate specimen immediately after collection unless transporting immediately. Alternatively, the specimen can be frozen at −70 degrees C; this requires a specialized freezer. Do not freeze in a regular freezer (−15 degrees C).
6. Refrigerated specimens should be transported on wet ice or cold packs to DHMH Virology Laboratory, 201 W. Preston Street, Baltimore, MD 21201. "Wet ice" is a mixture of ice with a small amount of water. Specimens should be placed into the water

Exhibit H–4 Respiratory Illness Resident Questionnaire for Pneumonia Outbreaks in Long Term Care Facilities

Name of facility: _____   Outbreak number: _____

Form completed by: _____   Date: _____

Demographics:

Name:	Sex:	Age:	DOB:
Wing and floor:	Room:	Admitted to facility:	

Vaccination history:

Influenza vaccine:	yes ❑ no ❑ refused ❑	Date:
Pneumococcal vaccine:	yes ❑ no ❑ refused ❑	Date:

Signs and symptoms:

Ill:	yes ❑ no ❑	Date of onset:		Duration:	
Fever:	yes ❑ no ❑	Cough:	yes ❑ no ❑	SOB:	yes ❑ no ❑
highest temp: _____		Nasal congestion:	yes ❑ no ❑	GI symptoms:	yes ❑ no ❑
Chills:	yes ❑ no ❑	Chest congestion:	yes ❑ no ❑	(specify) _____	
Myalgias:	yes ❑ no ❑	Sore throat:	yes ❑ no ❑	Other:	yes ❑ no ❑
Headache:	yes ❑ no ❑	Wheezing:	yes ❑ no ❑	_____	

Diagnosis and outcome:

Diagnosis: Pneumonia	yes ❑ no ❑	Causative agent:	Physician(s) name & number:
ILI	yes ❑ no ❑		_____
URI	yes ❑ no ❑		_____
Other:_____			
Hospitalized:	yes ❑ no ❑	Dates:	Hospital name:
Died:	yes ❑ no ❑	Date:	Cause of death:

Diagnostics:

Chest X-ray:	yes ❑ no ❑	Date:	Result:
Viral throat culture:	yes ❑ no ❑	Date:	Result:
Bacterial throat culture:	yes ❑ no ❑	Date:	Result:
Blood culture:	yes ❑ no ❑	Date:	Result:
Mycoplasma throat culture: *Mycoplasma* sputum culture:	yes ❑ no ❑ yes ❑ no ❑	Date:	Result:
Legionella sputum culture:	yes ❑ no ❑	Date:	Result:
Legionella antigen (urine):	yes ❑ no ❑	Date:	Result:

continues

Exhibit H–4 continued

Diagnostics: (continued)

Acute serum:	yes ❏ no ❏	Date:	Result:
Convalescent serum:	yes ❏ no ❏	Date:	Result:
Other:		Date:	Result:

If *S pneumoniae* isolated:

Penicillin sensitive: yes ❏ no ❏	*S. pneumoniae* type: _____	Isolate available: yes ❏ no ❏

Treatment: Antibiotic   Dosage   Dates

Other treatment: _____

Risk Factors: underlying illnesses, medications, etc.

_____

_____

_____

Comments:

_____

_____

_____

_____

_____

_____

_____

_____

_____

Exhibit H–5 Line-Listing for Respiratory Illness Outbreaks

Name of Facility: _____

Contact Person: _____

List for Residents ____ Employees ____ (check one)

Address: _____

Telephone: _____

NAME	Age (Optional)	Sex (Optional)	Room No. or Shift* & Unit*	Date of Onset	Shift of Onset	Duration of Illness	Signs and Symptoms								X-ray Results (if taken)	Influenza Vaccine this Season Y/N	Hospitalized Y/N	Death (Date)	Laboratory Results (if applicable)						Amantadine/Rimantadine (Date)	Pneumococcal Vaccine
							Fever (Record highest temp.)	Cough	Sore Throat	Runny Nose	Congestion—Nasal	Congestion—Chest	Muscle Aches	Vomiting or Diarrhea	Pneumonia					Viral Throat Culture (Date)	Bacterial Throat Culture (Date)	Rapid Antigen Detection	Serology—acute (Date)	Serology—convalescent (date)		

*List shift and unit (or ward) for employee cases

Exhibit H–6 Respiratory Illnesses in Long-Term Care Facilities: Outbreak Summary for Long-Term Care Facilities

DHMH Outbreak # _____
(Obtain from DHMH Division of Outbreak
Investigation @ 410-767-6677)

Name of facility: _____ County: _____

Person completing this form: _____ Agency: _____

RESIDENTS

No. Cases of Influenza/ILI _____ Total No. Residents in Facility _____

No. Cases of ARD _____ No. Case Hospitalizations _____

No. Cases of AFRD _____ Onset of First Case _____/_____/_____

No. Cases of Death _____ Onset of Last Case _____/_____/_____

EMPLOYEES

No. Cases of Influenza/ILI _____ Total No. Employees in Facility _____

No. Cases of ARD _____ No. Case Hospitalizations _____

No. Cases of AFRD _____ Onset of First Case _____/_____/_____

No. Cases of Death _____ Onset of Last Case _____/_____/_____

LABORATORY SPECIMENS

Type and number of lab specimens submitted:

Type of Lab Specimen/Procedure	Number Submitted	Results
Viral Throat Culture		
Rapid Antigen Test		
Acute Serology		
Convalescent Serology		
Other (specify:_____)		

Total number of laboratory confirmed cases: _____

Confirmed by:

Culture alone: _____

Rapid antigen test alone: _____

Serology alone: _____

Culture and rapid antigen test: _____

Culture and serology: _____

Serology and rapid antigen test: _____

Culture, serology, and rapid antigen test: _____

Causative Agent (if known): _____

portion of the wet ice. Specimens frozen at –70 degrees C should be shipped on dry ice.

Failure to follow the above procedures will render the specimens unsatisfactory and they will not be processed by the DHMH laboratory.

B. Rapid Antigen Detection

Techniques have been developed to allow the rapid detection of influenza type A antigen in as little as 15 minutes. These techniques vary greatly and include several different detection systems, such as the immunofluorescence assay (IFA) and the enzyme immunoassay (EIA). In addition, these systems are available as commercially sold kits. When compared to viral cultures, which are thought to be the "gold standard" for influenza detection, these rapid testing methods were able to detect from 87 to 99 percent of all positive influenza cases.

As with many laboratory tests, there is always a potential for a false-positive and false-negative results. However, use of rapid detection methods in conjunction with a viral throat culture should minimize false-positive results. In addition, use of both methods allows a more efficient administration of antiviral medications and infection control measures, while also permitting the identification and typing of circulating strains of influenza virus.

Decision regarding the choice of rapid detection method should be made in conjunction with the clinical laboratory used by the LTCF. Cost, technical support, and resources available for testing may all factor into the choice of rapid influenza detection methods.

DHMH will perform a rapid antigen detection test for influenza A on any viral throat kit specimen submitted for influenza detection between October 1 and April 30.

C. Serology

Serological specimens do not need to be routinely collected. If serological specimens are recommended by DHMH then two blood specimens (acute and convalescent) are needed to demonstrate a significant rise in anti-influenza antibody titer. The first specimen should be collected as early as possible after onset of

illness, and the second specimen three weeks later. In either instance, obtain 5 to 8 ml of blood in a *red top tube*. Do not freeze whole blood since this will result in complete hemolysis and renders the specimen unsatisfactory for testing. Serum or clotted blood specimens may be transported unrefrigerated to the laboratory.

SECTION 7. DATA COLLECTION AND SUMMARY

Pertinent information regarding each resident and employee case should be entered into the LTCF Infection Control Professional's surveillance log and up-

---

Exhibit H–7 Flow Chart for the Management of Respiratory Illness Outbreaks in Long-Term Care Facilities

Prevention Program: Influenza and Pneumococcal Vaccines and Antiviral Prophylaxis

⇓

Establish and Maintain Surveillance

⇓

Case Identification

⇓

Case Management

- restrict to room
- treat with antiviral drugs or antibiotics if appropriate
- vaccinate any unvaccinated roommate if appropriate
- observe others for symptoms
- report all cases of reportable disease to local health department (e.g., legionellosis)

⇓

Continue Surveillance

⇓

Outbreak Identified

⇓

Continue Surveillance and Place Cases on a "Line List"

- report outbreak
- implement control measures
- collect specimens
- maintain "line list"
- give outbreak information to LHD contact who will complete outbreak summary

dated daily. Once an outbreak has been identified, cases should be placed on a "line list" (see Exhibit H–5). A summary sheet should be filled out by the local health department at the conclusion of an outbreak and a copy should be forwarded to the Division of Outbreak Investigation (see Exhibit H–6). For each respiratory illness outbreak, indicate the number of residents and employees meeting case definitions for influenza, ILI, ARD, AFRD, *and* pneumonia.

Exhibit H–7 is a flow chart that outlines the recognition and management of respiratory illness outbreaks in long-term care facilities.

Courtesy of the Maryland Department of Health and Mental Hygiene, Baltimore, Maryland.

Maryland Department of Health and Mental Hygiene, Epidemiology and Disease Control Program. Guidelines for the Epidemiological Investigation of Gastroenteritis Outbreaks in Long-Term Care Facilities. November 1996.

INTRODUCTION

Outbreaks of gastroenteritis occur in nursing homes and other long-term care facilities (LTCFs) each year, most commonly in the winter. Risk factors in these settings include the close proximity of ill residents and staff in close living quarters and the decreased personal hygiene among some residents due to incontinence, immobility, or reduced alertness.

Viruses, such as Norwalk-like agents, are the most common agents causing nursing home outbreaks of gastroenteritis. Viral gastroenteritis is a self-limiting intestinal illness with symptoms of diarrhea and/or vomiting. Additional symptoms may include nausea, abdominal pain, headache, muscle aches, and low grade fever. The incubation period is 24 to 48 hours, and gastrointestinal symptoms usually last 24 to 48 hours. The virus is passed from person to person through the fecal-oral route (fecal matter to mouth); contaminated food and water have also been implicated as vehicles for transmission in outbreaks. Additional information can be found in the reference: Centers for Disease Control and Prevention (CDC), *Morbidity and Mortality Weekly Report (MMWR), Viral agents of gastroenteritis: public health importance and outbreak management.* 1990;39(RR-5).

For LTCF residents, gastroenteritis is important because it can lead to more serious illnesses and complications, such as dehydration, debilitation, hospitalization, and death. The symptoms, course, treatment, and control measures for gastroenteritis outbreaks in an LTCF will vary depending on whether the agent is probably viral or bacterial (such as *Salmonella* or *Shigella*).

In order to facilitate investigations of gastroenteritis outbreaks and implementation of control measures, the following guidelines have been established. These guidelines are divided into four sections:

- Section 1 provides a working case definition and an outbreak definition.
- Section 2 addresses the use of surveillance to detect cases.
- Section 3 outlines the management of an individual case of gastroenteritis.
- Section 4 outlines management of an outbreak.

SECTION 1. DEFINITIONS

A. Case Definition

A case of gastroenteritis is defined as a person with diarrhea or vomiting. Diarrhea is defined as two or more loose stools per day or an unexplained increase in the number of bowel movements.

B. Outbreak Definition

An outbreak of gastroenteritis is defined as three or more residents from a single ward or unit, or 3 percent or more of the entire facility, who develop diarrhea and/or vomiting within a seven-day period.

SECTION 2. SURVEILLANCE

Each LTCF should have its designated infection control practitioner (ICP) routinely maintain records on the occurrence of diarrhea and vomiting among all residents and staff. When a person meeting the case definition is identified, the case management procedures described below should be followed. Any employee with gastrointestinal illness should be instructed to report it to Employee Health or the ICP.

SECTION 3. SINGLE CASE MANAGEMENT

Each time a case of gastroenteritis is recognized in a resident or employee, the following measures should be implemented:

A. Residents

- Restrict the case to his/her room and restrict from participating in group activities for two days after the last episode of diarrhea or vomiting.
- Wear gloves. Direct patient care providers should wear disposable gloves when handling feces or fecally soiled articles or equipment (e.g., cleaning or changing an incontinent patient, cleaning feces from a bed or bedpan, etc.).
- Wash hands. Employees and residents must *wash their hands* carefully after contact with any feces or fecally soiled material. Employees should wash their hands after removing gloves.
- Dispose of feces or fecally soiled material in the sanitary sewer (toilet), or place in plastic bags for disposal as special medical waste.
- Clean environmental surfaces (toilets, bedpans, fecally soiled beds, etc.) with cleaning products and procedures normally used by the facility.
- Practice infection control precautions. Each LTCF should practice the Standard Precautions recommended by the CDC Hospital Infection Control Practices Advisory Committee at all times, regardless of the presence of an outbreak.

B. Employees

When a case of gastroenteritis is recognized in an employee, reassign the employee to non-patient care and non-food handling duties or exclude until two days after the resolution of diarrhea and/or vomiting. If sal-

monellosis or shigellosis is diagnosed, additional control measures may be recommended by the local health officer.

SECTION 4. OUTBREAK MANAGEMENT

A. Reporting

Code of Maryland Regulations 10.06.01.03 and 10.06.01.04 require LTCFs to report gastroenteritis outbreaks to the local health department within 24 hours. In the event of an outbreak on a weekend or holiday, please contact your local health department for the telephone number used to contact them at those times.

B. Outbreak Control Measures

Control measures for an outbreak of gastroenteritis should focus on stopping person-to-person spread and on removing any ongoing common sources of infection (ill food handler, ill patient care provider, or contaminated food or drink). When an outbreak is identified, the LTCF should institute the following control measures:

- Follow the recommendations for management of individual cases (Section 3, above).
- Assign employees to care for the same group of patients during a shift if possible.
- Stop new admissions; readmissions to the facility are allowed, preferably to an unaffected ward.
- Exclude symptomatic employees from direct patient care and food handling until two days after the resolution of diarrhea and/or vomiting.
- Restrict ill residents from group activities, including group dining, until two days after the resolution of diarrhea or vomiting.
- Institute visitor precautions (e.g., post a sign to alert visitors that an outbreak is occurring and that hand washing is recommended). A visitor ban is not necessary.
- Wear masks when cleaning areas grossly contaminated by feces or vomitus (since spattering or aerosols of infectious material of viral gastroenteritis may be involved in disease transmission).
- Handle soiled linen and clothes as little as possible; transport laundry in an enclosed and sanitary manner.

Unless otherwise indicated, all control measures for presumed viral gastroenteritis can be lifted when there are no new cases for four days after onset of the last case.

C. Specimen Collection

In all outbreaks of gastroenteritis, specimen collection for bacterial enteric pathogens should be done to rule out *Salmonella* and *Shigella* as causative agents. Stool specimens of no more than 10 to 12 residents should be collected. Process specimens through a commercial laboratory following their instructions, or use an enteric pathogen kit if sending the specimen to the DHMH laboratory. This kit is a jar containing buffered glycerol saline solution. Transport at room temperature to the DHMH laboratory.

If the outbreak is caused by *Salmonella* or *Shigella,* the epidemiologic and laboratory investigation will be different from an outbreak presumed to be caused by a virus. In outbreaks of salmonellosis or shigellosis, additional specimens and questionnaires from food handlers and patient care providers, as well as additional information on residents (e.g., food history) may be needed. The *Code of Maryland Regulations* also applies (COMAR 10.06.01.16 and .20).

Specimen collection for viral studies is not routinely indicated, as diagnostic capabilities are not readily available. There should be communication with the local health department and the DHMH Epidemiology and Disease Control Program prior to planning viral studies. When needed, viral studies of stool samples are coordinated with the Centers for Disease Control and Prevention (CDC), and it is the CDC who performs laboratory screening for Norwalk and Norwalk-like viruses. As a result, the CDC has provided guidelines for the submission of stool samples for viral studies (see Exhibit I–1). In addition to stool samples, the CDC requires paired serology. Serum samples should be collected in *red top tubes,* while stool samples should be submitted in a sterile stool jar. DHMH can provide stool collection kits, including stool jars, upon request. All samples should be delivered to the DHMH laboratory for processing and forwarding to the CDC.

Exhibit I–1 Guidelines for Collecting Specimens for Viral Diagnosis

STOOL

- **Collection in the first 48 hours.** Presently, viral diagnosis of a stool sample can be made only when the level of excretion is approximately 1 million particles/ml. For many viruses, this level of excretion is present only during the first two days of illness, and occasionally during the third. If specimens are not collected during the first two to three days of illness, an agent is unlikely to be detected. Thus, appropriate specimens should be collected as soon as an outbreak occurs. **Specimen collection should not await the results of epidemiologic and other investigations, since delay will almost certainly preclude a viral diagnosis.** If information gathered subsequently indicates that a viral etiology is unlikely, the specimens can be discarded before the cost of testing is incurred.

- **Ten diarrheal bulk specimens.** Bulk samples (enough to fill a large stool cup) are preferred, and only those specimens loose enough to assume the shape of their containers are likely to yield positive results. Serial specimens from persons with acute, frequent, high-volume diarrhea are particularly useful. The smaller the specimen and the more formed the stool, the lower the diagnostic yield. Rectal swabs are of little or no value. Specimens from at least 10 ill persons should be collected to maximize the chance that a diagnosis can be made. (The diagnostic yield is low when specimens from less than 10 persons are submitted.)

- **Storage at +4 degrees C.** Because freezing may destroy the characteristic viral morphology that permits a diagnosis by electron microscopy, specimens should be kept at +4 degrees C.

PAIRED SERUM SPECIMENS (essential for diagnosis)

- **Timing—** Acute: during the first week of symptoms
  Convalescent: third to sixth week
- **Number—** 10 pairs from ill person (the same persons submitting stool specimens)
  10 pairs from well persons
- **Quantity—** Adults: 10 ml; Children: 3 ml.
- **Storage—** Tubes containing no anticoagulant (tubes with red tops) should be used for collection. Sera should be spun off and frozen. If a centrifuge is not available, a clot should be allowed to form, and the serum should be decanted and frozen. If this step cannot be taken, the whole blood should be refrigerated, not frozen.

OTHER SPECIMENS

Viruses causing gastroenteritis cannot normally be detected in vomitus, water, food, or environmental samples. Although British researchers report electron microscope detection of virus in shellfish, no successful effort has yet been reported in the United States.

Source: Reprinted from *MMWR* 1990, 39(RR-5), Centers for Disease Control and Prevention.

Exhibit I–2 Line-Listing for Gastroenteritis Outbreaks

List for Residents _____ Employees _____ (check one)

Name: _____

Contact Person: _____

Address: _____

Telephone: _____

NAME	Age (Optional)	Sex (Optional)	Room Number	Onset and Timing of Diarrhea or Vomiting — Date of Onset	Time of Onset	Shift of Onset	Date/Time of Last Episode	Duration of Illness	Signs and Symptoms — Diarrhea	Vomiting	Abdominal Cramps	Nausea	Fever (highest temp.)	Blood in stool	Muscle ache	Headache	Chills	Hospitalized (Y/N)	Admission Date to Hospital	Discharge Date from Hospital	Death (Date)	Laboratory Results (if applicable) — Bacterial Stool Culture (Date)	Viral Stool Culture (Date)	Serology—acute (Date)	Serology—convalescent (date)

Exhibit I–3 Gastroenteritis Outbreak Summary

DHMH Outbreak # _____

Facility name: _____ County: _____

Residents

No. Cases	_____	Total No. Residents in Facility	_____
No. Cases Death	_____	No. Case Hospitalizations	_____
Onset of First Case	____/____/____	Onset of Last Case	____/____/____

Employees

No. Cases	_____	Total No. Employees in Facility	_____
No. Cases Death	_____	No. Case Hospitalizations	_____
Onset of First Case	____/____/____	Onset of Last Case	____/____/____

Laboratory Specimens

Type and number of lab specimens submitted:

Type of Lab Specimen	Number Submitted	Results
Bacterial Stool Sample		
Viral Stool Sample		
Acute Serology		
Convalescent Serology		
Other (specify:_____)		

Total number of laboratory confirmed cases: _____

  Confirmed by:

  Bacterial stool culture alone: _____

  Viral stool culture alone: _____

  Serology alone: _____

  Viral stool culture and serology: _____

Causative Agent (if known): _____

Exhibit I–4 Gastroenteritis Surveillance Form (for Employees)

**Name of Facility, Date: _____

Name: _____ Age: _____ Sex: _____

Address: _____

_____ Phone: _____

Type of Work: _____

Wing/Floor of Work: _____

Working Hours: _____

Do you work in any other facilities? _____ If yes, where: _____

_____

**Have you developed diarrhea and/or vomiting since _____ ? (Date)

_____ Yes _____ No   If yes, what date did the diarrhea and/or vomiting start? _____

Please check if you have or had any of these symptoms:

	Yes	No	
Diarrhea	_____	_____	
Vomiting	_____	_____	
Abdominal Cramps	_____	_____	
Nausea	_____	_____	
Fever	_____	_____	How high? _____
Blood in Stools	_____	_____	
Headache	_____	_____	
Chills	_____	_____	
Muscle ache	_____	_____	
Other	_____		

How long did your diarrhea and/or vomiting last? _____ days

Were you seen by a physician for the above symptoms?   Yes _____   No _____

If yes, by: Name: _____ Phone: _____

Did you take any medicine?   Yes _____   No _____   If yes, list: _____

Were you hospitalized for this problem?   Yes _____   No _____

If seen by a physician or hospitalized, was a stool culture taken?   Yes _____   No _____

**Note: Complete Name of Facility and Dates prior to distributing this form.

D. Data Collection and Summary Report

Data Collection

Pertinent information regarding each resident and employee case should be entered into the ICP's surveillance log. This log should be updated daily. Once an outbreak has been identified, cases should be placed on a line list (see Exhibit I–2).

Epidemic Curve

Plot an epidemic curve (epi curve) of the resident and employee cases (a graph of the number of cases by date of onset). The epi curve is a useful tool to track the progress of the outbreak and is helpful in determining whether a common foodborne source was present.

Summary Report

At the conclusion of the outbreak, the health department investigator and the involved facility should work together to complete a summary report. A copy should be submitted to DHMH. The report may be narrative in format or Exhibit I–3 may be completed instead of the narrative report. Regardless of which report format is chosen, please include the epi curve with the report.

E. Local Health Department Responsibilities

The local health department should act primarily as supervisors of the above operations, working in conjunction with the LTCF to ensure that indicated infection control and outbreak management procedures have been properly carried out, and that the appropriate data are collected.

Once notified of a gastroenteritis outbreak the local health department should take the following steps:

- Verify the existence of an outbreak of gastroenteritis by reviewing facility records.
- Notify DHMH (410-767-6677) of the outbreak.
- Verify that outbreak control measures have been properly implemented and residents with diarrhea have been cultured to rule out *Salmonella* and *Shigella*.
- Inspect the facility to assess:
  - General cleanliness
  - Availability of soap, towels, running water in rest rooms and in all patient care areas
  - Food preparation areas and food handling procedures when foodborne transmission is suspected
- Arrange for the collection of data on resident and employee cases as indicated in the line list (see Exhibit I–2).

When additional employee information is desired, Exhibit I–4 is a standardized questionnaire for investigation of gastrointestinal illness. It can be administered to all or only symptomatic employees at the facility, depending on investigation needs. The questionnaire may be modified as appropriate to the outbreak and facility, duplicated, and distributed as needed.

If the local health department or the LTCF distributes the questionnaire, be sure to fill in the LTCF name (on line 1 on the questionnaire) and the appropriate date for assessing symptoms (on line 10) before duplication.

Maryland Department of Health and Mental Hygiene, Epidemiology and Disease Control Program. Guidelines for Control of Scabies in Long-Term Care Facilities. September 1996.

INTRODUCTION

Scabies is a contagious parasitic infestation of the skin caused by the mite, *Sarcoptes scabiei* var *hominis*. Although not a reportable disease, scabies outbreaks reported from long-term care facilities (LTCFs) have increased in recent years. In Maryland, 61 scabies outbreaks were reported from 1986 to 1995, of which 57 percent (35/61) occurred in nursing homes. Both caregivers and residents of LTCFs are at increased risk of exposure to scabies. The increased risk is attributed to several circumstances of providing and receiving care in a LTCF.

Scabies in residents of LTCF may often be atypical in appearance and symptoms, causing a delay in diagnosis as well as heavy infestation. An additional factor contributing to the increased risk of exposure is the opportunity for direct skin contact between staff and residents or residents and other residents. Such contact is increased with LTCF residents who often require assistance with dressing or positioning as well as other nursing care. Further opportunities for transmission can occur through rotation of asymptomatic staff members to various units within the LTCF. Finally, environmental exposure to scabies can occur if residents mistakenly occupy another infested resident's bed.

DEFINITIONS

outbreak—an outbreak of scabies should be reported when an LTCF experiences two or more *concurrent* cases of scabies affecting residents and/or staff members. Two or more *consecutive* cases of scabies occurring within four to six weeks of each other should also be considered to be an outbreak.

case—a *confirmed case* of scabies is defined as a person who has a skin scraping with identified mites, mite eggs, or mite feces. A *probable case* of scabies is a person with clinical symptoms of a persistent pruritic rash.

contact—a contact is defined as anyone with whom a case has had skin-to-skin contact (e.g., staff member, physical therapy, phlebotomist, family member who is a regular visitor, or other residents with whom the case has had direct skin contact). Sexual partners and roommates are also contacts.

Incubation period: the time between contact with the mite and the appearance of the symptoms of the pruritic rash varies. If the individual has never had a previous infestation, the onset of symptoms occurs two to six weeks following the initial infestation by the mite. If the individual has had a prior infestation, symptoms can occur one to four days following mite infestation.

Period of communicability: the infested individual may be asymptomatic yet able to transmit the mite to others. After infestation occurs, the mite deposits eggs under the skin of the human host. After larvae hatch from the eggs, they travel to the surface of the skin. Transmission can occur as early as two weeks after the original infestation of the individual. A person is considered to be no longer communicable 24 hours after start of effective therapy.

Diagnosis of scabies: typical scabies lesions consist of papules, vesicles, or linear burrows containing the pinpoint mite; however, these may not be present on an elderly or immunocompromised infested person. Erythematous papules, excoriations, or occasionally vesicles are often located between the fingers, on the upper back, wrists, elbows, thighs, breasts, or genitalia. The lesions may also appear as eczematous plaques, pustules, or nodules located in skin folds under the breasts, around the naval, axillae, buttocks, scrotum, or at the belt line on the abdomen. Infested individuals usually complain of severe nighttime itching. The itching is often worse following a hot shower or bath. The location of scabies lesions also differs in the elderly or immunocompromised.

Residents and staff should have a skin examination by inspection. New residents or those accepted in transfer from another care facility should be examined on the first day of arrival. If a resident is undergoing treatment for scabies but requires transfer to another care facility, the accepting facility must be notified of the current diagnosis of scabies in this resident prior to transfer.

Residents of LTCF are at risk for hyperinfestation with the scabies mite. Crusted scabies, known as Norwegian scabies, is extremely contagious. If even a single resident has crusted scabies, the LTCF faces a significant risk of a scabies outbreak. Lesions resemble psoriasis with heavy crusting and scaling. Fingernails and toenails often appear discolored and thickened. Individuals diagnosed with Norwegian scabies may have one of the following characteristics: a history of treatment with steroids, an impaired ability to scratch caused by neurological or psychological illness, or an otherwise impaired immune response secondary to age or illness.

Confirmation of diagnosis: suspicious lesions should be scraped with a sterile needle or scalpel blade. Health care personnel can be trained to perform skin scrapings according to the following procedure:

1. Choose lesions without significant excoriation. A magnifying glass may be used to locate burrows. When a possible burrow is detected, mark with a wide felt tip pen. Apply an alcohol pad to remove the surface ink. If a burrow is present, the ink will remain within the burrow. The burrow will then appear as a dark, irregular line.
2. Apply sterile mineral oil to the surface of the lesion to be sampled.
3. With a glass slide held at a 90-degree angle to the surface of the lesion, scrape the lesion. Collect the scraping on the glass slide. Scrapings from several lesions may be collected onto a single glass slide.
4. Place a coverslip over the scrapings and examine with a microscope under low power. The pres-

ence of a mite, eggs of a mite, or mite fecal material confirms the diagnosis of scabies.

Treatment: The recommended treatment for scabies is 5 percent permethrin cream. Application of this cream to the skin of an infested resident should be supervised by the staff of the LTCF. Usually the cream is best applied prior to bedtime. The cream must cover all skin areas from the neck down. In the case of an incontinent resident, the LTCF staff must ensure that any cream that is removed during bouts of incontinence is promptly replaced. Following 8 to 14 hours of skin contact, the cream should be removed by shower or bath. Treatment may need to be repeated in seven days if there is evidence of persistant or recurrent lesions. An infested individual should be considered contagious until 24 hours after start of effective treatment. Itching often persists in spite of treatment and may require additional therapy for symptomatic relief.

Alternative treatments are occasionally prescribed. These may include 1 percent lindane cream or lotion, 6 percent precipitated sulfur in petroleum, or 10 percent crotamiton cream or lotion.

Environmental control measures: while scabies is readily transmissible with skin-to-skin contact, the mite can only survive in the environment for 48 hours without a human host. The bedding and clothing of an infested individual may contain viable mites, but exposure to a human host must occur within a short period of time for transmission to occur. In general, vacuuming and general cleanliness should provide adequate environmental control. Fumigation is not necessary; furniture should not be discarded.

Clothing or bedding that were used by an infested individual during the seven days before effective treatment should be laundered and dried with the hot cycle or dry cleaned. Items that cannot be laundered or dry cleaned should be placed in a plastic bag and sealed for seven days to allow time for mites and eggs to die.

Cohort measures: During an identified scabies outbreak, staff members who have been providing care to an identified case should not be rotated to other resident care units until 24 hours after completion of the staff member's scabicidal treatment. The case should also be isolated from other residents for 24 hours. Treatment of cases and contacts in a coordinated manner according to the attached protocol will minimize the inconvenience of these cohort measures.

PROTOCOL FOR ASSESSMENT AND CONTROL OF SCABIES OUTBREAKS IN LONG-TERM CARE FACILITIES

The following protocol provides guidance for surveillance, diagnosis, and treatment of cases and contacts in LTCFs and management of outbreaks.

General Actions

1. Make a line-list of all cases and contacts. Include roommates, staff members (permanent and rotating), providing care, and regular visitors as contacts (see Exhibit J–1).
2. Confirm the diagnosis when possible; refer to a dermatologist or physician for diagnostic evaluation.
3. Institute mass education regarding scabies outbreaks. Educate staff; consider community meetings for residents and family members, printed fact sheets (see Exhibit J–2) and newsletters to families of staff and residents.
4. Educate staff and residents (if possible) on:
   a. Mode of transmission
   b. Communicability
   c. Potential for widespread epidemic if prompt action not begun
   d. Need for prophylactic treatment of even asymptomatic contacts
   e. Need for coordinated timing of treatment
   f. Proper application of treatment medication
   g. Environmental control measures: Laundry, dry cleaning, or isolation of clothing in plastic bags for seven days
5. Categorize cases and contacts for treatment assignment as shown below.

Management

Group I: Confirmed or Suspected Scabies and Contacts

1. Action:
   a. Isolate case (Contact precautions) for 24 hours after start of effective therapy.
   b. Perform environmental control measures: laundry, dry cleaning, or isolation of clothing in plastic bags for seven days.

c. Exclude case from work (or school, day care center, if applicable) until the day after treatment.
   d. Do not transfer patient without notifying the accepting facility of the diagnosis of scabies.
2. Treatment:
   a. Day 1 (p.m.)   Clip nails.
                       Bath or shower.
                       Apply 5 percent permethrin cream to all skin areas from the neck down and under nails.
                       (Staff member should apply permethrin to the skin of the resident.)
   b. Day 2 (a.m.)   Bathe or shower to remove the cream.
                       Inform person that itching may persist for weeks.
   c. Day 14   Reexamine; retreat if persistent or recurrent lesions.
   d. Day 28   Reexamine; retreat if persistent or recurrent lesions.

Group II: Crusted Scabies or Norwegian Scabies (Hyperinfestation)

(Note: these individuals have a long term rash and are very heavily infested. They are very contagious. Repeat treatments with 5 percent permethrin cream are usually necessary.)

1. Action:
   a. Isolate case (Contact precautions) until dermatology consult determines that case's rash is no longer transmissible.
   b. Perform environmental control measures: laundry, dry cleaning, or isolation of clothing in plastic bags for seven days.
   c. Cohort staff so that only one group cares for a resident/inpatient case until case is no longer transmissible.
   d. Exclude symptomatic cases (those with a rash) from work (or school, day care center, if applicable) until dermatologist, in consultation with Health Officer approves resumption based on lack of risk of transmission.
   e. Do not transfer patient without notifying the accepting facility of the diagnosis of scabies.
2. Treatment:
   a. Day 1 (p.m.)   Clip nails.
                       Bath or shower.

Exhibit J–1 Line-List for Scabies Cases

Facility _____   Contact Person _____

Address _____

Phone Number _____   Fax Number _____

Name	Age	Sex	Room Number or Assignment	Date of Onset	Location and Description of Lesions	Duration (Days)	Results of Skin Scraping	Date and Type of Treatment

Exhibit J–2 Scabies Fact Sheet

Scabies is a highly contagious skin disease caused by a parasite.

The parasite that causes scabies is a mite that burrows under the skin.

Scabies is spread through personal contact.

Scabies is usually spread from person to person by close physical contact such as touching a person who has scabies or holding hands. It can also be spread during sexual contact. Clothes, towels, bed sheets, etc., can spread the scabies mite if the items were recently in contact with a person who had scabies. The mites will die within 48 hours if they are away from the human body.

The most common symptom is a rash that itches intensely, especially at night.

The rash can be anywhere on your body but is most common on the hands, breasts, armpits, genital area, and waistline. Often the rash looks like red bumps or tiny blisters, which form a line. Symptoms begin two to six weeks after the first exposure or one to four days after reexposure. Secondary bacterial infections of the skin may result from scratching.

See your doctor if you have symptoms of scabies.

Your doctor can check to see if your rash is due to scabies. Scabies is diagnosed by using a microscope to look for the mite in skin scrapings.

Scabies is treatable.

Creams or lotions that kill the mite (such as 5 percent permethrin, lindane, and crotamiton) can be applied to the skin. Follow your doctor's instructions for treatment. Itching may continue for up to one to two weeks after treatment; it does not mean that the treatment did not work or that you got reinfested. Sometimes, a second course of treatment is necessary. Clothing and bed linens worn or used in the 48 hours before treatment should be washed and dried on hot cycles or professionally dry cleaned. There is no need for treatment of rugs or fumigation of the house, other than vacuuming and general cleanliness. All household members and sexual contacts of a person with scabies should be treated at the same time as the person with scabies.

Scabies can be prevented.

Infested persons should be excluded from school or day care until 24 hours after treatment. No one should share clothing, bedding, or other personal articles with an infested person. Clothing that cannot be laundered or dry cleaned should be stored for several days to avoid reinfestation.

Apply 5 percent permethrin cream to all skin areas including scalp, temples, forehead, and under nails.
(Staff member should apply permethrin to the skin of the resident.)

b. Day 2 (a.m.) Bathe or shower to remove the cream after permethrin has been on skin for 8 to 14 hours. Inform person that itching may persist for weeks.

c. Day 7 (p.m.) Repeat bath or shower. Repeat application of 5 percent permethrin cream from the neck down.

d. Day 8 (a.m.) Bathe or shower to remove cream.

e. Day 14 Reexamine; retreat if persistent or recurrent lesions.

f. Day 28 Reexamine; retreat if persistent or recurrent lesions.

INSTITUTIONAL TREATMENT PLAN: SELECTIVE VS. MASS TREATMENT

Although scabies frequently presents as a widespread outbreak within a LTCF, there are circumstances in which a more selective treatment plan may be utilized.

Selective Treatment Protocol

If a single case of scabies (Group I, above) occurs within the population of residents or employees, a selective treatment protocol may be utilized:

1. Identify the case and make a line-list of all contacts (roommate, care providers including radiologists, physical therapists, etc., sexual contacts, family members, or regular visitors) for the previous two months. Check contacts for rash or itching symptoms.
2. Educate cases and contacts as prevously described. Emphasize the rationale for treatment of contacts.
3. Evaluate case and contact for assignment to proper treatment group (Group I or Group II, above).

4. Treat case and contacts to permit simultaneous treatment to prevent reinfection and spread of the infestation.
5. Emphasize the need for follow-up/reexamination at 14 and 28 days.
6. Employ environmental control measures for laundry and clothing as previously described.

Mass Treatment Protocol

A more extensive treatment plan should be utilized if any of the following occur:

1. A single case of crusted or atypical scabies (Norwegian scabies, Group II, above) is diagnosed within the resident population and at least one employee is symptomatic;
2. Two or more residents have positive scrapings and at least one employee on the same unit is symptomatic; or
3. One asymptomatic resident has a positive scraping and other residents or employees have exhibited symptoms of infestation for a period exceeding a month.

The following actions should be taken:

1. Designate an outbreak control officer. This should be a health care provider or infection control professional who is able to diagnose and treat cases and contacts.
2. Make a line-list of cases and contacts (see Exhibit J–1).
3. Institute a facility-wide screening to detect skin lesions or symptoms that may be present in residents, employees, or close contacts of cases.

4. Cohort employees to designated units until coordinated treatment is completed.
5. Educate the resident community, patients, employees, ancillary personnel, and family members or frequent visitors as previously described.
6. Make assignment to appropriate treatment group (Groups I and II, above).
7. Perform mass treatment within a 24-hour period of all residents and staff members employed within a defined area of the facility.
8. Perform follow-up examination and retreatment according to Group assignment.
9. Perform environmental cleaning as previously described.

Summary

Prompt identification and treatment of scabies cases and potential contacts remains the cornerstone of outbreak control. Education of residents, staff, and family members or regular visitors must be initiated immediately. Finally, treatment of cases, contacts, and the environmental control measures *must be coordinated*. If case and contact identification is not complete or if treatment of cases and contacts does not occur *at the same time,* transmission of the mite will continue. Strict surveillance for possible cases should be performed at time of resident admission or during times of skin care or bathing assistance. The unique circumstances of the LTCF provide a population that is extremely susceptible to outbreaks of scabies. Vigilant and ongoing surveillance for cases is of paramount importance within this setting.

Courtesy of the Maryland Department of Health and Mental Hygiene, Epidemiology and Disease Control Program, Baltimore, Maryland.

Alphabetical Reference of Resources for Literature Searching and Outbreak Investigation

Resource	Access Method(s)
APIC	http://www.apic.org or Phone: 202-789-1890
CDC Home Page	http://www.cdc.gov
CDC Home Page, Data and Statistics Section	http://www.cdc.gov/nchswww/fastats/infectis.htm
CDC, Hospital Infections Program, Investigation and Prevention Branch	Phone: 404-639-6139
CDC Voice Information System	Phone: 404-332-4555; Fax: 404-332-4565
Emerging Infectious Diseases	http://www.cdc.gov/ncidod/eid/eid.htm
HazDat	http://atsdr1.astsdr.cdc.gov:8080/hazdat.html
Internet Grateful Med	http://igm.nlm.nih.gov
Medical Matrix	http://www.medmatrix.org.
Medscape	http://www.medscape.com
NIOSH Investigations	Phone: 800-356-4674.
National Library of Medicine	http://www.nlm.nih.gov/mesh/meshhome.html
PubMed	http://www.ncbi.nlm.nih.gov/PubMed
Regional Medical Library Service	Phone: 800-338-RMLS (7657) Monday through Friday 9:00 AM to 5:00 PM
WHO	http://www.who.ch

Index